Occupational Therapy without Borders

To my mom Nellie Kronenberg, a true survivor,
whose spirit continues to enlighten and
invigorate my life's journey.

To my wife, Linda.

To my parents, Salvador and Maria Dolores.

For Churchill Livingstone:

Commissioning Editor: Susan Young
Development Editor: Catherine Jackson
Project Manager: Ailsa Laing
Designer: Judith Wright
Illustrator: Richard Morris

Occupational Therapy without Borders

Learning from the Spirit of Survivors

Frank Kronenberg BSc OT BA(Ed)

International Guest Lecturer in Occupational Therapy
Joint Founder of Spirit of Survivors – Occupational Therapy Without Borders (NGO)

Salvador Simó Algado BSc OT

Lecturer in Occupational Therapy, Universitat de Vic/Catalunya, Spain
Joint Founder of Spirit of Survivors – Occupational Therapy Without Borders (NGO)

Nick Pollard BA DipCOT MA MSc(OT)

Senior Lecturer in Occupational Therapy, School of Health and Social Care,
Sheffield Hallam University, UK

Forewords by

David Werner BSc

Director, HealthWrights (Workgroup for People's Health and Rights), Palo Alto, California, USA

Kit Sinclair PhD

President, World Federation of Occupational Therapists, Department of Rehabilitation Sciences,
Hong Kong Polytechnic University, Hong Kong

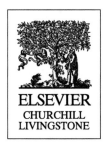

ELSEVIER
CHURCHILL
LIVINGSTONE

EDINBURGH   LONDON   NEW YORK   OXFORD   PHILADELPHIA   ST LOUIS   SYDNEY   TORONTO   2005

ELSEVIER
CHURCHILL
LIVINGSTONE

An imprint of Elsevier Limited

First published 2005

ISBN 0 443 07440 2

British Library Cataloguing in Publication Data
A catalogue record for this book is available from the British Library

Library of Congress Cataloging in Publication Data
A catalog record for this book is available from the Library of Congress

Notice
Knowledge and best practice in this field are constantly changing. As new research and experience broaden our knowledge, changes in practice, treatment and drug therapy may become necessary or appropriate. Readers are advised to check the most current information provided (i) on procedures featured or (ii) by the manufacturer of each product to be administered, to verify the recommended dose or formula, the method and duration of administration, and contraindications. It is the responsibility of the practitioner, relying on their own experience and knowledge of the patient, to make diagnoses, to determine dosages and the best treatment for each individual patient, and to take all appropriate safety precautions. To the fullest extent of the law, neither the Publisher nor the author assumes any liability for any injury and/or damage.

The Publisher

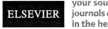

ELSEVIER your source for books, journals and multimedia in the health sciences

www.elsevierhealth.com

Transferred to Digital Printing in 2011.

Printed in U.K.

The Publisher's policy is to use **paper manufactured from sustainable forests**

Contents

Contributors

Judith Abelenda MS OTR/L
*Occupational Therapist, Illinois Early Intervention
Program; Chicago, Illinois, USA*

Denise Dias Barros PhD (Sociology) Master
(Social Sciences – Anthropology) OT
*Professor of Occupational Therapy, Universidade de
São Paulo; Member of the Metuia Project; Member of
Casa das Áfricas Project, Brazil*

Valdo Bomfim BA(Linguistics) MSc(Anthropology) student
*University of Perugia, Italy; International
Co-ordinator for Children's Forum 21 (International
Center for Research, Practice and Policy Analysis);
Founder of Association 'Sem Fronteiras'*

Helen Buchanan BSc(OT) MSc(OT)
*Lecturer in Occupational Therapy, Department of
Health and Rehabilitation Sciences, University of
Cape Town, South Africa*

Imelda M. Burgman MA PGDipSc BAppSC(OT) OTR BCP
*Doctoral Candidate, School of Occupation and Leisure
Sciences, University of Sydney, Australia*

Cesar Estuardo Cardona MD Master(Public Health)
*Postgraduate in Peace Culture, Doctoral candidate in
Political Sciences, Universidad Autónama de
Barcelona, Spain*

Lynn Cockburn MEd BSc(OT) BComm OT(C) OTReg(Ont)
*Lecturer, Department of Occupational Therapy,
University of Toronto, Canada*

Madeleine Duncan MSc(OT) BAHons(Psychology)
*Senior Lecturer, Occupational Therapy Division,
School of Health and Rehabilitation, Faculty of Health
Sciences, University of Cape Town, South Africa*

Mary Egan PhD OT(C)
*Associate Professor, School of Rehabilitation Sciences,
University of Ottawa, Canada*

Hetty Fransen BSc(OT) MSc(OT)
*Lecturer in Occupational Therapy, Ecole Supérieure de
Sciences et Techniques de la Santé Tunis, University of
Tunis El Manar, Tunisia*

Hiroko Fujimoto BA OTR
*Graduate Student, Master of Science in Occupational
Therapy, Faculty of Health Professions, Dalhousie
University, Canada*

Beth Fuller MPH BOT
*Senior Program Development Officer, Australia
International Health Institute, University of
Melbourne, Australia*

Sandra Galheigo PhD(Social Sciences) MEd OT
*Professor, Faculty of Occupational Therapy, Pontificia
Universidade Católica de Campinas, Member of the
Metuia Project, Brazil*

Roshan Galvaan BSc(OT) MSc(OT)
*Lecturer, Occupational Therapy Division, School of
Health and Rehabilitation, Faculty of Health Sciences,
University of Cape Town, South Africa*

Débora Galvini BSc(OT)
*Occupational Therapist, Universidade de São Paulo,
Brazil*

Maria Isabel Garcez Ghirardi PhD(Social Psychology)
*Professor of Occupational Therapy, Universidade de
São Paulo, Brazil*

Barb Hooper PhD OTR
*Visiting Assistant Professor Occupational Therapy
Learning Center at Carolina, University of North
Carolina at Chapel Hill, North Carolina, USA*

Michael K. Iwama PhD OT(C)
*Associate Professor, Faculty of Health Professions,
Dalhousie University, Canada*

Gary Kielhofner DrPH OTR FAOTA
*Professor and Wade-Meyer Chair, Department of
Occupational Therapy, College of Applied Health
Sciences, University of Illinois at Chicago, Illinois,
Chicago, USA*

Kimberley Kielhofner
Student, McGill University, Montreal, Quebec, Canada

Abigail King BOccThy
*Occupational Therapist, Mater Children's Hospital
and District Child and Youth Mental Health Service,
Brisbane, Australia*

Debbie Kramer-Roy BSc(OT) MA (Education and
International Development: Health Promotion)
*Senior Instructor/Occupational Therapist,
The Aga Khan University, Pakistan*

Frank Kronenberg BSc OT BA(Ed)
*International guest lecturer in occupational therapy,
Joint Founder of SPIRIT of SURVIVORS–
Occupational Therapy Without Borders (NGO)*

Paul Kronenberg
Joint Founder of Braille Without Borders

Barbara Lavin NZROT MOT
*Co-ordinator, Occupational Therapy Program,
Bethlehem University, Palestine*

Roseli Esquerdo Lopes PhD(Education) MEd OT
*Professor, Department of Occupational Therapy,
Universidade Federal de Saõ Carlos, Member of the
Metuia Project, Brazil*

Theresa Lorenzo BSc(OT) MSc(Disability Studies)
*Senior Lecturer, Division of Occupational Therapy,
University of Cape Town, South Africa*

Elise Newton BOT(Hons) BA(DevptStudies)
*Occupational Therapist, ACT Health, Canberra,
Australia. Joint Founder of the Occupational Therapy
International Outreach Network (OTION)*

Suzanne M. Peloquin PhD OTR FAOTA
*Professor, Department of Occupational Therapy,
School of Allied Health Sciences, University of Texas
Medical Branch at Galveston, USA*

Nick Pollard BA DipCOT MA MSc(OT)
*Senior Lecturer in Occupational Therapy, School
of Health and Social Care, Sheffield Hallam
University, UK*

Elelwani L. Ramugondo MSc(OT)
*Lecturer, Division of Occupational Therapy,
University of Cape Town, South Africa*

Melina Simmond BSc(Hons)(OT)
*Australian Youth Ambassador (Nepal), Australian
Agency of International Development (AusAID)*

Salvador Simó Algado BSc OT
*Lecturer in Occupational Therapy, Universitat de
Vic/Catalunya, Spain, Joint Founder of SPIRIT of
SURVIVORS–Occupational Therapy Without
Borders (NGO)*

Pat Smart
*Outreach Co-ordinator and Adult Basic Education
Workshop Leader, Yorkshire, UK*

Yolanda Suarez-Balcazar PhD
*Associate Professor, Department of Occupational
Therapy, College of Applied Health Sciences,
University of Illinois at Chicago, USA*

Sabriye Tenberken
Joint Founder of Braille Without Borders

Rachel Thibeault PhD OT(C)
*Associate Professor, Occupational Therapy
Programme, University of Ottawa, Canada*

Elizabeth Townsend PhD OT(C) RegNS FCAOT
*Professor and Director, School of Occupational
Therapy, Dalhousie University, Canada*

Barry Trentham MES BSc(OT) OTReg(Ont)
*Lecturer, Department of Occupational Therapy,
University of Toronto, Canada*

Reg Urbanowski EdD OT(C)
*Associate Professor, School of Occupational Therapy,
Dalhousie University, Canada*

Gail Elizabeth Whiteford BAppSc MHSc(OT) PhD
*Professor and Chair, Occupational Therapy; Director,
Research into Professional Practice Learning and
Education (RIPPLE), Charles Sturt University,
Australia*

Jennifer L. Womack MSc(OT)
*Clinical Assistant Professor, Division of Occupational
Science, University of North Carolina, USA*

Wendy Wood PhD OTR/L FAOTA
*Associate Professor, Division of Occupational Science,
University of North Carolina at Chapel Hill, USA*

Cover photo by Gervasio Sánchez

Born in Córdoba (Spain) in August 1959, Gervasio Sánchez achieved his degree in journalism in 1984. Since then he has worked as a freelance reporter in over two dozen armed conflicts. His publications include:

El cerco de Sarajevo (*The Siege of Sarajevo*) 1994

Vidas Minadas (*Mined Lives*) 1997 in collaboration with the NGOs Intermón, Manos Unidas and Médicos Sin Fronteras, and Editorial Blume

Kosovo, Cronica de una deportación (*Kosovo, Chronicle of a Deportation*) 1999
Niños de la Guerra (*War Children*) 2000

La Caravana de la Muerte, las víctimas de Pinochet (*The Death Caravan, Pinochet's Victims*) 2000

The Press Association in Aragón gave him the award of *Best Journalist of the Year* in 1993. In 1994 he won the *Award for the Best Photographic Work of the Year* for his coverage of Bosnia. In 1995 he was awarded with the *Andalucia Culture Award*, for 'his generous humanitarian vision, committed to the highest journalistic vision – an example of new journalism that should inspire future generations of photographers'. In June 1996 he won the *Cirilo Rodriguez prize*, the most prestigious Spanish Award for reporters. In December 1997 the Pro-Human Rights Association in Spain awarded him the *Human Rights Award* for his book *Vidas Minadas* and for his personal commitment.

The Zaragoza City Council designated him *Adoptive Son of Zaragoza* in September 1998, 'in recognition of the exceptional merits gained in his work as a photographer, in which his social sensitivity and his efforts to denounce the horrors of war stand out'.

The United Nations Education, Science and Culture Organization (UNESCO) designated him as UNESCO *Artist for Peace* during the celebrations of the 50th Anniversary of the Universal declarations of the Human Rights, in December 1998, 'for the extraordinary testimony he offers through his photographs of the suffering undergone by victims of antipersonnel mines and for his untiring support of culture for peace'.

In July 2001, the Zaragoza provincial government awarded him the *Gold Medal of Saint Isabel* for 'his career in journalism and his dedication to the support of victims of war'.

The editors of the book want to thank and acknowledge Gervasio Sánchez, for his extremely generous collaboration with this book, sharing his amazing and touching photographs that perfectly reflect the essence of this book, the strength of the human spirit.

Foreword I

Nearly every field of human endeavor can be approached in ways that are narrow and disempowering, or in ways that are expansive and enabling, even liberating. Despite their ideology of 'service', the health professions today tend to be dominated by the narrow, disempowering approach. The prevailing biomedical model focuses on illnesses of individuals rather than on collective wellbeing. Also it tends to be elitist: its costly interventions are least accessible to those whose needs are greatest.

Where does occupational therapy fit into this larger picture? Because occupational therapy deals with how people function in their environment and community, it strives to take a more comprehensive, holistic approach. Rather than emphasizing biomedical intervention, it focuses on underlying social and community concerns, at least in theory.

In practice, however, the occupational therapy profession too often falls short of its more holistic, egalitarian goals. And as with the other health professions, the poorest and neediest often fall between the cracks. In our increasingly globalized free market economy, there is no such thing as a free lunch. You get what you can pay for.

Occupational Therapy without Borders challenges this neo-conservative trend. The book's inspiring articles present a far-reaching, socially responsible and potentially revolutionary challenge to the profession. Although the book centers on occupational therapy, its reach is so all-embracing that it is an invaluable resource for anyone in the helping professions who is concerned with the wellbeing of people, both individually and collectively.

Occupational Therapy without Borders in some ways calls to mind *Pedagogy of the Oppressed*[1] and other groundbreaking writings by the iconoclastic Brazilian educator, Paulo Freire. Freire's work grew out his pragmatic (some would say subversive) learner-centered approach to adult literacy training. But because it facilitated awareness-raising for collective social action for change, his revolutionary methodology has been adapted to every field from health and agriculture to civil rights and peace movements.

Like Freire's writings, *Occupational Therapy without Borders* embraces the human struggle to build healthier communities – and ultimately to build a civilization – which both celebrate diversity and provide equal opportunities for all. It envisions a society that excludes no one, regardless of race, religion, gender, orientation, age, socio-economic class, or level of ability. Through a cycle of analysis, reflection, and action, Freire's methodology aimed to enable concerned and disadvantaged people to discover their self-confidence and work together to 'change the world'. *Occupational Therapy without Borders* shares a similar vision: its scope extends from the personal to the global.

This book is subtitled *Learning from the Spirit of Survivors*. Indeed, it emphasizes the importance of spirituality in the pursuit of personal and societal transformation. But 'spirituality' is used in its broadest (least doctrinaire) sense, to imply 'the discovery of meaning in our day-to-day lives'.

Meaning, in its existential sense, involves actively realizing the link between our personal health, our collective wellbeing, and our small but vital place in the universe.

Martin Luther King had a dream: a far-reaching dream of a kinder, fairer, more inclusive world. The authors of this book have an equally grand and challenging dream. They realize that our current age of globalization, far from promoting equal rights and opportunities for all, is widening the gap between the over-privileged and the under-privileged. In such a regressive social climate, the book comes like a breath of fresh air in a dungeon. Its many practical examples and inspiring stories bring its global vision gracefully down to earth.

To occupational therapists, especially those working or tempted to work in disadvantaged communities, *Occupational Therapy without Borders* presents a daunting challenge. It is a gold mine of methods, practical alternatives, and thought-provoking discussion for anyone working in the fields of health care, community mobilization, alternative education, people-centered economics, human rights, environmental protection, social justice, or sustainable development.

In sum, this book is an indispensable tool for anyone who sides with the underdog. It is a treasure chest for agents of change and community-based facilitators in every field related to equitable and sustainable development.

Palo Alto, CA 2005   David Werner

Reference

1.   Freire P. Pedogogy of the Oppressed. New York: Continuum; 1970.

Foreword II

A shared vision for those who work in caring professions is of a world in which every disabled and disadvantaged person who can benefit from it has ready access to the right kind of support. That perfect world is still a long way off but in many societies dedicated therapists, social workers, and doctors are working to bring succor to people who live on the edge.

Four years ago, on 8 September 2000, the United Nations in its Millennium Declaration[1] set goals to improve the lot of humanity. In the face of rapid globalization, the United Nations proposed a commitment for all nations to strive for economic and social development for the common good. This laudable commitment asked governments to meet certain basic targets. But even as the delegates were voting in the United Nations, there were dedicated individuals and movements working in many places to achieve the same aims. What was being done by these pioneers in many ways foreshadowed or paralleled what was called for in the United Nations resolution.

Quietly, without fanfare, largely without publicity, and with no widespread public acknowledgement or recognition, these movements have gained significant momentum. Over the past 20 years they have helped spearhead a significant change in social thinking; from an emphasis on treating people with impairments or disabilities in institutions, the focus has switched to promoting participation within their communities.

During that time, globalization has led to enormous and sweeping changes. In wide areas of the world economic growth has affected the lives of many millions of people. New technologies such as the internet have made people much more aware of modern trends. Better preventive medical systems, new drugs and improved medical care have led to an increase in life-expectancy in many societies. The changes add up to great opportunities and vast challenges. But in some instances they have also led to socio-economic inequalities and political instability. Two years after the historic call for action by the United Nations, the World Health Organization published its annual health report, *Reducing Risks, Promoting Healthy* Life.[2] It stated the obvious, reiterating the close and self-evident links between poverty and disease. It added that disease often meant people could not work, which in turn led to a lack of food on family tables with the inevitable results: malnutrition and other health issues. Global statistics tell the stark facts. More than half of the world's people suffer from malnutrition and substandard health-care.[3]

So where should we occupational therapists and others in the caring professions place our priorities? How should we be addressing the awesome challenges? How best can we use our knowledge, skills and dedication to bring about lasting improvements? Much is being done. In communities around the world, proactive therapists have been addressing issues at the heart of these global concerns, looking at ways we can effectively tackle the problems of occupational deprivation caused by social injustice.

This book is an inspiring collection of how occupational therapists are facing the problems of today and the challenges of tomorrow. Each chapter examines the fundamental belief of occupational therapy, that occupation is essential for life and health. It is a basic human right. We all know that occupational therapy can realize a tremendous unfulfilled potential,[4] using a diversity of vision and practice to help people and communities. These chapters stress again and again that participation in meaningful occupation has an important positive influence on health. The lack of such participation leads almost inevitably to poor health, and the absence of a feeling of wellbeing.

Disruption of life patterns and the loss of meaningful occupation exist widely in today's world. But there are some groups who suffer to a far greater degree: the unemployed, refugees, minorities, people with disabilities, and those who live in places where conflicts rage and safety and security are absent.

The service focus of occupational therapists guides people to choose, organize and perform daily life activities that are meaningful and useful. It helps people explore opportunities to gain greater control over their health and destinies.[5]

Being present and interactive with people in their natural everyday lives puts occupational therapists in an excellent position to gain first-hand knowledge and understanding about the needs and interests of those they seek to help, and to support their clients to make changes in the community; society as a whole benefits, as well as the individual. Occupational therapists must develop their roles as agents of social change, taking the profession to a new level that makes a difference to entire communities as well as to the individuals we treat and encourage. To enable them to become effective agents of change, the way in which occupational therapists are educated must come under sweeping review. The future trend in professional education must include a strong component on enablement, advocacy and social reform.

In many under-developed areas, the difficulties with prevention and rehabilitation have a lot to do with general economic issues. With widespread poverty, creaky infrastructures, poor education and a total absence of democratic structures, the outlook is grim for therapists seeking to improve the life and health of their clients and the community. Occupational therapists as facilitators can highlight and help make public the problems faced by disabled and disadvantaged individuals. They can challenge invisibility, discrimination and poverty. They can lead people with disabilities to develop their full potential and enable people on the fringes of society to take part in different spheres and activities.

This book is a call to action for our profession. These chapters show what we should and could be doing. They guide occupational therapists down a path of activism and opportunity, showing how we can understand the challenges facing us and, awesome as these problems may be, outline how they can be confronted.

This book orients future actions based on current understanding and perspectives of enablement, justice, caring, and participation. Not only does it report narratives of therapists who have taken risks to improve the lives of others, it also provides a foundation for making change. It illustrates how to use the training and resources of our profession to apply principles of occupational justice.

Hong Kong, 2005   Kit Sinclair

References

1. United Nations. UN Millenium Development Goals. New York: United Nations; 2002.
2. World Health Organization. World Health Report: Reducing risks, promoting healthy life. Geneva: WHO; 2002.
3. Smith DJ. If the world were a village. Toronto: Kits Can Press; 2002.
4. Townsend E Occupational therapy's social vision. Can J Occup Ther 2003; 60(4):174–184.
5. Kronenberg F. Draft Position Paper on Community Based Rehabilitation. World Federation of Occupational Therapists; 2003.

Preface

If we reduce the population of the Earth to a village with 100 people, keeping the existing proportions, it looks like this:

57 Asians, 21 Europeans, 14 Americans (northern and southern) and 8 Africans
52 women, 48 men
70 are people of colour, 30 are white
89 heterosexuals, 11 homosexuals
6 people own 59% of the whole world's wealth and all of them are from the USA
80 live in substandard housing
70 are illiterate
50 are undernourished
10 are disabled
1 is dying
2 are newborns
1 has a computer
1 (only one) has higher education.[1]

If you look at the world from this point of view, you will see how great a need we have of solidarity, understanding, patience and education.

Why this book was written

This book has arisen through a coming together of the editors' personal and professional views and experiences, but its basis lies in the genesis of the Dolphin Association. In 1997 Salvador Simó Algado launched his humanistic vision and mission of occupational therapy, reaching out to groups of people who our profession appeared to neglect or under-serve, such as survivors of war, prisoners, immigrants, prostitutes, people living with HIV/AIDS. Disillusioned that his occupational therapy training did not include the possibility of working with these populations or inform him about their needs, he started his own initiative, searching for and connecting with like-minded colleagues through the internet.

Soon after he was invited by occupational therapy programs internationally to share his views and experiences of working with immigrants and female prisoners in Spain, with children in situations of armed conflict in Bosnia and a community of returning Mayan refugees in Guatemala (*see* Chapter 25). In 1999, while giving presentations in Belgium and the Netherlands, he met Frank Kronenberg and invited him to join him in building the Dolphin Association, which at that point only represented Salvador plus some hundred occupational therapy students and teachers worldwide who had e-mailed their interest in working for the Dolphin Association or had requested information concerning occupational therapy in marginalized contexts. After practice and research experiences with survivors of war in Kosovo and street children in Mexico and Guatemala (see Chapters 18 and 19), in 2002 Salvador and Frank decided to rename the Dolphin Association 'SPIRIT of SURVIVORS – Occupational Therapists without Borders', abbreviated to SOS-OTwB for the website.

'SPIRIT of SURVIVORS' refers to the people we aspire to work with, and their inherent strengths. The people we engage with as occupational therapists are experiencing conditions that we often only know about through what we have seen or read; we have not actually lived that experience. When you realize that your survival may be at stake, your energies are focused. If you listen carefully and exercise your critical faculties, you can greatly enhance your chances, which is powerfully and compellingly illustrated by the accounts in the opening chapters of the book.

The title 'Occupational Therapists without Borders' is to be understood beyond its geographical meaning. Traditionally, occupational therapy (and healthcare and rehabilitation) thinking and practice appear to be exported from westernised cultures to most other parts of the world. 'Occupational Therapists without Borders' aims to foster dialogues and (multilateral) collaborations between occupational therapists and other professionals from 'developed countries' and 'developing countries'. The book's rich diversity of contributions from established as well as emerging occupational therapy leadership from all over the world is an expression of this vision. If occupational therapists are about emancipation and enabling the participation in everyday meaningful occupations of *all* people who experience disabling conditions, in order to live up to that promise they must think and act critically, become aware of the value patterns and assumptions embedded in our theories and avoid contributing to the oppression of the very people we intend to help.

SOS-OTwB can be viewed as a catalyst for a movement within the international community of occupational therapists, a kind of global new millennium version of the 'National Society for the Promotion of Occupational Therapy' (1917), whose objectives were 'the advancement of occupation as a therapeutic measure; the study of the effect of occupation upon the human being; and the scientific dispensation of this knowledge'.[2] SOS-OTwB aims to develop, implement and promote occupational therapy practice, education and research initiatives with marginalized people, inspired and guided by a vision of overcoming occupational apartheid and working toward occupational justice (*see* Chapters 1, 6, 18, 19, 31), while raising critical awareness about and facing up to the political nature of occupational therapy.

Since 1997 Salvador and Frank have held occupational therapy courses and workshops about their experiences at universities in Spain, Belgium, the USA, Canada, Georgia, Portugal, England, Wales, Germany, the Netherlands, Guatemala, Mexico, Sweden, Norway, Denmark, the Czech Republic, Slovenia, and South Africa and presented at national and international congresses in many of these countries. They were met with great interest and enthusiasm, but students and practitioners often commented that their professional education was insufficient to equip them for this field. This book is a response to their repeated calls for a comprehensive portrayal of occupational therapy theory, methodology and practice examples related to working with underserved and neglected populations.

Nick Pollard joined the OTwB book project after exchanging messages with Frank during an occupational science listserve debate on the subject, 'The political nature of occupational science and occupational therapy', back in January 2003. It appeared that Nick's views, experiences and hopes for the profession of occupational therapy are very much akin with those of SOS-OTwB. He was a natural fit to the project and his contributions to this project have been essential.

Occupational therapists believe that human occupation is central to human existence, and that occupation is an element of all human activity, not just work. The book will use this expanded definition of occupation to explore the new idea of occupational apartheid, which refers to the separation between those who have meaningful, useful occupations and those who are deprived of or isolated from such occupations, or otherwise constrained in their daily life. The ideas and examples that will be presented are matters of justice – occupational justice.

What this book is about and who it is for

In the original proposal and guidelines for this book,[3,4] the editors invited contributors to exchange ideas and engage in a critical debate around 'the development and implementation of occupational therapy initiatives with marginalized populations from an occupational justice perspective of health'. All the chapters were submitted to a peer-review process in which they were refined and developed through often-lively on-line discussions. This has enabled authors to come into contact with each other, as well as working with the editors.

Through this interaction a community of writers has emerged with passionate voices and practical proposals for changing the living conditions of those people who are marginalized by society, whose capacity for meaningful daily occupation is constrained by conditions of poverty, violence, or confinement. It introduces occupational therapy students, educators, practitioners and researchers to areas little covered in occupational therapy literature and opens the door for others to connect with the huge potential offered by our profession. It addresses a philosophical basis, applied methodologies and practice examples related to intervention, education and research outside medical contexts with these under-served and neglected populations.

As our profession is just starting to reconsider what we ought to do for marginalized people, this book offers many opportunities for occupational therapists to consider the larger sociopolitical and cultural issues surrounding the human condition. Perhaps the sparse availability of literature in this field contributes to the lack of inclusion of occupational justice in education programmes.

The discussions presented in this book challenge occupational therapy students, educators, researchers and practitioners (members of a still small and rather invisible profession) to more fully realize the profession's social vision of a more just society. Disability, old age, and other marginalizing conditions and experiences are addressed by involving people in helping themselves to obtain the capacity and power to construct their own destinies through their participation in daily life.

In line with the importance that we attach to the role of critical debate within and outside the profession as a vehicle of social change and human development, this work is presented mainly for open deliberation and critical scrutiny. If our arguments arouse interest and lead to more public discussion of these vital issues, we would have reason to feel well rewarded.

We would very much welcome comments from readers with a view to improving the next edition. A form is available on the book's interactive website for this purpose.

Frank Kronenberg
Salvador Simó Algado
2005   Nick Pollard

Note:
All royalties from this book will go to a special fund that supports the initiatives of SPIRIT of SURVIVORS – Occupational Therapy without Borders.

References

1. Smith DJ. If the world were a village, Kits Can Press, Toronto, 2002.
2. Wilcock AA. An Occupational Perspective of Health, Slack, Thorofare, New Jersey, 1998.
3. Kronenberg F, Simó Algado S. Spirit of Survivors: Occupational Therapy Initiatives with Marginalized Populations Occupational, book proposal, Elsevier Science, Oxford, September 2002.
4. Kronenberg F, Simó Algado S. Contents specific guidelines for the contributing authors of the book, Venray, December 2002.

Acknowledgements

The first challenge of the book project was the writing of a proposal. Since we had never before written or edited a book, putting together such a document presented a daunting task. It was accomplished during the summer of 2002 in the inspiring and supportive company of good friends at *Cal Cases*, a gorgeous rustic farmhouse (formerly housing the first therapeutic community in Spain for persons with a history of substance abuse) situated in the beautiful countryside of Catalonia. We would like to express heartfelt gratitude to the late Frederic (Fede) Boix; to Cesar, Clara and Genís Martí Cardona-Melendez; to Maria Boix and to Maria Isidora Herrero Garcia for encouraging us to believe in the journey that we were to convincingly describe and explain in detail to the publisher. Companyeras, os agradecemos un monton!

We would like to also express a very special thanks to Elsevier's commissioning editor Susan Young, development editor Catherine Jackson and project manager Ailsa Laing for their relentless support, their sustained patience with and acceptance of our urges to 'draw outside the lines', and for their appreciation of the personal touch and humour which coloured the coming into being of this book. Annie Turner – our friend, colleague, seasoned writer and editor – stood by us from day one with invaluable technical and content-related advice and she provided morale boosts at times when our batteries ran low. It must also be mentioned that all the contributors to this book greatly appreciated and benefited from the sensitive and conscientious feedback and modifications from our copyeditor Linda Sharp. Going beyond the technical aspects of her job, her engagement was characterized by a touch of personal care. It's been great working with you all, and should the chance to work on another book arise, we would be happy to go for a rerun.

We consider ourselves very fortunate for the opportunity to engage in open dialogues with a wonderful group of some 60 individuals who wrote or otherwise contributed to the chapters in this book, including our colleagues Mady Reekmans, Birgit Heuchemer and Staffan Josephsson. Together they represent perspectives and experiences from countries from every continent (except Antarctica). They were generous with their time, investing their energies in the project pro bono and waiving their royalties in support of future SOS-OTwB initiatives.

Finally, we wish to thank the many people whose names are not mentioned here, all the children, adults and elderly persons far away and nearby who allowed us to walk with and learn from them, and to our colleagues, students and teachers of occupational therapy.

Frank Kronenberg It continues to amaze me, how events that at the time when they occurred seemed rather mundane, later led to encounters and opportunities that without doubt broadened and enriched the contents of this book. 'Tack' to our colleagues Frida Lygnegård, Kristina Alinder and Rebecca Persson who presented a Dolphin-Sweden poster at the WFOT 2002 in Stockholm, which featured the concept occupational apartheid. This led us to encounter our colleagues Madeleine Duncan and Ruth Watson from Cape Town University, which led to a number of contributions to this book by colleagues from South Africa. 'Dank je wel' Annelies Feelders for making that lunchtime phone call in September 2002, inviting me to join a powerful 2-day workshop with David Werner during an *International Course in Management of Disability and Rehabilitation* in Utrecht organized by Huib Cornielje (www.enablement.nl). This experience helped facilitate the start of and my involvement with the WFOT-CBR project team. Many thanks also to Kit Sinclair for inviting me to represent the WFOT at the WHO international consultation on the review of CBR in Helsinki in May 2003. Participation in these meaningful events led to the inclusion of important CBR perspectives in this book.

A special word of thanks goes out to Sarah Thomas de Benitez, for her openness and willingness to listen to an occupational therapy 'without borders' vision on and approach to working with street children. Her constructive critique and her encouragement to keep believing in the book project were of great help.

My parents, brothers, sister, in-laws and my nephew Luc and niece Milou so often had to accept that I had to give the book priority over staying and spending (play) time with them. Without their patience, understanding and unconditional support, this book would hardly have eventuated.

Nick Pollard   First of all I wish to thank my wife Linda and our children Emma, Sally, Molly, Joshua and Daisy for their love, patience and support during the development of this book.

I must also thank: Auldeen Alsop, Susan Walsh, Colette Fegan, Melanie Bryer, Nick Hall, Margaret Spencer, Joan Healey and my friends and colleagues in occupational therapy and the Faculty of Health and Wellbeing at Sheffield Hallam University, and at Doncaster and South Humber Healthcare NHS Trust, particularly Sue Sparks and Kathryn Deighton at the RED Centre, who have all generously given support and allowed both me (and also Frank) crucial time and resources for this project. Their interest in our progress has often been valuable in enabling the thinking through of problems and ideas, and many have been flexible in enabling the exchange of tasks around deadlines in the book's progress. I would also like to thank my students for their encouragement and lively interest.

Thanks also to the members of the Federation of Worker Writers and Community Publishers, and Heeley Writers Workshop, Sheffield, and staff and service users at the Assertive Outreach and Community Rehabilitation Teams and the Fieldside Centre, Loversall Hospital, and People Who Rely on People, Doncaster, for their inspiration.

My brother Simon, for his continued interest and wise advice, thank-you.

Frank and I should also mention the restorative support of the Wharncliffe Arms on Burncross Road, Chapeltown.

Salvador Simó Algado   To my parents, Salvador and Maria Dolores, without them none of my dreams would have become a reality. To Nadia for her inspiration. To all my soul friends.

To all my teachers, the Mayan Indians of Guatemala, the refugee community of Bosnia, the men and women of the prison and the immigrant community in Spain, the children of Gjakova: to Zeca, Bolito, Tere, José and Claudín, Krenora and Herden.

To all my colleagues in the occupational therapy world who believed in me when I had no support and gave me breath to keep on walking: Mary Egan, Rachel Thibeault, Liz Townsend, Mary Law, Reg Urbanowsky, Lynn Cockburn, Barry Trentham, Mady Reekmans, Luc Vercruysse, Lena Borell, Hans Johnson, Stephan Josephsson, Lena Haglund, Gary Kielhofner, John Chacksfield, Clara Sanz, Maria Jesus Calvo, Marta Perez de Heredia, and Silvia, Alberto, Paco, Noelia, Beatriz, Javi and many more.

To the friends and colleagues of the Universitat de Vic, for believing in my work and helping me to achieve my occupational dreams. Especially to all my students.

Chapter 1

Introduction
A beginning ...

Frank Kronenberg, Nick Pollard

OVERVIEW

There is a new focus in occupational therapy, a drive to sharpen up the profession's thinking about its relationship not just to the people we engage with, but to the environmental realities we share and participate in. This rethinking of professional values is, as is evident from the diversity of the contributors to this book, occurring around the world.

This chapter describes the origins of the book, and the focus which we have developed around ideas attributed to the sociologist Herbert de Souza by Molinas Maldonado and Monroy Peralta.[1] Formulated as a set of guiding principles, these ideas are explored as a tool for examining the philosophy, values, and beliefs of occupational therapy in its applications to the individuals, groups, and communities with whom we work.

This critical process addresses the political aspects of facilitating meaningful and empowered occupation through negotiated outcomes. It explores the implications of changes that can facilitate a new basis for working with people with disabilities, and at the same time, empower therapists. Finally, it offers a fundamental approach that enables both therapists and the people they work with to consider what they should do as citizens of the world.

INTRODUCTION

In the preparation of this book and through the discussions between the editors and the contributing authors we have sensed a growing awareness of a need for a new and progressive focus in the occupational therapy profession. This is evident in the readiness of both survivors and so many writers in the field of occupational therapy at all levels to engage in the critical dialogues which have generated these chapters. By the term *survivors* we mean people who endure chronic disabling conditions through which they are marginalized or socially excluded. The term survivors can refer to both individuals and communities. The explorations that follow investigate new areas of work for occupational therapists and revisit founding principles; they discuss new paradigms for research and education, even new models, and suggest, we hope, a profession in the act of rediscovering itself and breaking the mold at the same time.

As the editors of this project we have also tried to break a few molds. Throughout the writing of this book we have been engaged with our contributors and collaborators in critical feedback, to question and explore further the arguments both we and they were unfolding. As we will explore below, this is in line with the emphasis we wish to place upon a participatory, 'transformative'[2] process rather than outcomes. This is an inclusive process in which we ask the readers to consider themselves and recognize the people they work with as participants, as activists for an occupational therapy which seeks to recognize and overcome situations of occupational apartheid (see Ch. 6) and occupational injustice (see Ch. 9).[3]

WITHOUT BORDERS

We should first explore how the book came about. The initial proposal was developed by Frank Kronenberg and Salvador Simó Algado who had founded SPIRIT of SURVIVORS–Occupational Therapists without Borders (SOS–OTwB, formerly known as the Dolphin Association) in 1997. The first part of the name 'SPIRIT of SURVIVORS' refers to the inherent capacities of the people with whom they collaborated,[4] and provides a point of departure which guides the occupational therapy process, enabling the therapists to walk the talk of 'people-centered practice'.[5,6] The second part, 'Occupational Therapists without Borders' emphasizes occupational therapists as citizens[7] working in and outside of mainstream, medically-oriented thinking and practice contexts, purposefully not setting borders for the people they work with, enabling them to challenge the limits imposed on them through disabling conditions, and combining local actions with global perspectives. To do this effectively entails that occupational therapists learn from the spirit of survivors.

A border is a political frontier which requires a passport to cross. It can be the line of a geographical feature, such as a river, or an arbitrary line, such as the twenty ninth parallel, but the fact of its presence is that people on either side of it have different rights, destinies, and histories – even if they speak the same language or share the same culture. If we stand exactly aligned with either foot on each side of a border it does not follow that the bisection runs through our minds. Once we have seen over the border and experienced whatever lies there we are not then able to 'not-see' and 'not-experience' what we have seen and experienced. People make borders, therefore they can be unmade or renegotiated. In the development of health and social services there has been a distinct border between those who deliver the service and those *upon* whom – not *with* whom – the service is delivered. In a profession which talks of empowerment it is evident that the fortifications along this border have to be demolished. This does not mean the destruction of expertise, of clinical competence, but is about enabling expertise and competence to be shared and to work to the needs of those who are excluded from the privileges expertise offers. Therefore we ask:

- What are the 'borders' that deny or restrict people from exercising their human right to meaningful participation in daily life?
- What are the 'borders' that deny or restrict occupational therapy from walking its talk, and fleshing out its potential as a people-centered occupation?
- What is the nature of these 'borders'? Who sets them?
- Do occupational therapists set 'borders' for others?[8]

Finding answers to these stinging questions entails taking on the full cross-border connection of the profession, with its bases in art *and* science, realizing the potential of this position to determine *how*, with *whom*, *where* and *what type* of work we do. Not setting borders for the people we work with, challenging borders that deny or restrict people's access to dignified and meaningful participation in daily life, thinking globally, acting locally, going beyond occupational therapy's limited grasp of 'holism',[9] and recognizing and acting upon our interdependence,[5,10] is our 'ethical responsibility'.[7] (p. 296) Our ethical responsibility must also recognize that there are, none the less, borders limiting what can be realized. All expertise has limits, which are necessary to the functioning of society, but this does not suggest that these are immune to question.[11]

If we aim to collaborate with others to contribute to building communities in which all people can realize their potential, don't we need to challenge those 'borders'[8,12] and through this discover the freedom (creative energy) to enable a person, group, or community to liberate themselves from the disabling conditions that they experience? Liberation, rather than a restricted and conformist normalization or rehabilitation, then becomes the goal of the occupational therapy process.

FIVE PRINCIPLES

To guide the writing process for this book we considered five principles attributed to the Brazilian sociologist Herbert de Souza,[1] which are described below in relation to the philosophy, values, and beliefs of occupational therapy. We were introduced to and worked with these principles during an occupational therapy project with street children in Guatemala (see Ch. 19), where they proved to be helpful in untangling the diverse and often conflicting interactions between the project's stakeholders.

Chomsky said: 'You may not know in detail – and I don't think that any of us *do* know in detail – how those principles can best be realized at this point in complex systems like human societies. But I don't really see why that should make a difference: what you try to do is advance the principles.'[11] (p. 201) We challenge ourselves and all our readers to advance these principles, particularly in relation to the often intangible, blurry, and almost invisible roles fulfilled by occupational therapists as they mold themselves not just to the needs of the 'client', but even more to the other actor groups in the multidisciplinary context of care. Imagine these principles as 'sparring partners' in the reasoning and decision-making processes that inform and guide daily practice with people. If the starting point for intervention is the Hippocratic ethic 'first do no harm', then the principles of moral reasoning should also extend into other areas of practice concerning occupation. We would also argue that a person-centered approach to occupation should recognize choice, or if this is not possible, give sound reasons. As Chomsky[11] (pp. 201–202) explains: 'People have the right to be free, and if there are constraints on that freedom then you've got to justify them.' If we are to uphold an evidence-based practice, then, as he also says:

> *The burden of proof for any exercise of authority is always on the person exercising it – invariably. And when you look, most of the time these authority structures have no justification: they have no moral justification, they have no justification in the interests of the person lower in the hierarchy, or in the interests of other people, or the environment, or the future, or the society, or anything else – they're just there in order to preserve certain structures of power and domination, and the people at the top.*

This exercise in moral and ethical reasoning is aimed at awakening our understanding of the political dimension of who we are and what we do in the world as occupational therapists *and* citizens. As occupational therapists, how do we realize the roles which we proclaim with our holistic all-encapsulating models and approaches, and at the same time meekly fit within the constraints of a social system that enables only as far as limitations prescribe? As front line workers, is the future role of occupational therapists that of apologists for the barriers interposed continually in the face of a people-centered practice, when the department is closed because of hospital building work, there are not enough staff to facilitate home assessment, clinical time is eroded by demands for quality assurance paperwork and attendance at meetings to discuss evidence-based practice, and no more disability aids can be issued in the current financial period? As allied health professionals working to principles of clinical accountability from medicine and hospital accountants, how often do we find that the people-centered principles under which occupational therapy operates are secondary to organizational and hierarchical demands?[13] If the outcomes we seek for the people we work with are freedom and liberation, then we have to reconstruct the basis on which we are enabled to achieve those outcomes.

Through SOS–OTwB (see Preface) and this book, along with a growing number of occupational therapists and survivors,[3,5,14–18] the editors propose rethinking our traditional occupational therapy roles, in some respects revisiting our professional origins in social action[19] (see Chs 7, 9, 11). We've been hemmed in for too long. When we begin to look at the world without borders we will be enabling ourselves to revise the basis for the work we do with other people, to live the process described by Mary Reilly: 'Man [sic], through the use of his hands, as they are energized by his mind and will, can influence the state of his own health.'[20] We will have begun to explore different social and cultural forces, realize different political contexts, and re-articulate our aims for occupational therapy. The following principles, attributed to de Souza by Molinas Maldonado and Monroy Peralta,[1] offer a basis:

1. Everybody is responsible for everything.
2. Think globally, act locally.
3. Nothing changes if nothing is done to change.
4. The aim is not to attain the goals proposed, but the processes above all.
5. There is no public ethic without a personal ethic.

These require us to address 'the fact that far reaching improvements in health depend more on social, economic, and political factors than on either medical breakthroughs or health care interventions per se, and that a key to widespread improvement in health is strong political commitment to equity in meeting all people's basic needs.'[21] (p. 129)

RETHINKING OUR APPROACH TO WORKING IN COMMUNITIES

Like the fundamental ideas behind occupational therapy, these principles may appear disarmingly simple,[22] but they entail the rethinking of our approach to acting in the communities with whom we work.[1,2,5]

Everybody is responsible for everything

The first principle calls us, both as professionals and as citizens, to rescue *responsibility* from the dilution which has occurred through the development of society.[1] This responsibility was acknowledged by occupational therapy pioneers at the turn of the last century;[23–25] our *'ability to respond'* connects with our primary role of 'enabling occupation'.[26] Responsibility is inextricably linked with occupation as a means by which we interact with the environment and other people, as we take ownership for what we do, or are able to do. As participants in society we have to negotiate the nature of our occupation according to our ability. Successful participation depends on being able to cooperate with others in a way that reflects occupational ability. In the framing of disability as 'those who are different from a non-disabled us', there is a supposition that knowledge of how to respond appropriately is held not by those who experience disabling conditions, but by those who are 'able'. The caring professions are often popularly constructed as 'people who are *more* capable'. If occupational therapists are seduced by the ethics of *Animal Farm*[27] in which 'some are more equal than others' (p. 114), differences in ability or disability become medicalized, and the people who possess them are excluded and presented as having no connection with the rest of society. They become invisible, or else curios, something different from the normal experience, objects for the technologies of care.[28] As a consequence, we do not think that we are in some way responsible for them. It appears that the sense of responsibility has become diluted, thus as people-centered *allied* health professionals we are reluctant to ally ourselves with the grassroots elements of disability rights and other social movements. Those who do cross this border are the exception.[5,14,29] Perhaps it is unreasonable, even unethical, to expect that all occupational therapists can actively engage politically,[2] but we are bound to interrogate and justify the basis of our alliances, as we have already noted from Chomsky.[11] It is *irresponsible*, in terms of the first principle set out here, to overlook this.

Martin Luther King's statement, 'Whatever affects one directly, affects all indirectly. I can never be what I ought to be until you are what you ought to be. This is the interrelated structure of reality,'[30] (p. 70) appears appropriate to the context of health and wellbeing. In our field of practice, in the new millennium, the infamous excuse that was heard after the Holocaust, '*Wir haben es nicht gewusst*' ('We did not know about it') does not hold up. Technological improvements are giving an ever-increasing number of people around the world access to a wider range of information. This facility adds to our personal and collective responsibility for what goes on in the world,[31] as the possession of knowledge makes it more difficult to ignore social justice issues and raises questions about the basis for inequalities. All of us are participants in history, nothing excludes us, every action or non-action involves a moral choice concerning the potential outcome through this interdependence. However, while knowledge is a determinant of wealth, health, and wellbeing, many people lack access to education and information, and to the empowerment and participation these offer. Thus enlightenment involves a realization of the need to think globally and act locally, the second of our five principles.

Think globally, act locally

The second principle talks about the need to take a global perspective toward the conditions that we hope to influence. It is useful to know who is doing what, with which methods, the extent of their contributions, the results, the mistakes that were made, and the means of overcoming them, in whatever field we hope to make a difference. We need to recognize a state or quality of being 'other' or 'otherwise'. Put simply, one might use the 'relative' test: 'is the service I am providing as good as I would want for my partner, child, parent, or myself to receive? What changes would they, or I, want?' Through this we can establish a context for our actions and make connections between what we do and what others do.[1] Whether or not we are experiencing disabling conditions, we construct ourselves through our occupational interactions with others.[32,33] This underlines our interdependence. The construction we make of ourselves depends on others to facilitate and enable it. Empowerment is a mutual consent. Each individual's achievement rests upon the support of others, just as people support their children in achieving developmental milestones. We may recognize the child's achievement, but we might also recognize the assistance given by others.

Rather than focusing on occupation within the framework of individual lives, Goldstein[34] addresses the importance of occupation in an international context. He argues that, just as occupational therapists recognize that 'persons shape and are shaped by their environments',[26] the world of international relations produces scripts for daily life experiences and vice versa; everyday occupational choices affect the course of international politics. Goldstein's work requires us to think about both the occupations of the people that we work with and our own activities in a global and political context. Human occupation does not take place in a vacuum.

However, it is impossible to take in the whole sweep of history and a global view of human activity simultaneously. While it seems necessary to take into account the whole picture, we are only practically able to work with a portion of it. 'Thinking globally, acting locally' in an occupational therapy without borders demands a critical awareness of the political nature of who we are and what we do, and encourages dialectic discourse which recognizes that we could be either or both survivors and professionals and respect the positions of the other. Although Goldstein[34] refers to political science issues, his points may also inform therapists in negotiation with their patients toward their reconstruction of meaningful lives. According to Goldstein, the choices that individuals make in their daily experience have powerful and potentially international significance. Therapists using an occupational science perspective will be interested in analyzing the impact of international and global issues on their patients' valuing of activity. For example, an interest in macrobiotic gardening might be engendered in a patient through reference to global environmental concerns. Patients may choose to join a political movement as a way of dealing constructively with tensions between society's expectations and their disabling conditions or sexual orientation. Goldstein's work alerts us to think about our own patients' occupations in an active global and political context.

As Chomsky[11] remarks (pp. 191–192):

> I don't think any sane human being can look around at the world and not figure out things that have to be done – take a walk through the streets, you'll find plenty of things that have to be done. So you know, you get started doing them. But you're not going to be able to do them alone. Like, if you take a walk down the streets and say, "That ought to be done," nothing's going to happen. On the other hand, if people become organized enough to act together, yeah, then you can achieve things. And there's no particular limit to what you can achieve. I mean, that's why we don't still have slavery. ... you start by saying: **"Look, here's where the world is, what can we begin to do?"** Well, you can begin to do things which will get people to understand better what the real source of power is, and just how much they can achieve if they get involved in political activism. And once you've broken through the pretense, you just construct organizations – that's it. You work on things that are worth working on. If it's taking control of your community, it's that. If it's gaining control of your workplace, it's that. If it's working on solidarity, it's that. If it's taking care of the homeless, it's that.

Nothing changes, if nothing is done to change

As Lyotard put it: 'The nineteenth and twentieth centuries have given us as much terror as we can take. We have paid a high enough price for the nostalgia of the whole and the one experience.'[35] If this is so, the search is on for 'fresh ideas and practices for a more promising millennium'.

However, in the uncertainty of this new millennium we have to work out a number of questions: what do we hang on to, what do we abandon from the past; *what is worth doing?*[36] (p. 4) '*What exactly are we trying to change.*'[37] (p. 234) We have to know this in order to be able to facilitate others in achieving the being and doing of what they value.[38]

The third principle calls us to act, to 'walk the talk', to make the transition proactively from discourse to concrete practice. Of all the principles, this one connects explicitly with occupational therapy's core construct, occupation, which refers to 'groups of activities and tasks of everyday life, named, organized, and given value and meaning by individuals and a culture'.[26] Equally, it connects with the profession's primary role of enabling occupation, which refers to collaborating with people to choose, organize and perform occupations which they find useful and meaningful in their environment.[26,39] However, the central question is whose value and meaning are occupational therapists committed to in everyday practice?

One of the most debilitating issues for many people in so-called developing societies is that they do not live long enough to see significant changes in their lives.[1] Grand political discourses do not deliver practical and lasting implementation. Similarly, development agencies (e.g. NGOs, the UN) continue to make promises for a tomorrow that never seems to become a reality, consequently many community groups no longer believe them.[1] Changes are not just given or done to people, but need to be encouraged and advanced in collaboration with them. We need to evaluate, with those with whom we have been working, whether the processes we engage in generate visible and desirable changes. These steps are clearly within the remit of occupational therapy's person-centered approach to enabling occupation,[16,40] and are in collaboration with inclusion movements.[5]

The aim is not to attain the goals proposed, but the processes above all

The fourth principle calls us to rethink the way we propose and carry out our projects, interventions, and programs.[1] Besides measuring the success of activities through outcomes, we should give importance to the processes that have articulated the work, including a participatory occupational justice framework (see Ch. 9),[3] in other words, we should clearly recognize the collaboration between the therapists and those they work with. Outcomes represent fixed points in time. Working with people on the development of a project suggests and often demands a continuity that the processes are geared to enable,[40] yet in concluding the evaluation, the voices of people with experiences of disability are 'often the missing piece of the puzzle'.[5,16,41] (p. 116), Evaluating processes tells us what progress our work has enabled, and allows learning from mistakes through reconstructing the lived processes and experiences of collaboration and interdependence irrespective of our roles.[5] Mistakes are inevitable, people-centered collaboration involves taking and sharing risks and responsibilities, as the earlier principles have described. However, in the story of the change processes on which we have embarked, we must recognize that there is no public ethic without a personal ethic – the last of our five principles.

There is no public ethic without a personal ethic

Equally, there is no personal ethic without a public ethic, and people are judged by their actions. This last principle takes us to the theme of ethics. According to de Souza people have equal rights. 'All types of poverty are unacceptable. All types of misery are intolerable.'[42] Consequently, human beings should take precedence over government: 'It is imperative that ethics stands over politics and that politics stands over economy.'[42]

Our professional codes of ethics articulate values such as equity, equality, and justice; for example, 'occupational therapists are committed to providing services for all individuals who are in need of these services, regardless of ability, gender or other defining characteristics.'[43] That is what we say, but often we are addressing these values to a group of people we refer to as consumers.[44] This suggests a unidirectional provision of services rather than a collaborative process of occupational justice which benefits all the actors in the community. Consumers are people who have the resources to buy services such as occupational therapy and products that come with it such as meaningful occupation. Thus the term consumer does not represent a holistic view of people, but focuses on one aspect of a limited occupational function – not even, for example, the relationship between productivity and consumption. It does not recognize the complexities of a person who interacts with the natural environment and is a social being with a human right for dignity and reciprocity, expressed through community,[45] nor does it suggest that 'the need for love, friendship, home and meaningful occupation are universal human needs, irrespective of age, class, race or disability.'[5] (p. 84)

Bockhoven, a psychiatrist, considered that 'acknowledgement of the critical moral importance of occupation in human life demands an in-depth review by the health professions of their own value judgements and practices with respect to identifying which are the means and which are the ends of our endeavours.'[46] He further argued that occupational therapy is 'a neglected source of community re-humanization' which was 'blocked from perceiving either the depth or the breadth of its role as a moral and scientific force. This role has even more central importance to future human development than could possibly be claimed by any existing scientific specialty which neither has nor claims a moral basis.'[46] (p. 222)

Given this, how do we return to the social concerns which motivated pioneer occupational therapists? In questioning and reflecting upon the meaning of our work, what are the personal ethics that underpin what we do, and as Molinas Moldonado and Monroy Peralta ask, 'are the means we use as dignified, correct and honest as the results that we hope to achieve?'[1] (p. 45) In a world of public corruption in daily life, moral values appear to have lost their usefulness, and prominent individuals are able to distort information and manipulate attitudes and public opinions. Truths have become uncertain, the difference between right and wrong is blurred. The perception is more valuable than the fact, thus it is important to be seen to be doing good. People experiencing disabling conditions are both the victims of this rupture of values and at the same time offer a valuable opportunity to those who need to demonstrate their worth as good citizens. This may include people who genuinely feel a need to restore right to a wronged world, acting from a wish simply to help others (and thus 'therapize' themselves). Pity motivates working out of an individual need for forgiveness,[29] because it is seen as a duty to do something for people with disabilities. Therefore, we have to question our motivation to become therapists; we might otherwise find ourselves in a strange profession, whose existence was enabled by a dependence on pity for others, yet holds onto values of enabling and empowering them. Such a profession would be unable to find an arena for collaborative work, because pity does not recognize the mutuality of responsibility suggested by the first principle; instead, it depends on the unequal distribution of wealth and opportunity without offering reciprocity.

This is something we need to confront to empower ourselves to work with people, as Sen proposes[38,47] for wellbeing based on the freedom to be and do, which correlates with Wilcock's[46] occupational perspective of achieving health through 'doing, being and becoming'. These concepts demand we pay attention to enabling sustainability. This work requires a 'conviction and commitment' to human rights in which there are rights holders (i.e. people experiencing disabling conditions), and duty bearers (i.e. the professionals working with them).[48] (p. 8) As de Gaay Fortman argues, if the rights holders are unable to effect their fundamental entitlement to justice, then the duty bearers have to enable them to exercise their political and legal rights.[48] The role of occupational therapists is thus concerned with enabling active participation in the first principle of shared responsibility as a consequence of enabling meaningful occupation (see Ch. 6).

CONCLUSION

This book is about a process; it is not a total view, not an attempt at holism. The process is one of critically re-evaluating what occupational therapy has to offer human society and how it can effectively address the political aspects of facilitating meaningful occupation. The process cannot be fixed in time, but involves the continuous recognition of useful components, their refinement, and their application on locally negotiated bases. From this a diversity of practice is inevitable, but fundamental to it all will be – just as is evident from the diversity in this book – the recognition of occupational needs and the application of the occupational right to do, be, and become: 'the need for love, friendship, home [community] and meaningful occupation are universal human needs, irrespective of age, class, race or disability.'[5] (p. 84)

This statement comes not from an occupational therapist, but from Micheline Mason, a disabled activist for inclusion rights. Who are to be our role models in our quest for a society based on rights to meaningful occupations? We have given the first section of this book to the voices of survivors, i.e. people who have demonstrated their capability to find a why, despite adverse conditions, despite society's restrictions. All these people have, like Mason, turned situations of disadvantage into 'an opportunity to create a new response which will lead to learning and growth for the whole community. If we take this attitude towards our unsolved problems, then the life of anyone who presents such 'problems' has a value – a meaning.'[5] (p. 82)

This also implies a concern with dignity through meaningful occupation. In Chapter 6 we will explore meaningful occupation as a need and a right which is denied through occupational apartheid and occupational absurdity. The value of occupation is perhaps first perceived by the person engaged in it. Something has, as we have already mentioned, to be worth doing. As occupational therapists, who have traditionally prescribed occupation to others, we have sometimes been criticized for getting people to perform inappropriate, embarrassing and boring activities.[26,39,49] To fulfill our professional role, and manifest our expertise in occupation, we have to acknowledge that successful occupational therapy requires informed consent, and a negotiated basis around need. A repositioning of occupational therapy is therefore required which, as we have been arguing here, asks searching questions of the nature of needs, and political questions about the formation and development of needs and the means to address them. Along with over 50 authors, many of whom are well established in the field, from northern and southern hemispheres, from wealthy and impoverished countries, who have contributed to this book, we have for the last 2 years been engaged in a continuous dialogue around the dialectic of occupational needs and rights, which goes further than existing models of human occupation. This book introduces a number of new concepts, not only occupational apartheid and occupational absurdity, but new and updated models, new approaches to education and fields of practice. The contributors who follow are challenging and redefining our professional borders, critically refining the art *and* science of occupational therapy, and emancipating practitioners in determining *how*, with *whom*, and *where* we work.

Acknowledgement

We would like here to express our gratitude to Michael Iwama and Reg Urbanowski for their valuable critical comments during the development of this chapter.

References

1. Molinas Moldinado MM, Monroy Peralta JG. *Sistematizacion de experiencias: una invitacion para la accion una propuesta para instituciones y/o prograganas que trabajan con el Sector de la Infancia.* Guatemala City: Childhope; 1999.

2. Duncan M, Watson R. Transformation through occupation: towards a prototype. In: Watson R, Swartz L, eds. Transformation through occupation. London: Whurr; 2004:301–318.

3. Townsend E, Wilcock AA. Occupational justice. In: Christiansen C, Townsend E, eds. Introduction to occupation: the art and science of living. Thorofare NJ: Prentice Hall; 2003:243–273.

4. McKnight J. The careless society – community and its counterfeits. New York: Basic Books; 1995.

5. Mason M. Incurably human. London: wORking Press; 2002.

6. Turner A. Patient? Client? Service User? – What's in a name? Br J Occup Ther 2002; 65(8):355.

7. Swartz L. Rethinking professional ethics. In: Watson R, Swartz L, eds. Transformation through occupation. London: Whurr; 2004:289–300.

8. Kronenberg F. Overcoming occupational apartheid: enabling people to celebrate their differences. (Paper) Cape Town: OTASA; 2004.

9. Watson R, Lagerdien K. Women empowered through occupation: from deprivation to realised potential.

In: Watson R, Swartz L, eds. Transformation through occupation. London: Whurr; 2004:103–118.

10. Lorenzo T. Equalizing opportunities for occupational engagement: disabled womens' stories. In: Watson R, Swartz L, eds. Transformation through occupation. London: Whurr; 2004:85–102.

11. Chomsky N. Understanding power: the indispensable Chomsky. Eds Mitchell P, Schoeffel J. New York: The New Press; 2002.

12. Kronenberg F. In search of the political nature of occupational therapy. MSc OT paper. Linköping University, Linköping, Sweden. 2003.

13. Watson R, Fourie M. International and African influences on occupational therapy. In: Watson R, Swartz L, eds. Transformation through occupation. London: Whurr; 2004:33–50.

14. Kronenberg F. WFOT Draft position paper on community based rehabilitation (CBR). Online. Available: www.wfot.org link Archives.

15. Kronenberg F. WFOT report Helsinki review on community based rehabilitation (CBR). Online. Available: www.wfot.org, link International Liaison.

16. Kronenberg F. WFOT Position paper on community based rehabilitation (CBR). Online. Available: www.wfot.org, link Document Centre.

17. Wilcock AA. Reflections on doing, being and becoming. Can J Occup Ther, 1998; 65(5):248–256.

18. Watson R. New horizons in occupational therapy. In: Watson R, Swartz L, eds. Transformation through occupation. London: Whurr; 2004:3–18.

19. Wilcock AA. Occupation for health, vol. 2. London: College of Occupational Therapists; 2002.

20. Reilly M. Occupational therapy can be one of the great ideas of twentieth century medicine. Am J Occup Ther 1962; 16(1):1–9.

21. Werner D, Sanders D. Questioning the solution: the politics of primary health care and child survival (with an in-depth critique of oral rehydration therapy). Palo Alto, CA: Healthwrights; 1997: p. 129.

22. Hagedorn R. Tools for practice in occupational therapy. Edinburgh: Churchill Livingstone; 2000.

23. Frank G. Opening feminist histories of occupational therapy. Am J Occup Ther 1992; 46:989–999.

24. Townsend E. Muriel Driver lecture: occupational therapy's social vision. Can J Occup Ther 1993; 60:174–184.

25. Thibeault R. 2002. In praise of dissidence: Anne Lang-Etienne. Can J Occup Ther 2002; 69(4):197–203.

26. Canadian Association of Occupational Therapists. Enabling occupation: an occupational therapy perspective (*revised edn.*). Ottawa, ON: CAOT Publications ACE; 2002.

27. Orwell G. Animal Farm. Harmondsworth: Penguin; 1951.

28. Foucault M. Discipline and punish. Harmondsworth: Penguin; 1991.

29. Marks D. Disability: controversial debates and psychosocial perspectives. London: Routledge; 1999.

30. Luther King M. Strength to love. Philadelphia: Fortress; 1963.

31. Kronenberg F. Occupational therapy without borders: occupational justice education. Paper presented at the 9th European Network of Occupational Therapy in Higher Education. Prague. October/November 2003.

32. Sumsion T. Overview of client centred practice. In: Sumsion T, ed. Client centred practice in occupational therapy. Edinburgh: Churchill Livingstone; 1999:1–14.

33. Snow J. What's really worth doing and how to do it. Toronto: Inclusion press; 1994.

34. Goldstein J. International perspectives in occupation. In: Zemke R, Clarke F, eds. Occupational science, the evolving discipline. Philadelphia: Davis; 1996.

35. Lyotard J. The postmodern condition: a report on knowledge. Minneapolis, MA: University of Minnesota Press; 1984.

36. Gergen K. An invitation to social construction. London: Sage; 1999.

37. Sloan T. ed. Critical psychology: voices for change. London: Macmillan Press; 2000.

38. Sen A. Development is freedom. Oxford: Oxford University Press; 1999.

39. Townsend E. Reflections on power and justice in enabling occupation. Can J Occup Ther 2003; 70(2):74–87.

40. Watson R. A population approach to transformation. In: Watson R, Swartz L, eds. Transformation through occupation. London: Whurr; 2004:51–65.

41. Barnes C. Theories of disability and the origins of the oppression of disabled people in western society. In: Barton L. Disability and society; emerging issues and insights. Harlow: Longman; 1996:43–60.

42. de Souza H. Speech at the Plenary of the United Nations during the second session of the Preparatory Committee for the Social Summit. New York, August 23, 1994.

43. American Occupational Therapy Association. Code of Ethics. 2000. Online. Available: http://www.aota.org/general/coe.asp

44. Council of Occupational Therapists for the European Countries. Code of Ethics. 1996. Online. Available: http://www.cotec-europe.org/

45. Garrett T, Baillie H, Garrett R. Health care ethics: principles and problems. Englewood Cliffs, NJ: Prentice Hall; 1989.

46. Wilcock AA. An occupational perspective of health. Thorofare, NJ: Slack; 1999.
47. Sen A. Inequality reexamined. Oxford: Oxford University Press; 1992.
48. de Gaay Fortman B. Persistent poverty and inequality in an era of globalization: opportunities and limitations of a rights approach. Economic, Social and Cultural Rights Workshop. Nairobi:14–16 April 2003.
49. Hawking S. Striving for excellence in the presence of disabilities. In: Zemke R, Clarke F, eds. Occupational science, the evolving discipline. Philadelphia: Davis, 1996.

SECTION 1

Voices of survivors

INTRODUCTION

Perhaps one of the first questions the reader might have about this book is the significance of the subtitle *'Learning from the Spirit of Survivors'*, and why it is we have started with 'Voices of survivors'. First, we should explain that the term 'survivors' was arrived at from the experiences of two of the editors, who worked in Mexico, Guatemala, and Kosovo with the survivors of extreme situations and conflicts who were also survivors of trauma and disabling conditions at an individual and at a community level. This experience led to the formation of the small organization which became SPIRIT of SURVIVORS – Occupational Therapy without Borders (see Preface). Subsequently, we became aware of other ways in which people with disabilities were referring to themselves as 'survivors', (see Useful websites), as part of the process of identifying themselves as empowered individuals who make decisions about their own lives.

Enablement, and the promotion of this capacity, is becoming central in occupational therapy.[1,2] Sharing people's narratives of their experiences of health-related problems and concerns in their lives and communities enables links to be made between their everyday realities and policy-making and global politics, and allows inclusion of their own analyses of causal factors, their own initiatives, their successes and failures, and their proposals for the future. If we are only concerned with the work of the therapist, the most we can achieve is a partial history of occupational therapy which ignores the most valuable evidence.

Any occupational therapy *without borders* has to learn from the spirit of survivors if it is to offer an individual, group, or community centered approach, negotiating on the basis of people's needs, rather than an imposed approach. Most of the survivors in this section have sustained their achievements outside the borders of occupational therapy's territories. Despite this, the lessons that can be derived from their testimony and spirit are centered around a familiar core: the right to engage in meaningful occupation (see Chs 1 and 6).

The stories shared in this section by Valdo (Ch. 2), Sabriye and Paul (Ch. 3), Barbara (Ch. 4), and Pat (Ch. 5) traverse the world, being located in places as far apart as Brazil, Tibet, Palestine, and England. The 'borders' we are 'without' are not geographical features, and the 'maps' described in these personal histories offer no boundaries between human beings, between the therapist and the recipient. Instead these writers, reporting back from terrae incognitae, offer a cartography of the potential of meaningful occupation, whether, for example, in the curfew-confined washing of Barbara's kitchen floor, or in blind children's robust confidence in their new skills.

These lands were not just unknown, but were forbidden possibilities, which the writers have had to gain the right to explore. This driving determination is evident throughout. Valdo's determination that he should survive the streets of the *favelas* eventually makes it possible for him to become a university student of linguistics and anthropology, who also runs a support organization for children and families in Brazil;

Sabriye's insistence that despite being a blind woman she could travel to Tibet carries her and Paul Kronenberg through to the establishment of a project which is unique, not only in what it offers blind children, but as an example of local cooperation.

If our souls dream, and there are moments when we realize who we are and the mission we have, then these stories are an inspiration to seek those peak experiences[3] beyond the borders of perception. Whenever we are faced with a task and we understand what we have to do – write a book, start a project, do anything – immediately our minds start to throw obstacles in the way, and we doubt ourselves. We become afraid of our real potential. This is why, as Pat Smart says in her chapter, we have an obligation to publish our testimonies: 'we need to take responsibility for the way our memories are recorded for others to have'. To do this, we have to enable people in their capacity for activity; in the full sense of social, political, and economic dimensions to the purpose of action, the key words, as the World Bank says, are 'participation and equality in distribution of the benefits'.[4] We have to facilitate a process in which people find the means to grow and develop, and to voice, affirm and reflect on the part they are playing, i.e. to recognize their enactment of occupational justice. Whether this is enacted through the process of developing community publications or the distribution of financial support for families, the achievements of people such as Valdo, Sabriye and Paul, Barbara, and Pat have not come about through passivity and acceptance. The Catalan poet Marti Pol, a survivor of multiple sclerosis for more than 30 years, wrote:

> *We have just what we have, and it's enough*
> *The space of concrete history that we hold*
> *And this minuscule territory to live in*
> *Stand up again*
> *Be all the voices, solemnly and clearly*
> *Shout out who we are*
> *And that the whole world should listen*
> *And that in the end each one will see their place*
> *And say louder*
> *That everything has to be done*
> *And everything is possible …*

> (L'ambit de tots els ambits)[5]

References

1. Canadian Association of Occupational Therapists. Enabling occupation: an occupational therapy perspective (revised edn.). Ottawa, ON: CAOT publications ACE; 2002.
2. Sumsion T, ed. Client centred practice in occupational therapy. Edinburgh: Churchill Livingstone; 1999.
3. Maslow A (1970) Religions, Values and Peak Experiences, Harmondsworth, Penguin, http://www.google.co.uk/search?q=cache:-hjPVliArngJ:www.druglibrary.org/schaffer/lsd/maslow.htm+Maslow+peak+experiences&hl=en
4. De Gaay Fortman B, Persistent poverty and inequality in an era of globalization: Opportunities and limitations of a rights approach, Economic, Social and Cultural Rights Workshop, Nairobi, 2003.
5. Farres P. *Miquel Martii Pol. Antologica Poética*. Barcelona: Edicions 62; 1999.

Useful websites

The Landmine Survivors' Network
www.landminesurvivors.org
Survivors' Poetry http://66.102.11.104/search?q=cache:gFP841WuaZUJ:groups.msn.com/survivorspoetry+survivors+poetry&hl=en

The World Network of Users and Survivors of Psychiatry
http://www.wnusp.org/

Chapter 2

Once a street child, now a citizen of the world

Valdo Bomfim
(From an interview with Frank Kronenberg, translated by Nick Pollard and Christina Szanton Blanc)

I'm from Independencia, a little town that's part of Belo Horizonte, a big conurbation and state capital of Minas Gerais in the south east of Brazil, 500 kilometers from Rio de Janeiro. I was born in 1972 into a really impoverished home. My mother was very happy with her two children, a girl and a boy, but my parents hoped for another son. When they had twin boys, they had to worry about feeding four children, not three. However, even when the others arrived our family of seven children was still not very big compared with those who had fifteen children in one family.

My first eleven years were pretty normal. Though there were many difficulties, and we had no toys and nothing much to play with, we were very happy. We were a very loving family, particularly us boys. Like many working people in Brazilian society, my parents had no opportunity to learn to read or write. They worried about how to educate their children and put them on the right road. I was a normal child, studious, intelligent, very interested in history, but with a growing tendency to be critical of the inequalities and injustices that history produced. It was difficult for me to accept that other children would have toys and bikes to play with, while my parents could not afford to buy these things for us. I have known kids who ran away from home because there were toys to play with in the organizations for street children where they could find refuge.

One thing that sums all this up for me is the particular smell of my own childhood, the smell of the red earth on which I walked to school, and which was always on my school uniform. The red earth also reminds me of football games, and of the little plastic toy cars that people gave poor boys. At that time it was common for church people, both Catholic and Protestant, to give gifts to families who lacked a regular income, in the hope of attracting them to their church or toward a change in their religious affiliation. These things played an important role in small towns like ours. They created a kind of second religious colonization that made things worse for me. Unfortunately, our town didn't have any Protestant organizations giving handouts to poor people, so because I was Protestant (and have remained Protestant up to now) rather than Catholic and did not belong to a Catholic organization, I could not receive handouts.

My Catholic friends, who could easily get clothes from the 'padres' (Catholic fathers) and from the people in the Catholic organizations, were thus much better dressed than me. This made me very bitter. The roots of my disillusionment were planted in those first eleven years.

I wanted to leave home, not because my father, mother, or family mistreated me, but because of the many good things I had seen on television, in the soap operas, and the films made in Rio de Janeiro. Although I was only a boy I wanted adventure and to know the world.

A GIRL, AND THE BEGINNING OF MY TROUBLES!

All this came to a head when I got to know a very pretty girl while walking to school. She was about 9 years old, I was 11 years old, and I wanted to make her fall in love with me. She was my first dream girl, blonde with blue eyes, totally perfect, and I wanted to be like her. However, she was related to one of the most important and better off families in the neighborhood, and she did not seem to have any interest in me, a poor black boy.

I tried very hard to win over this girl. First of all, in order to obtain some money to buy snacks to share with her from the street vendors outside the school gates who sold poor kids' popcorn and other items, I stole from my dad when he was asleep. It was only a small amount, his bus fare for work. This went on every week for 5 months. The theft was all the more sinful because I stole in order to capture the attention of a girl who paid no attention whatsoever to me; but she was very pretty and I was attracted to her and everything she represented.

To win her over I needed something else up my sleeve. Her boyfriend was in the same social class as her, well dressed and with clean clothes, in contrast to me. Unlike my mother, his mother didn't work from seven in the morning till nine at night, then return home and have no time for him. Likewise, his father was not out at four in the morning until five in the afternoon every day, working for a minimum wage (150 reales, reais or 70 euros a month). I made friends soon afterwards with another boy who always sat at the back of my class. He did not like my girl's boyfriend. He offered to teach me the ways of the world and how to win over this girl. We started by smoking a cigarette together. Later we roamed the streets. Years later I found out that he'd been killed by the police.

As you might imagine, these 5–6 months were a crucial time of my life. I had started doing bad things. One day, for the first time in many generations of my family, a policeman arrived at my house, looking for me. He had caught me out on the streets and took me home. For many years the government had a strange policy of 'social cleansing', like cleaning up rubbish. Rather than having the streets full of poor kids at Christmas time, they ordered the police to arrest all the kids and take them back to their homes. For my poor yet very honest family this was a great humiliation. My father was at work. My eldest sister pleaded with the policeman: 'Please, this isn't a street kid, he attends school.'

She said nothing to my parents, but in a small neighborhood the neighbors gossip among each other, especially when something bad happens.

Eventually a neighbor spoke to my father when he was coming home from work: 'Why does a hard-working man like you have a son who is a delinquent?' Having heard what happened my father understood why his money had been stolen. I felt very bad that day because it was the only time in my life that my father ever beat me. He and my mum are very good people, who have stayed together despite very difficult and sad times. They had not chosen our social conditions; it wasn't their fault that I was misbehaving. I had actually only done so for a few months.

I decided that loving this girl was impossible. I also decided not to study any more but to escape, to leave home for the first time. I left when I was 12 years old and did not return until I was 18 years old. I left a card for dad and mum saying that I was leaving to make or break my fortune. I didn't want to make them suffer any more. Because my actions had led to gossip my father felt he had to sell the house he'd built with his own hands on our little piece of land. It was my fault because the police had arrested me. He bought a small piece of land in another struggling town, called Betim, 50 kilometers further south. They still have a house there. Betim is where I have based the project that I describe toward the end of the chapter.

ROAMING THE STREETS IN THE 1980s: THE PENAL CODE FOR MINORS

The years 1982–1983 were very difficult in Brazil. At that time everyone from the poorer classes, but particularly the kids, lived under a rigid penal code, the Minors' Code. This was established in 1979 and replaced the Assistance Service to Minors (SAM) created in 1941, whose methods were already correctional and repressive. Under the Minors' Code, any young people found roaming the streets and thus presumably in 'an irregular situation' involving need or crime became wards of the court.[1] They fell under the authority of state judges who could take them from their families and imprison them until the age of 18 years in the Fundaçao Naçional do Bem-estar do Menor (National Foundation for the Wellbeing of Minors), known as the FUNABEM, first established in Rio de Janeiro and gradually duplicated in all the states through the creation of State Foundations for the Welfare of Minors or FEBEM. These juvenile prisons were dreary institutions where often quite deserving poor young people were literally 'parked' without the benefit of school education, in the company of some very tough kids. Under the pressure of local non-governmental organizations (NGOS), which were increasingly aware of the plight of these children, and after the First National Congress on Street Children held in the federal government building in Brasilia in 1986 with the participation of more than 500 street children (including myself), there was a popular swell of support for these disadvantaged children together with a push for democracy. The Minors' Code was replaced in late 1990 with a Children's and Adolescents' Act, after the country had drafted a new democratic Constitution in 1988, with a whole chapter on children patterned on the Convention for the Rights of the Child ratified by the UN General Assembly in 1989. This new Act included important provisions at the federal level that were supposed to be adopted by each state, together with a general trend toward decentralization of control over social services and related resources. Many of these options promised disadvantaged Brazilian kids the dismantling of the FEBEM system and a better hope for the future.[1,2]

It should be added that these FEBEM juvenile prisons operated quite differently in different places. The FUNABEM in Rio de Janeiro was considered the most dangerous. It was closed down in 1989. Today there is a public school for the kids who live in the neighborhood, but the school has an annex called Padre Severino that is again a prison for minors. The kids under 18 years are placed right next to older tougher boys of 18 or 19 years, who are still there because the adult prisons don't have a place for them. In my opinion this puts the futures of these under 18 kids at risk.

The continued existence of the FEBEM in Sao Paulo also tells us that this state hasn't fully implemented the Children's and Adolescents' Act of 1990. Of the 5507 municipalities and 26 states in Brazil, so far only just over 100 municipalities and two states have fully adopted the provisions of the Children's and Adolescents' Act of 1990, i.e. Children's Councils and Participatory Budgeting.[3] The political downfall in the late 1990s of President Fernando Collor De Mello, who strongly supported the Act, has delayed its enforcement.

Where the FEBEM remain repressive there are protests and frequent killings of young kids who thus never reach adulthood. Crime-hardened older kids continue to use and abuse the smaller ones.

SURVIVING AS A CHILD ON THE STREETS

After running away I spent 3–4 months on the streets of Belo Horizonte. While my parents searched for me I was learning how to live on the streets. There are many ways to survive. First you need to learn one of the many street languages, which use different consonants, such as f, ch, p, r, ls. The 'p' language is the easiest to learn and in fact because of this the Belo Horizonte street kids never spoke it. Instead, their street language is similar to how the kids talk in Sao Paulo, but different to kids from Rio, where they use the dialect from the *favelas*. To use the 'p' language, you always insert the consonant *p* into the words you're saying, so *'qualè meu irmao'* ('hey my brother') becomes *'qualepe meirmaopao'*. We used this language to identify our group and stay together, for example when we were using marijuana or ether, or at other times to let others know we were a little high.

If I wanted to speak with my friends from the streets, perhaps to sort out how we might rob someone without anyone else understanding what we were going to do, we'd use this street kids code. This has often saved me from the bandits. They would ask me, 'Are you a street kid?' and I'd say, 'Yes, yes,' then speak in my back-slang. There was a second language that was much more difficult because we added two consonants in the middle of the words. For example, we'd use *ch* so that in Portuguese 'Hey my friends, do you want to be my street brothers?' sounded like '*Qualècheche mechecheu amichichigo, voçecheche quecheche secheche mechecheu irmacamchao di rucuchua?*' On the basis of my own personal experience I'd say these street languages were particularly common in the three regions of Sao Paulo, Salvador, and Belo Horizonte. In Rio and Mato Grosso del Sur, where I also lived, I encountered street languages that were more directly influenced by regional dialects.

I liked the 'double f' language which was usually used in the FUNABEM. We used it to plan an escape from the FEBEM of Belo Horizonte. My subsequent interest in studying linguistics and socio-linguistics was a result of this emphasis on language construction.

Language was the first means of survival on the street, but I also developed many other skills that I still use today, such as sociability (I am a very sociable person), perseverance (when I love something I want to defend it to the finish), and leadership (I showed leadership qualities from my first day on the street).

That first day I was suffering. I'd nothing to eat, no place to sleep, no sleeping bag or blanket, and no goodnight kiss from my mum. That was the first consequence of my running away from home. But I knew my life had changed and I didn't want to go back because, as I'd written on that card, I was going to make or break my future. It was terrifying. I didn't sleep all night. I was afraid. I sniffed a little glue to keep out the cold, holding my shirt around it like the other kids. Belo Horizonte is in the mountains, and it gets very cold. It was the longest night of my life.

I began to learn about survival. Three things helped me. First was resourcefulness. There were a lot of gangs on the streets, each with a leader. I was a natural leader, and I wanted to succeed. I rescued the little brother of one of the most dangerous gang-leaders on the streets from a brawl with another gang. I intervened, stayed calm, and said that he'd done nothing and wasn't looking for any trouble. They let us go. Several days later when the boy's brother's gang found me alone on the street they thought I was part of this rival band of kids. The gang-leader accused me of wanting to hurt his little brother, and was going to kill me with a big knife, but then his brother stopped him and explained. So I entered the street gang hierarchy. It was the biggest thrill I'd had since learning to use street language.

My second survival skill was generosity – this went down well with the other kids. Some kids wouldn't beg because they were too proud. I'd look after cars for people. When they came back I'd ask them for a sandwich. They'd come back with two or three, which I gave to these other kids. This way I won them over to me, and they thought of me as their leader.

The third skill was that I was honest. I came through when I committed myself to doing something, and I still do. Between the ages of 12 and 18, these skills that I either possessed or developed were my passport. These tactics enable survival wherever you are.

After leaving my family, I initially lived in a central area of Belo Horizonte called Plaça da Savassi where the incident with the gang-leader and his brother took place. I was taken repeatedly to the FEBEM of Belo Horizonte by the police but always managed to escape. At the end of

1983 I escaped again with three friends, but this time we stole a car and took the highway to Rio de Janeiro. However, we were on drugs and the car overturned as we approached a small town.

I just got a little scratch but my friends had several broken bones. When the police came they thought that we were beggars and took us to the local lock-up. We told them we didn't know where we were, and that we'd taken a wrong turn, hoping that they wouldn't find out that we'd stolen a car. After our wounds had been treated we were placed temporarily in an institution for boys, since the penal code at the time still didn't allow kids like us to be cooped up with hardened criminals. However, we all managed to escape into the woods and ran in different directions. I hid for the whole night in the forest and hitched a lift by hiding in a car when a transporter full of Fiats stopped for a toilet break. The next week I was in Sao Paulo, where I stayed on the streets for 4 months. There I met a friend, a fantastic thief, who had a family on the streets. He taught me to break into houses and burgle them.

Later I moved thousands of kilometers away to the city of Campo Grande, capital of the state of Mato Grosso do Sul, but 3 months later the police caught me again. This place didn't have a FEBEM, but something very similar called the Delegacia Especializada para Menores (DEM). They knew nothing about me, and I had no documents, nothing to identify me. They asked me where I came from, how I had traveled so far, and why I was on the streets. They threw me on a bus for Rio de Janeiro, as I told them that was where I was from, and sent me to the FUNABEM there.

When I arrived I gave a false address in a *favela* run by one of the main gangs controlling drugs in Rio. This was an area the police never entered. Various gangs are at war with each other for the control of the drug trade in the *favelas*. Poor people who live in these areas have to cooperate with the gangs for fear of their lives or the lives of their children, since the Government seems to have no control in those *favelas* and the police cannot enter them. In some areas one can be shot by gangs for simply passing through. Other *favelas* are less dangerous and can be entered. The gangs that control most of the narcotics business in the territory of Rio are recognizable by their initials and by their tattoos. The children of the *favelas* respect them more than they do the police.

The FUNABEM sent me to the *favela* I had mentioned, accompanied by an educator recruited from the streets. When he asked me where the precise street was, I told him not to worry about it, and walked into the *favela*, which happened to have lots of gunmen. It was similar to a scene in the film *City of God* where people who were black in color were free to come and go in dangerous locations because they looked as if they belonged. As in their case, my black face fitted the situation so I didn't have any problems. My companion, however, started getting frightened and left, saying it was too dangerous to be there. I stayed on. The *favela* we had entered was called Canta Galo because whenever the police entered it a cockerel called out the alarm.

Survival on the streets of Rio was again very difficult. Things often got hot between the police and bandits and shootouts would take place. We younger kids would then seek refuge in the streets of the city center or at

Copacabana, but there too there were dangers lurking, especially at night. Sometimes I would lie awake all night, afraid of being captured or killed by the police, by the so-called death squads, or by drug traffickers from other gangs looking for the money we had stolen during the day. Street kids tended not to sleep at night for fear of being killed. I often spent the nights in cinemas. The last showing was at half-past six and I slept there to be safe. If I fell asleep during the day it was also OK because people would spot me. This way I wasn't in danger from the death squads.

As mentioned in numerous publications on street children in Latin America[4] and described in the *Report on the Situation of Human Rights in Brazil*[5] submitted to the Inter-American Commission on Human Rights in 1997, summary executions of children on the streets either by the police, or by professional killers who call themselves '*justiceiros*' and are called 'death squads' by others, unfortunately were and still are common in Brazil and also other Latin American countries. Crimes such as the death of six children shot while they were sleeping in front of the Candelaria Church in Rio in 1993 gave rise to an investigation of the 'death squads' by the National Human Rights Council. Some of the children killed were my friends and acquaintances.

THE SAO MARTINHO EXPERIENCE

I missed my family, I was trapped in this way of life, it was my own fault, and I had no hope. In the end I was able to escape thanks to Roberto Jose dos Santos, the director of the Sao Martinho organization, which was operated by the Carmelite Order of Saint Elias. He gave meals to street children but couldn't offer us anywhere to stay because the law (which was in force until 1990) said no lodging could be provided to minors without the intervention of a judicial authority. After the adoption in Brazil of the United Nations Charter for the Rights of Children and Adolescents[6] (1989) and of the Children's and Adolescents' Act[7] (1990) these conditions changed.[1,2]

We street kids came in to the Sao Martinho institute around 8 a.m., having slept near the entrance so that we could be the first to go in. We would shower and breakfast, play football, then break for lunch. At 5 p.m. there was a *merenda* (snack) and then we would leave again. Some kids came at lunchtime because they slept in the mornings when there was less likelihood of being hurt since there were more people around.

The best times at the Sao Martinho were when I was asked to work in the kitchen. I would get more to eat, because I'd get the tidbits, and I could also learn a few things. I liked to be at the center of what was going on because I was eager to find opportunities for myself. Eventually I found a way to win a study fellowship for the upper school through an unexpected acquaintance at the expensive private Catholic school, Santo Ignacio de Loyola. Even though my fees were fully paid, because of my situation and different social standing the priests there still asked me to wash the school's bathrooms and stairs three times a week in exchange for their teaching.

Working as an ex-street child in institutions like this had its problems. I will always be thankful for the help I received at such a critical time in my life, but most kids in such institutions will never have the chances I got through sheer good fortune and through my enterprising nature. It seemed to me that too much time could be spent by an institution's staff making lists of attendees or attending meetings in order to satisfy the quotas on which funding depended. I felt that older kids often did the work with the younger ones that should have been done by the salaried experts. It felt to me as if the better-paid experts, such as the psychologists or social workers attending to an institution's children, were more often than not using ex-street kids like me to do their work. They would promise that good kids who worked could become educators on a salary.

When institutions like this make ex-street kids into models for the other children to follow it seems to me that they are exploiting their past experience, rather than training the other kids for a different future. I held such a position of ex-street child helper from 1989 to 1992. Something that highlights the institutional power structure for me is that while the experts might ask for my help when they were confronted with particularly violent or troubled kids, they didn't invite me to official meetings, claiming that I could not understand their technical discussions.

The Sao Martinho was started by Roberto Jose Dos Santos. An ex-educator in the FUNABEM, he saw how bad things were for the children on the streets. He then started giving out sandwiches twice a week in Cinelandia Square, and I took advantage of it at times, though sparingly because I feared meeting kids from other gangs. Then the church gave Roberto the use of a high floor room in the buildings of the famous cathedral in Rio and he started his regular work with children. We would assemble there to play with the billiard machines or to play soccer, then eat. A few years later Roberto received from the municipality a large open space in the center of Rio. A building was put up with money donated by the Italian Caritas organization and by other organizations from Holland and Belgium. At the inauguration of the building there was a large and well attended celebration that marked the birth of an important new NGO. This NGO became very well known; it was visited by many illustrious people. Many additional donations were received, including other houses and farms purchased by the *Zecchino d'Oro*, a popular Italian TV show that did fund-raising.

By 1996 a major struggle had started regarding the intended sale of some of these properties. There is an ecclesiastical legal inquiry going on into this matter, to which I was asked to give my testimony. It is still not fully resolved.

Roberto Jose Dos Santos has created another small NGO called *Amar* (Love) but he is still saddened by the events described above. The new Sao Martinho now works predominantly for better-off kids, rather than for street children.

In 1989, I had to leave the Sao Martinho because I was no longer a minor. It was a rude awakening to my difficult situation in the world! One Sunday morning, as I was walking through Copacabana in Rio de Janeiro, without any prospects for the future, I saw outside a cinema a bright sign saying 'Rambo film show – free entry'. Inside, instead of a film show, I found a Baptist Church meeting. I wouldn't have gone in if

I'd known. As I tried to sit down, with my dirty clothes and my shoeshine box, the congregation thought I looked like a thief. An old lady next to me suddenly embraced her handbag. I finally blurted out: 'Lady, I'm not here to steal your handbag or watch, but to find something better in my life. In fact, I came to see a movie!' At the end of the meeting, however, I met some friendlier people. I returned every Sunday.

Soon after that a rich member of the church offered me his small yacht on which to live and sleep, provided there was no evidence of my presence when he used it on weekends. This was much better than sleeping in the streets.

The Baptist congregation disbanded 2 months later, due to the lack of a following. I would have been back on the streets but for another church member, a musician who let me sleep at night in his recording studio despite the misgivings of his fellow musicians, who thought me a thief. I stayed there until 1994, when I left for Italy where I now live. In exchange for this trust I helped my musician friend to transport his instruments to concerts, slowly making a place for myself in his heart, a place I still have today.

CONTACTS WITH MY FAMILY

While in touch with the Baptist Church, I was able to trace my parents' and family's whereabouts through them, and I went back to Betim to ask forgiveness from them and to tell them that I was working hard to find a living and make them proud of me. This was around 1989–1990. I had decided to stay in Rio de Janeiro because I had somewhere to sleep. I was working as a trainee-educator at Sao Martinho, and I was studying at night at the Santo Ignazio de Loyola High School. I was becoming a bona fide citizen, despite frequent provocation by the police. They would sometimes stop me in the streets and ask me for money, or, when I was coming back from night school and got caught in some shoot-out between police and bandits, they would accuse me of belonging to a gang and beat me up. They would always tell me 'once a crook, always a crook' and emphasize that I would never change. When the police had identified me in one area I would cautiously move to another, trying at the same time not have the local bandits think I belonged to a rival gang.

Once I was coming home after a day's work and study when the police stopped my bus. Seeing me with the nice Italian bag given to me by some friendly Italian priests who had visited the Sao Martinho, they called me a thief. One of the cops drew his gun, a KL38, and placed it against my head, in front of all the women and children in the bus. He didn't want me to explain. I really thought I was dead. Was it worth suffering this humiliation while working so hard to become a proper citizen?

BECOMING A MESSENGER OF PEACE

One morning in 1992 a lady was driving a car into the Sao Martinho courtyard when some street kids hanging around outside the gate armed themselves with a broken bottle and tried to rob her. I told them to leave off. Since they knew me well, they obeyed and she was able to enter the compound unharmed. She was Mrs Sonia Maria Drivis, ex-secretary of the Norwegian consul in Rio and one of the local organizers for ECO RIO 92 (the United Nations International Conference on the Environment in Rio in 1992).

A few days later she called Sao Martinho and invited me to be one of the Rio de Janeiro youth representatives collaborating in the construction of a green park in Manaus, the capital of Amazonia, in connection with the conference. There were 145 of us, young people from 45 countries, under the sponsorship of Queen Silvia of Norway and under the supervision of the Norwegian embassy.

Thanks to Sonia Maria Drivis I became an ambassador for peace in the Amazonian region, and on returning to Rio was one of the youth representatives for ECO RIO 92. The participants were surprised by my life experiences and my presentations. There were NGOs from all around the world, including some representing the United Nations. Some people envied all the fuss about a street kid, asking what I'd got that they didn't have. Hearing this comment a few times made me feel uncomfortable. I felt that people expected a lot from me! I worked for the United Nations Children's Fund (UNICEF) as a kind of unofficial ambassador, and I represented Sao Martinho during some children's rights conferences. My story was all the rage and I was the 'top dog' in children's rights. Current and past representatives of UNICEF in Brazil as well as popular TV personalities were talking about me. My photo and story appeared in many newspapers and magazines, attracting funding for Sao Martinho, but no one ever informed me of it. My actual life did not change much.

By 1996, upon a sudden and unexpected change of leadership of the Sao Martinho and the departure of the people in the organization who had helped me so much during my earlier years on the streets, I started expressing progressively harsher criticism of the new directors. At that point, I felt that I became 'disposable'. The street children, who knew me personally and whom I had never abandoned, were on my side. I believe that I had become potentially dangerous because I asked too many questions. I think this is why they sent me away. I wasn't an expert or scholar, but I'd identified some of the problems that I believed the Sao Martinho was going to face in the future.

A CITIZEN OF THE WORLD

At present I live in Perugia, Italy, under the eyes of a loving Perugian family who have taken me under their wing. My most important work is with Children's Forum 21 (CF21), an international NGO working with volunteers, set up in Italy and Greece by a group of UN-based individuals and in particular Cristina S Blanc. We work and research together, and she has enabled my participation in international conferences to talk about the experiences of children. CF21 is determined to help children and adolescents develop their creativity and sense of self by informing them about the society within which they live, and about how everything is connected globally, thus helping them to become more responsible and critical human beings. Through this work I am learning about using self-evaluation techniques to make sense of my own experiences and I can pass on aspects of these techniques to young people with similar dreams to those I had in my early years.

In addition to my work for CF21 and my studies (I am finishing an MA in Anthropology at the University of Perugia) I am a volunteer in an institute for older people, I visit schools to talk about street kids and other unfortunate children in Brazil, and I assist Sem Fronteiras (Without Borders), an NGO I helped to set up because I felt strongly that I should do something for the new generation in Brazil, the children of people like me who were born during the decade 1970–1980. I also felt that, after my expereince of privilege, I could help European people (who are so used to wealth that they often do not even realize what they have) to go as volunteers to help Brazilian NGOs and learn from direct experience the harsh realities of Brazilian daily life. In the long-term they may end up adopting a family from the *favelas* in the area where I was born. Not everyone has the chance to go abroad and experience what I did. I wanted to channel my energies into creating a form of solidarity between the North and the South, greater understanding across borders between the haves and the have-nots. Once I'd started with my friends, both in Italy and in Brazil many went along with me and helped me realize this dream.

I'm now in regular contact with my own family, whom I try to visit as often as I can. I kept my promise that they would become proud of me. So far, 89 Brazilian families have been sponsored through Sem Fronteiras. People sponsor a child but in that process help to support and improve the conditions of the whole family, often through better housing and enhanced education. It is very important that these families and children do not learn dependency on external aid, but realize their own strengths. We must nurture their sense of dignity, and encourage their self-determination so that they can find hope and joy in the difficulties of their lives. Most of our investment is in education because we are convinced that this will enable Brazil to become a stronger country.

Thanks to the generosity of many people working together, Sem Fronteiras hopes to buy some land in an appropriate location in Brazil and build a center to be managed by the sponsored families themselves, with a house for the volunteers who come to Brazil to work. We are currently engaged in talks with the municipal authorities of Betim, in the state of Minas Gerais. What is lacking at this point are the funds to start the project.

With my varied life experience I could not close my eyes to the conditions of my own people. Once I had no ideals. Now I communicate with important people, but life in the streets has taught me that it's not only important people who can make something happen for the children and 'poor people' who suffer. Life in the streets has taught me to survive with whatever little I have. If I receive a smile I can survive in any part of the world. What is important to children, especially those who are suffering, is the sincerity of our love for them. Any child searches for support amongst the grown ups around him, just as I did and was unable to find easily in my childhood. In working with children it is most important not simply to consider them as the object of our work, but to remember that they have dreams that can come true. In this spirit, when I use the phrase 'once a street child, now a citizen of the world' I am referring not only to the various stages of my own life, and everything that has led me to where I am now, but also to these other children. We must enable them in all ways possible effectively to claim and shape their own citizenship.

References

1. Rizzini I, Munhoz-Vargas M, Graleano L 1994 Brazil: A New Concept of Childhood, In Blanc C. et al. Urban Children in Distress: Global Predicaments and Innovative Strategies. Gordon and Breach: London. p. 77, p. 81–87.
2. Blanc CS et al. 1994 Urban Children in Distress. Global Predicaments and Innovative Strategies, Gordon and Breach London.
3. Unicef 2003. Human Rights-Based Programming Case Study. United Nations, Geneva.
4. Dimenstein G 1993 A Guerra dos Meninos: assassinatos de menores no Brasil, Editora Brasiliense: Sao Paulo, Brasil.
5. Report on the Situation of Human Rights in Brasil 1997 Submitted to the Inter-American Commission on Human Rights, Chapter V. pp. 5–7.
6. United Nations 1989 United Nations Charter for the Rights of Children and Adolescents.
7. Estatuto da Criança e do Adolescentes 1990.

Chapter 3

The right to be blind without being disabled

Sabriye Tenberken, Paul Kronenberg

INTRODUCTION

It is a sunny day and we are walking through the city. We sit down on a terrace beside the river and wait for the waiter. He arrives and asks for my order. I order a soup and wait for him to ask Sabriye the same question, but he addresses me: 'What does *she* want to eat?' This often happens to us. In other situations people ask, 'Does *she* want something to drink?' or 'Does *she* want a candy?'

Why do people ask things in this way? Most are insecure, some are just ignorant, others feel an incredible pity. I keep wondering *why* people behave this way towards those who are blind. Blind people hear and speak wonderfully well, so verbal communication shouldn't be any problem.

Over the past 6 years Sabriye and I have been working to develop a rehabilitation and training center for blind people in Tibet. Since we are also responsible for fundraising we travel a lot. It's funny that the 'Does she…' factor appears in every country. What causes it? To create more equality for blind people we are trying to change the 'Does she…' factor by showing the world what blind people are capable of.

I have been working with blind people for 6 years. For me it has been a real eye-opener to '*see*' what is possible. I have met many blind people whose accomplishments might seem impossible. Eric Weihenmeier climbed Mount Everest and several of the other highest peaks in the world. Anne-Mette Bredahl won five special Olympic gold medals for downhill skiing. Even in my home town there is a blind guy who repairs pianos, working with a lathe, milling machine, drills, and other power tools. I learned that this all has to do with self-confidence in combination with mastering the right techniques.

Eighty percent of our perception comes through our eyes; the idea of 'not seeing' scares us and makes us believe that it is the worst thing that can happen to us. The best way to see or, maybe more accurately, to feel, smell, taste, and hear how the other senses can give you impressions of your surroundings once the sight fails, is to experience it yourself.

In Germany I had the great experience, together with several of the Tibetan project teachers, of training in orientation, mobility, and daily living skills at the rehabilitation and training center for the blind in Marburg, the Blinden Studien Anstalt (BLISTA), Sabriye's former school. For much of the training my eyes were covered so I had to compensate for the loss of sight. At first it is not that easy but the longer your eyes are covered the more you appreciate the function of the other senses. You suddenly feel what kind of pavement you're walking on with the soles of your feet, you smell and taste the air and notice things you don't normally register, you listen to sounds you don't normally hear.

Of course, sight cannot be compensated for completely by the other senses but it is amazing to discover how perception changes. During these weeks I learned several special techniques which helped me to orient and to perform some daily living skills without sight. I realized how important it is that the surrounding world is confident in you. No borders or limits should be set, you need support to find out your own borders.

I met Sabriye in the summer of 1997 in Lhasa. She told me the story of how she became blind, went to a special school, learned to read and write Braille, developed the Tibetan Braille script, travelled alone to Tibet, and how she was planning to start a project for blind people in Lhasa. I was very interested and decided to join her to realize this goal. Now 6 years later, the training and rehabilitation center (website: http://www.braillewithoutborders.org) has 4 component parts:

- preparatory school for blind children
- vocational training center
- Braille book printing house
- re-integration program.

In the center blind children, adolescents, and adults are being prepared to live their lives as independently as possible. The main goal is to give them a chance to develop self-confidence, to be able to stand up in society and claim the right to be blind without being seen as disabled.

In the next section Sabriye tells her own story, interspersed with comments from some of the young people she works with.

SABRIYE'S STORY

'We are not afraid to walk through the city by ourselves, … it's just….' Nyima hesitates. Bungzo adds, *'It's sometimes so, so embarrassing.'*

'What is so embarrassing?' I ask the two girls who are standing in front of me nervously twitching their fingers. 'It's the people talking about us and their pitiful comments,' Bungzo sighs. 'Why can't they just leave us alone and accept us the way we are?'

'Maybe they don't know any better,' I say, realizing that this was maybe not comforting them very much. *'You have to show them that you don't want their pity but that you need their acceptance and acknowledgement. You have to show them who you are. You are blind, so what? You just take different paths to reach the same goals! Just think of all the things you are capable of doing!'*

> *'We can speak English,'* shouts Yudon, *'and much better than the kids that go to regular schools.'*
> *'I'm learning Aikido,'* says Tenzin. *'Who among the sighted children is learning that?'*
> *'And besides,'* Kyla says, *'we can read and write and we don't need a light!'*

It was a sunny afternoon during the autumn holiday, which was too short to have sent the children home to their villages all over the Tibet Autonomous Region, the South West province within the Peoples' Republic of China. Together with the children I sat in the courtyard drinking butter-tea, the main daily drink, and discussing what is important in order to cope with daily life as a blind person.

Survival in a society which sees blindness as a punishment, and degrades blind people through pity, requires the confidence and power to accept blindness as a positive quality. And this acceptance, as I discovered in my childhood, is the starting point in the fight for dignity and recognition in a sighted world which is full of prejudice. This fight is a long and exhausting process in which blind people recognize that they are being disabled and limited by sighted society and by their blindness itself.

All of our students will have to experience this process for themselves. They cannot avoid it, and in fact *we don't want them to miss out on it*, since this struggle will prepare them for a life of dignity. They will become survivors in a world full of obstacles and borders, but these students will have the power to overcome obstacles and cross borders and will not allow society to set them new ones.

> *'You are not alone,'* I say, since many of our students until a few months ago believed they were the only ones in this world who were different. *'There are many blind people, not only in Tibet but world-wide, who all have to experience what you are going through.'* The children ask me to tell them how I coped with my life, and this is my story.

The day my feet sank into a frightening cold nothingness and my forehead hit the sharp edge of an ice-hole it suddenly became very clear to me that I was different to all the others, since they had seen the ice-hole and had gracefully avoided it. The result of this fall wasn't only shock and a concussion that never really healed, but also an increasing insecurity in my mobility. I no longer trusted my eyes. I became more and more insecure in my contact with other people, mainly due to the suspicious attitude of my classmates, many of whom had until then been friends. Both they and I sensed that something had changed, but it was not clear to anyone exactly what.

My sorrow about the loss of acceptance and friendship began when teams were chosen in physical education. Several students were chosen by the teacher to pick their teams. In this merciless procedure the last ones to be selected were always the outcasts: the fat ones, the unsporty types, the useless ones, and those who would ruin the team's chance of victory. I belonged to this last category. For a long time I didn't relate this to my loss of sight.

The teachers' behavior towards me slowly changed. They either approached me with great caution or completely ignored me during class and so gave me free reign to become disobedient. With my deteriorating sight, I saw the blackboard as a dirty green surface that didn't surrender any secrets of mathematics or grammar. The teachers put me in the last row where, through boredom, I became a troublemaker.

The teachers' response to my behavior was in every way extreme, probably due to their insecurity. Some treated me like delicate china and I was allowed to get away with anything. Others punished me with exaggerated force. Some of them humiliated me by telling me that I should be happy that I was tolerated in this school at all, and several others treated me as if I was a little child or mentally retarded. All these different reactions were discriminatory and humiliating. I wasn't simply one child amongst others, who happened to have bad sight, but I was looked upon as a strange creature whose needs, wishes, and talents weren't taken seriously.

> 'That's the worst,' expresses Kienzen, a very cheerful boy most of the time, who became blind at the age of 9 years through an eye infection. 'Suddenly you lose your friends, and everybody is treating you as if you were stupid!'
> 'And what about your parents?' asks Ngudup, a boy who was locked away in a dark room most of his life. 'What did your parents do?'

My parents seemed to be the only ones who responded to the changes in my sight in an easygoing way. They had trust in me and my perseverance. They were confident I would find my own limits and overcome my personal problems by myself. For as long as I still saw colors, and could orient myself to the sidewalk or to the green edge of the road, they let me ride my bicycle. And as long as I trusted myself, they let me do everything that other children of my age did, so I wouldn't become even more isolated from my peer group. However, they couldn't protect me from the increasing aggression and humiliations of my former friends and my classmates. When you become an outcast amongst fellow children, you don't like to run to your parents for help. I fled into a lonely world in which I learned to entertain myself and to avoid any upsetting confrontation. I often tried to analyze what exactly caused the changes in the behavior of those around me. Their reactions suggested there was something odd about me.

One afternoon, an incident while I was going home on the school bus finally destroyed my last bit of confidence. I had just lost a good friend to some of the most relentless classmates. This friend had supported me for a long time, but in the end he also gave in to the group pressure and rejected me. He was sitting a couple of rows behind me. One of the girls sent him some hand signals. I realized that they were exchanging information and making fun of someone and I guessed that the object of their non-verbal communication was me. Eventually I stood up and said, 'When you talk about me I wish you would address me directly and tell me how stupid I am.' The girl started to laugh. 'Who is talking about you then? Don't fancy yourself so much! Nobody wants to deal with you anyway! Be happy you can't see yourself because you are not only stupid, but also very, very ugly!'

Years later I came to appreciate this verbal attack. By crushing the last bit of my self-confidence she brought me to a turning point in my life. I was discriminated against for something I couldn't understand and above all couldn't change. I lost all my joy and my will to live. My mother told me later how powerless she felt during this period in which I was suffering so much. She realized that I had reached the point where I would either give up or start afresh.

I decided on a new start. This began when I met a girl like me who didn't see much, only enough to recognize colors and landscapes. She could also identify people by their jackets. She said, as if it were the most natural thing in the world, 'I am blind.'

'You are blind?' I asked, astonished. 'But you use your eyes like me!' The girl smiled and said, 'I am blind, I read Braille like a blind person, and use a cane even though I can still see a bit. I use the rest of my sight to find my way around.'

This self-confident blind girl opened up a new world to me, in which I could identify myself with blind people despite still being able to see a little. The word 'blind,' which had previously seemed eerie, black, and final, suddenly developed a new definition in my new awareness, different to the one I had created out of the prejudice caused by darkness and fear. It opened up a world of new methods and techniques.

Up to this point ophthalmologists had overloaded me with many state-of-the-art visual aids. I had to try different colored glasses, magnifying jam jar-like glasses which made me look a mockery, hard as well as soft lenses which I always lost during sport, and finally giant video reading machines which were supposed to create an appetite for reading books.

While I sat, suffering migraine attacks, at a flickering video reading screen (named 'TV magnifying screens') deciphering a word at a time, experiencing reading as a total torment, I wondered about the perseverance of those around me who were trying to make me into 'a sighted person' although I had not been one for a long time and *did not want to be one anymore!*

When I discovered the ease of reading and writing with the help of Braille I stated with increasing relief that I did not have to be a sighted person any longer. I was now a blind person with a little bit of sight which, from now on, I would use for relaxation. I recognized that Braille had changed my life completely. It gave me a chance to develop self-confidence and independence. Together with my mother I learned the Braille alphabet. I was so fascinated by the logic of this captivating six dot system that wherever I went I was busy learning it. At first I kept this achievement my secret since I feared further humiliating attacks, for which I wasn't yet ready, from my classmates, but instead of teasing me as I had feared, the girls to whom I finally explained the system were suddenly respectful. They admired my tactile capabilities, since they could only feel crumbs when they touched the Braille on paper.

In this way I started to reveal my blindness to those around me and I developed pride in describing my complex situation with the three simple words 'I am blind'. Before I had found the right words, I once walked across a playground and accidentally destroyed a child's sand castle. The angry mother attacked me: 'Don't you have eyes in your head? *Look* where you are going!' I didn't know how to react. I had eyes and was even able to see a little, but how could I explain this to the furious mother of a sighted child. Now, however, I found how easy it was to explain my situation with my new label. Now, when I was running across the street to catch my bus and jammed my head into someone's stomach, I didn't have to wait to be yelled at by the stomach's owner but could immediately say 'Sorry, I am blind!' and everything was clear.

I found a name for what made me different from other people and I enjoyed trying out this newly discovered magic word in different and in the most absurd situations. I once enthusiastically explained to a neighbor that I was now blind and had to learn Braille. She was shocked. As I heard her pitying sigh and reply, I jumped on my bicycle, waved at her, and shouted with a laugh, 'See you later!'

My favorite hobby is horseriding. Once I was walking through the stables to get to my horse when I got in the way of a rider who immediately shouted, 'Hey, are you blind?' Over the past months I had got used to these salutations and immediately replied simply, not without some pride, 'Yes!' At first the rider was astonished, but then, annoyed by my big mouth, she screamed at me, 'Smart-ass as well, right!' When I was 12 years old I heard about a grammar school (a *gymnasium*) for blind and partially sighted people in Marburg, close to Frankfurt, and decided to go with my parents to check it out. I discovered that it was a boarding school and that I would only be able visit my family once a month and during the holidays, but this didn't bother me at all. On the contrary, I guessed that this school would be a gateway to freedom and independence. I soon found this to be true.

Another great advantage of this institute occurred to me. I would live and learn together with other students who had had to overcome similar obstacles in life. They were all blind or partially sighted and had similar stories to tell. After a long time I had friends again, was accepted for the way I was, and the teachers in the school treated me as an equal. I was a child amongst other children, a feeling I hadn't had since my early childhood.

Most of my blind friends had also had painful experiences of discrimination, pity, and exclusion. I admired those who had lots of self-confidence and enjoyed their cynical, quick-witted ripostes to assaults by sighted people. 'When a sighted person acts silly towards me,' said Manuel, a classmate who was born blind, 'then I just turn around and say: better blind than moronic!'

Kienzen giggles. *'He is right, we don't have to put up with such comments, we are blind, but we are not brainless!'* Kienzen was one of our first students who very soon learned not to put up with discriminatory comments. Half a year after he entered the rehabilitation and training center he collided with a nomad walking across the Barkhor, the famous pilgrims' street in the center of Lhasa. This nomad started to make fun of Kienzen's infected, pulpy eyes and called him a *'blind fool'*. As the other blind children quickly tried to get out of sight of the nomad, Kienzen turned around and asked his tormentor, *'Have you ever been to school? Can you read and write? At night, can you find the way to the toilet without a torch?'* This left the nomad speechless, but it also made a great impact on him because about 6 months later the same man brought a blind child from his region to our project.

'Did you have blind teachers in your school as well?' Bungzo, who wants to become a teacher, asks curiously.

In my school I had both blind and sighted teachers. However, we were very cautious of the blind ones because they knew our special blind tricks, which they had used to fool their own teachers. During examinations they sneaked up to our desks and touched our opened books or crib sheets as if by chance, and sometimes also caught our hands on the work of the neighboring student.

Some of the school's sighted teachers impressed me even more. Most of them weren't specially educated teachers for the blind, which appeared to be a great advantage. Many of them joined the school out of pure fascination. The idea of teaching a special group of people attracted and motivated them to develop and try new methods. Whereas the specialist teachers always reckoned they knew the capability of a blind child exactly, or rather what a blind child was *not* and never would be capable of, the non-specialist teachers were much more flexible in letting us try out many things, which enabled us to explore our own potential and also our limits.

'It is important that you master the techniques,' said a sports teacher who was showing us how to do an Eskimo roll with a white water kayak. 'If you master the technique, then you will be able to rescue yourselves from danger.' Our teachers' considerable trust encouraged us to try to solve most of our problems by ourselves. Whether practicing white water kayaking, horse riding, or downhill skiing, maneuvering with the cane through street traffic, or later during travels, it always came down to adopting the right techniques.

Life away from my family and my familiar surroundings gave me the feeling I could travel the entire world by myself. Later on I discussed the advantages and disadvantages of boarding school with an established development organization. The organization believed that taking children away from their families was the most dreadful thing to do. But my personal experiences, and those I collected from my time in Tibet with blind children, showed me how valuable a boarding school can be for social development and independence. Compared with the five students from Lhasa who are brought to school in the morning and picked up in the evening every day, the other 24 students who live in at the school are very independent, active, and socially skilled.

Often I've thought how different my life would have been if a rehabilitation worker had come to my home in Morenhoven. He would have

Figure 3.1   Walking independently on the roof of the world: students outside the Potala, Tibet's famous winter palace (© Paul Kronenberg, reproduced with permission).

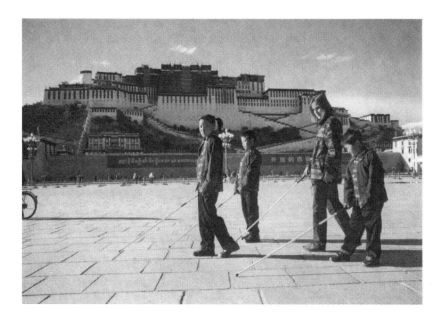

showed me how to use a cane to find the way to the baker's and the butcher's; the local people would have been astonished since I never needed a cane to get around my little village before. My world would not have been so expanded, I wouldn't have learned so much more and, especially, I would not have had the opportunity to build up confidence and any experiences outside my village borders.

'When we now return to our village,' Kyla says, *'we are different children. Now we are respected and some people even ask us things that only we know since we have lived in the big city. Most people from our village have never even visited Lhasa!'*

Indeed, the behavior of the Tibetan community towards our blind students did change quite a bit. Whereas once blindness was seen as bad karma, and the blind were hidden away or were sent on the streets to beg, the community now recognizes and acknowledges that these children have more to tell about the world than they have ever experienced within their isolated surrounding (see Fig. 3.1). 'The world is round,' they are told by our students because they were able to explore a relief globe, something the villagers have never seen. 'After dinner you have to brush your teeth,' says Tendsin, and teaches the villagers the art of cleaning teeth.

CONCLUSION

Based on our own experiences and those of the blind children in our project, *Braille* opens a door to an independent and self-determined life. Only those who have access to information can take their lives into their own hands! More important than techniques and knowledge is the passing on of self-confidence, the basis for not being ashamed any longer of being blind, for being bold and assertive in the fight against exclusion from our efficiency obsessed society and for fighting for the right to be blind without being disabled!

Our newly founded organization 'Braille Without Borders' is fighting for this. The name 'Braille Without Borders' stands for our newly developed philosophy. 'Without borders' on the one hand means that anywhere in the world, blind people can be prepared for a self-determined and independent life in training centers such as the one in Tibet. But 'without borders' has another very important other meaning: we don't want to set any borders or limits for blind people. Blind people should have the chance to live their lives according to their own talents, possibilities, and wishes. They should not be forced into the mostly very monotonous blind-oriented career plans which are implemented by many institutions for the blind world-wide.

Our organization is about the dignity of blind people, about the power of each blind person to stand up and say, 'I am blind, but I am part of this society and have a right to be treated equally to other people.'

An example of this power is a 5-year-old student in our center in Tibet who, because of her lack of sight, was screamed at by her mother and abused by her father. This child didn't respond directly when asked whether her parents had any reason for their behavior. She stood in front of me thinking. Then she said, first hesitantly, but then firmly: 'I don't know why they hit me, but now I know that they don't have a right to do so!'

Chapter **4**

Occupation under occupation
Days of conflict and curfew in Bethlehem

Barbara Lavin

I have lived in the Palestinian town of Bethlehem for the past 5 years, working at Bethlehem University and developing a program in occupational therapy. This was a challenging task from the outset given the embryonic level of development of occupational therapy within the existing rehabilitation system. But somehow both the students and I survived, learned from each other and by June 2000, when the first group graduated, were feeling positive about the future for our profession, the program, and ourselves. Certainly I had a lot of plans and ideas which I looked forward to developing. Instead, for most of us, the last 2 years since the start of the *intifada* (the popular uprising against the Israeli occupation of the West Bank and Gaza Strip) have been spent adapting our personal and working lives to meet the demands of a dangerous, constantly changing, and unpredictable situation.

Bethlehem, like other Palestinian towns, has been the setting of intense military activity that has resulted in deaths, injuries, psychological disturbance and considerable damage to private and public property, including the university. It has also been repeatedly invaded by the Israeli army and placed under curfew, meaning that the entire population is confined to their homes, for extended periods of time. When not under curfew, exit and entry to Bethlehem is difficult, time consuming, humiliating and, for most of the Palestinian population, impossible. Every aspect of daily life including education and employment has been and continues to be disrupted in the extreme.

Suffering is relative. In comparison to many people living in these same circumstances my hardships are minimal and I frequently remind myself of this when I am in danger of feeling excessively sorry for myself. My position as a foreigner gives me the option of leaving at any time, should I choose to do so. However, in comparison to the lives of most of the people who will read this book, I am suffering. I am deprived of my liberty and freedom of movement. I am deprived of all my normal occupations save those I can carry out in isolation in the confines of my home.

I am deprived of social contact and companionship. I cannot easily access regular health care services should I need them.

My story is not one of surviving unendurable hardship, at least not in the usual sense of lacking access to food, water, and shelter, or lacking adequate financial resources because I am denied access to the means of earning my living. Nor is it about having to cope with circumstances that are threatening either to my life or to my property. Other people have and are having such experiences on a daily basis. Some of these have been reported, many not. The media records and reports the dramatic aspects of the conflict – the assassinations, killings, house demolitions (sometimes) – and occasionally makes reference to the harassment suffered as people attempt to go about their daily lives. These are not my experiences, and as terrible as they are, they are not what I intend to write about. I want to share particular aspects of my experience of living under occupation, aspects that are mostly left unrecorded because they are not the stuff of headline news or breaking television news, aspects that relate to daily life and the actions, thoughts, and reflections that help make sense of what is a very abnormal situation. In doing so I have had to resolve a dilemma of my own: is it not just a little frivolous to write about occupational deprivation in the context of people dying, being disabled, and losing their homes and their livelihoods? Perhaps. But taking the perspective that the survival of individuals, families and communities, be they towns, workplaces or schools, depends largely on the degree to which people can adapt and respond to their circumstances, then it becomes anything but frivolous. This story is about what it is like to be deprived of choice, of freedom, of opportunity to work, socialize, and participate in leisure activities as well as in the essential daily activities, all of this in a context that at best does not make sense and at worst is punishing and oppressive. The experience takes on a more universal application as it is the lifestyle not only of those of us in conflict situations but also of those who are deprived by reason of illness, disability, lack of resources, displacement, and incarceration.

From where I sit to write this I have a view that spans most of the town of Bethlehem down to the valley of Beit Sahour and across to the hills of Beit Jala. It is a beautiful sight, especially at certain times of the day when the light catches the stone of the buildings and turns everything a rosy pink. There is a glow to the light that is unique to the region. Ordinarily, I am content to sit on my balcony and watch the world go about its business. The streets are usually busy with traffic and people. While it is a reasonably quiet area, some of the noise floats up so that there is always a sense of lives being lived, of people going about their daily activities, of something happening out there – reassuring when you live alone. Now I look out and there is nothing, not a car, not a child on a bicycle, not a man on a donkey, nor a shepherd with his sheep and goats. The only sound is the sound of tanks and jeeps racing up and down the main road not far from my house. From time to time there is an explosion and I assume that a house is being demolished. In the late afternoon, as in the early morning, there is the sound of the curfew being announced or reinforced. The jeeps cruise the town, broadcasting their messages through megaphones. The sound echoes over the valley, the words recognized by the smallest child. (My neighbors' children take great delight in announcing curfews when they see me venture outside the yard: 'It is forbidden to go out! Stay inside! Curfew! Go home!') But mostly there is overwhelming silence and a sense that life has stopped, been put on hold, and that perhaps everyone is sleeping. At such times the days seem interminable and I am frequently overwhelmed by an inertia from which it is difficult to rouse myself.

It may sound absurd, but somehow it seemed easier to cope during the periods of active fighting. I can say that because I live in an area that is relatively safe and it was always reasonably unlikely that my house would be directly attacked. In that sense I was privileged to be able to feel that my home was a source of safety and protection. Diversion and distraction became very important, as I did not need to use my resources to cope with and control extreme fear and anxiety. Some days and nights were filled with the sounds of missiles being fired from helicopter gunships, tank shells, machine gun fire and the screaming of F–16 fighter planes with their cargo of bombs. On those days and nights it made perfect sense to stay at home and distract myself with music, videos, and books. The whole concept of diversion became a very meaningful and important one. There was something out there that was, variously, frightening, disturbing, or just plain intrusive, that would not go away and could not be avoided. It became imperative to focus on something that engaged my mind or my hands, or preferably both. A combination of new and familiar activities seemed to work the best for me. The former required more effort and discipline to initiate, whereas the latter were essential when the energy was low. The end result was similar. I am equally pleased that I can now (almost) touch type (new) and have (almost) completed my second 'curfew' embroidery.

To be diverted implies that there is something to be diverted from, naturally. But when all is quiet, when the only sounds are those you make yourself, when nothing is moving in the street, the concept flounders. When there is nothing then the issue becomes one of fighting the nothingness. I have discovered that this is not only different, it is much more difficult.

My capacity to cope with this nothingness varies from day to day, as do the strategies I use. Sometimes I feel totally in control and other days I seem to have succumbed to a 'what's the point of all this' and 'nothing's any use' mentality. On such days, getting out of bed is an effort and once out of bed I don't know what to do and the day is something to be endured, not enjoyed. My background as an occupational therapist has been both helpful and a hindrance in this respect. Having an awareness of the organizing nature of activity and the importance of finding meaning in everyday life, and the process of consciously thinking about these issues as I lived each day, was helpful. The hindrance arose mostly from my own belief that as the 'expert' in occupation I should be able to rise above the feelings of helplessness and hopelessness, the lack of interest and motivation, and the sense that how I spent the day was not important. It has been quite a process to learn and accept that sometimes it is perfectly okay not to cope.

I have discovered that it is easier to cope if the space to be filled with detailed plans is small – an hour, an afternoon, no more than the present day. With the loss of the predictable future in work, hobbies, and social contact, I assert control over what I can and orchestrate my time in an almost obsessive way. I write a lot of lists, lose them, and start over. In the afternoons I make a careful search of the cookbooks, mostly already known by heart, in order to find something I may have overlooked that will not only challenge, interest, and occupy me for a time, but will be achieved using whatever ingredients I happen to have left. I am in no danger of starving or even going hungry, unlike many others, but I wonder what to do when the stocks are so low that I cannot use this activity to structure part of my day. The preparation, and to a lesser extent the consumption of food has assumed a greater magnitude in order to replace other activities.

I wash the floors. A lot. There is something about the combination of the physical effort and the sloshing of water that is eminently satisfying. And yet, from time to time when I am washing floors or cleaning cupboards or sorting my wardrobe for the umpteenth time I have to stifle the little voice that says, 'Why are you doing this? Is this the most important and productive activity you can think of?' What is it about this experience that pushes me toward the mundane and the mindless when I could be doing something creative? These questions are the impetus to reflect on what I know about the need for meaning in everyday experience, particularly when the usual sources of meaning are out of reach for the moment. There is no work, no face-to-face social interaction, and no opportunity to enjoy a film, a walk in the forest, a swim. So, in the absence of all the activities that I find meaningful, I must create meaning where I can and attach it to the activities that are available to me. And sometimes that is washing the floor. As I reflect I think of how complex these issues are and how we have been guilty of simplification, as if it were all a question making an effort.

A disconcerting feature of being confined in one place and deprived of regular routine is that of a certain disorientation. I find myself consulting the calendar frequently, sometimes several times a day. The rhythm of the week has disappeared. Saturday (or Monday or Sunday) no longer feels the way it always has. One morning I lay in bed trying to work out what day it was. If it was Friday, where had Thursday and Wednesday gone? I could identify Tuesday quite clearly as that was the last day the curfew was lifted and I went to work. It disturbed me. More than that, it made me angry. Apart from feeling slightly unhinged because I couldn't place myself in time, I felt that part of my life was being stolen from me.

Like most people from privileged societies, my life has had, at least until recently, a fair degree of predictability. Barring absolutely unforeseeable events, I have never been in any doubt that not only was I the person in charge of my life and the one responsible for planning and organizing it, but that I could also count on my world remaining relatively stable and predictable. I had no idea just how much I was privileged in that respect. An extract from my diary illustrates in a small way how maintaining a climate of unpredictability is a strategy used by those in power to maintain control and authority and to undermine order, effort, and morale.

December 10, 2002 – 19th day of current occupation. It is cold and wet – the sort of gray winter's day that begs to be spent around a fire with a book, or some music. But I can't wait to get out. Long before the curfew is to be lifted I am standing at the door, impatiently counting off the minutes and doing a quick checklist in my head. Stop and buy fruit and vegetables before the shop gets too crowded, perhaps something from the grocery store, stock up on library books. I wonder how many of the students will make it and how I should best spend the time with them. How are they going with their assignments? I am looking forward to seeing the students and my colleagues. It has been 9 days! But now we have a whole 6 hours.

The morning flies by. Almost all the students managed to make it to the university and we spent some time talking about ways to encourage each other. They are making connections between the materials we discuss in the classroom and their own situations. I encourage them to try to apply themselves and commiserate with them about the difficulties of doing this. They are finding it difficult to work alone, especially to do the reading. They seem to cope better with the structure of an assignment. We toss around ideas. The Jerusalem students suggest meeting as a group to discuss what they have been reading. The Bethlehem students are scattered and cannot meet each other because of the curfew but think they will try phoning each other more often. I hastily hand out some material to be copied and distributed. It is almost 1 p.m. and they are getting anxious to leave. I spend some time with one student who is catching up a course and hope that she is clear about what she needs to do. I structure it as much as possible. She leaves.

I change my library books and settle to a few outstanding tasks. Then I hear the familiar sounds of the curfew being announced. It is not yet 2 p.m. and it was announced that the curfew would not be lifted until 4 p.m. Sometimes the soldiers like to amuse themselves in this way so we are not really sure what is happening but then the word goes around that the curfew is on and so there is no option other than to troop home. I am glad I got the fruit and vegetables on my way this morning, the groceries will have to wait. I feel an overwhelming upsurge of anger. I am angry because my working day has been cut short. More than that, because this small amount of stability and predictability – to be able to stay out of the house until a specified hour, and carry out a few planned activities – has been taken from me without justification.

I feel manipulated and controlled. This manipulation has to be one of the worst abuses of power over an entire community, affecting, as it does, not only the psychological state but also the occupational life of the entire community.

This was not an isolated incident, merely one I happened to have documented in some detail. What is really extraordinary is that in spite of these frequent power plays, on again/off again curfews, the minute the opportunity came to snatch even a few hours of normal life, it was seized without exception. I think of the society I have come from and I am not sure we could be as resilient and adaptable.

I look back on what I have written and am dismayed by all that I have neglected to mention. It would take a book to cover all the aspects of this experience in sufficient detail to do them justice, and to include the experiences of others so that a truly representative story emerges. Such a short account is invariably somewhat superficial. In spite of that, I hope that a sense of the impact of conflict and curfew on the occupational aspects of our lives, using my own life as an example, has emerged. I also hope that a sense of the extent to which maintaining as normal a life as possible, when possible – going to work, to school, shopping, visiting – becomes a form of resistance to being oppressed, stifled, marginalized, is apparent. This resistance is a powerful aid to survival of individuals and communities.

I have wrestled with this closing paragraph. What kind of conclusion to present when nothing is concluded or resolved, in spite of the early days of the implementation of another plan for peace? The Israelis have withdrawn from Area A, the area under full Palestinian control, and, after a long absence, the Palestinian police are back on the streets of Bethlehem. Some of the usual summer activities are happening – weddings, picnics, summer camps for children. Like many others, I find myself anxious to make the most use of every day and every opportunity, to really live in the present moment, as though it may not last, as though the repressive and restrictive circumstances of the recent months could return at any time. I am not sure if this attitude is pessimistic, realistic, or a sign of adaptation. Regardless, the small signs of life that are returning to the streets of Bethlehem are a tribute to the resilience of its people. It has been a privilege to share this experience.

Chapter 5

A beginner writer is not a beginner thinker

Pat Smart

> *Sowing the Seeds*
>
> *Sow the seeds of words in fertile minds,*
> *scatter them on the wind far and wide.*
> *Words are life*
> *never fear of giving them to others.*
> *Once the seeds are sown,*
> *feed often with encouragement.*
> *Watch as the seedlings unfold*
> *and the words are caressed by eager ears.*
> *What a wonderful feeling when you see*
> *the stem of knowledge blossom.*
> *Spring, Summer, Autumn or Winter,*
> *whatever the season, sow those seeds.*

© Pat Smart (1992)

Everyone has the right to some sort of education. I say 'some sort' because I'm a firm believer that not everyone can learn or be taught in the same way. 'Teachers' need to be more aware that often just a different approach is needed. In my case this was never found. I don't have any memory of learning to read, I only know I've always been able to. My late father encouraged me and my brothers by buying children's comics. Books were never an essential item when finding work and filling bellies was my painter and decorator father's first priority.

At school I was often told I was a 'stupid girl', and to 'stop asking questions and just get on with it!' I didn't just accept what the teachers said like the other kids. I just wanted to know more, to know why things worked the way they did. So 'stupid girl' I was, and I left school at 15 years old.

Between the ages of 8 and 15 years I would look after other people's children, and tell them stories. They seemed to love it. I never thought of writing them down though; after all, I was a 'stupid girl'.

Years later, married with four kids, I 'gained' some inherited ailments and disabilities from my parents, such as angina, asthma, and arthritis, and was diagnosed with diabetes. This was not enough to disable me fully but enough to have me reliant on others for some help with personal care and to make me steer clear of stairs and hills. Although I had to slow down considerably because of pain and exhaustion, my mind was still as fast as it had ever been. After bringing up three sons and one severely disabled daughter, I realized I couldn't be all that stupid.

My daughter wasn't as defeatist as her mother. She was always strong and independent, and never asked for help unless she really couldn't do it. She would insist people spoke *to* her and not *about* her to me, especially the doctors and therapists she had to see often because of her ataxic cerebral palsy. Her school therapist soon found out that Helen was going to be one of their stronger more independent pupils.

As my children grew up, I must have slowly realized that achieving what I wanted was still in my own hands! I'd told my children often that they should push for what they wanted in life, go for the things they felt they were good at. Although this worked with Helen, two of my sons tended to take after me and didn't make as much of their lives whilst at school as they could have. My eldest son decided, because he was getting top marks in exams, coming top in his class each year, that he didn't have to put in extra work. So it wasn't until he was 32 years old that he enrolled at university to study prosthetics. Maybe that trait is inherited as well. From things my father used to say, it seems this happened a lot in our family. My second son didn't like being held up to his fellow classmates as a very clever boy who they should be like! He became the class rebel, as he wasn't going to have his school friends calling him names.

My youngest son found it very hard to learn to read and write. When he was 6 years old the school he had just started attending only 9 months previously was to be torn down and all pupils moved to other schools in the area. He never quite recovered. I was told when he was 8 years old his reading age was only 5.5. When I threatened to go to the newspapers and show the school up, they got in an extra tutor. They tested his whole class and found 10 of his classmates were of a lower reading age. After a year of extra lessons, his reading age was reclassed as 10.5 and he was still only 9½ years old! Now 28 years old, he reads well but has great trouble spelling. His father is an unassessed dyslexic, and his own 7-year-old son is having difficulties learning to read and write. (I believe it can run in families and more often than not down the male line.)

After the death of my mother in 1984 I decided to improve my education, or lack of it. I enrolled in night classes, and had almost the same bad experiences I'd had at school. However, here I heard about 'writers' workshops', where ordinary people write stories (and much more).

This is when I found the Federation of Worker Writers and Community Publishers (FWWCP), a network of groups who simply write and publish community based books. The FWWCP's aim is 'to make writing and publishing available to all', not just by making books, but, for example, by performing their work at venues around the country. After joining a local writers' workshop, I volunteered to go to one of the FWWCP meetings on behalf of the group as no one else seemed interested. I was terrified, but determined this time nobody was going to put me down!

At first I felt others were picking up on my lack of confidence and my poor vocabulary, but I soon decided that if I came across any negative attitudes or criticism I would treat this as a challenge not to give up. (I have learned now not to worry about this. These days I can blame it on the change of life and get away with it!)

I began to understand the ethos of this organization, and found it was all the kinds of things I'd been thinking about over the years, and had been preaching to my children, without realizing what it all really meant. As I got involved in the FWWCP I felt I was doing something that was useful.

The majority of people I met seemed to me to be very clever, yet they didn't look down their noses at me, they allowed me to speak and encouraged me. If I got in a tangle with my words it didn't matter, somebody knew the word I was looking for and would say it for me. I never felt stupid.

At the same time I'd been getting involved in the Merseyside Association of Writers' Workshops. Many of these were also members of the FWWCP. I began putting my computer knowledge to some use by typing up and 'publishing' anthologies of the workshop writers and, later on, individual writers. These took the form of A5 sized 10–60 page 'books' with thin glossy card covers. These were cheap to make, you could even knock them up on a typewriter; that's how I did my very first one. I volunteered to run a 'publish a book in a weekend' workshop at FWWCP events. These went down well. I also found the confidence to run a 'writing for children' workshop.

Most of my courage came from other people's praise and help, in particular people who belonged to the FWWCP. A couple of years ago two published writers sent me their thanks! They both said I was the inspiration that put them on the road to becoming published writers of children's books. But I know they were both brilliant writers anyhow and just found an avenue they hadn't explored before.

This was why I wanted to be involved with this organization; I wanted to be able to give a similar kind of help and encouragement to other people.

Soon I got involved with other groups of writers, such as Pecket Well College (PWC), founded and run by people working on their basic reading and writing in West Yorkshire. I met them at a performance of writers from workshops across the North West of England. I was amazed, astounded, and very humbled. Men and women, some of them grandparents, were standing up in front of an audience and saying, 'I can't read or write properly yet.'

They read, hesitantly, and were prompted or told the words from a piece they had prepared with another person, their 'write hand' (to outsiders a 'scribe'), about their lives as adult learners, about their struggle to raise money to have their own college, a place where they could plan and deliver courses for themselves and other adults in the community, and be able to learn what they wanted in their own time and at their own pace, using their own lives as material.

PWC asked for my help in teaching other participants, as well as some of their paid workers, to use computers on their courses, so I became a volunteer. I brought my own computer (one my brother had cobbled together from bits and pieces of old computers and nailed up in a box of old plywood with holes cut in the front to accommodate the twin floppy drives) as they had only one or two of their own.

I had no formal qualifications, yet found myself passing on what I knew to others, to people who had no other way of speaking out, who had no voice in the community; people who wanted to find work, write letters, be able to fill in forms, and help their children with school work, but who had been let down by the education system. They believe, quite rightly, that it isn't their fault that they lack reading skills. A sizeable number of people attending courses and involved in running them have degrees of disability. These include cerebral palsy, mental heath problems, reading/writing problems, dyslexia (usually undiagnosed), dyspraxia, learning disabilities, and lack of confidence and/or self-esteem, and this is probably what has prevented them gaining access to education.

PWC had been struggling for a few years. Members had raised money from raffles, holding all sorts of charity events, and with the help of some tutors who'd broken free from the main adult and basic education system they wrote letters to raise funding for their own building. These letters were dictated by the learners and written in their own way of speaking – not 'poshed up' by the tutors.

They began to meet in each others' homes. Those with cars would pick up those who couldn't access public transport; others came on buses and trains. This was all taking place in a quiet, rural area where buses were few and far between and often finished running by 6 p.m.

They made plans whilst running courses. For example, they would decide to have a 4-day course, run over 4 weeks on Saturdays – the course could be 'Writing about your life'. They photocopied leaflets at the local library and sent them to local day centers and adult educational centers. The leaflets told people that the college would pay for or provide transport, supply lunch and refreshments, pay for children to be looked after, or that they could be brought along and 'we will share looking after them to allow you to take part'. They would also visit places to talk to those to those who couldn't yet read.

The first day of the course would be a planning day for all those attending to plan what they wanted to do; the next 2 days would see the writing being done, either by the participants themselves or by them telling their story to a 'write hand'. Great care was taken to respect people's words and their own particular dialect.

The fourth day would be the 'follow-up day', which didn't always happen on the fourth Saturday, but often 2–3 months later. It gave participants a chance to discuss what a difference the writing and other activities had made in their lives: did they have a different outlook in their learning, were they considering looking for a job, had they got one, etc. From this a longer and more structured course would then be planned by the participants.

These courses were held in rural villages around West Yorkshire, with such titles as 'You're a good writer – don't let your spelling get you down', 'New directions', and 'A Pecket chance to learn'. The 'college' (they called themselves a college even before they acquired a building) went along to local groups to publicize these courses by word of mouth: 'Come and write about your life, write stories and poems – we can help you write your words down,' or 'Have a go at computers.' Members encouraged participants with statements like, 'A beginner reader is not a beginner thinker!' and actually ran a course with that title.

The founder members were two basic education tutors, one of whom was no longer working in mainstream adult education, a typist, and four people, some of whom were disabled, who were working on their reading and writing. One of the issues being confronted was that people with disabilities were able to learn, to teach, and to think.

Some of the founders and other members contributed to a writing resource pack entitled *Opening Time*,[1] written by students in basic education. This was edited and compiled by Gillian Frost, who was one of the leading forces of PWC itself, and Chris Hoy. It was published by the Gatehouse Project, Manchester (now known as Gatehouse Books), themselves members of the FWWCP.

People who heard about and came along to PWC in the hope they might be able to improve, or, in some cases, begin their reading and writing, found there was more to it than they thought!

Florence was born in Ghana, and after many years as a volunteer and director of the college she became employed as the first paid Outreach worker for PWC. The fact that she had great problems reading and writing was no matter. She was brilliant with people, helping and encouraging them and spreading the word about the college. A support worker for her was employed to help her keep her records about her work, her visits and various events, and her diary and meeting appointments in order; this enabled her to do what she was best at.

One of the college's ex-directors, who has cerebral palsy, literally had no voice. She couldn't speak at all due to her 'disability'. She would teach people knitting to help raise funds for the college. She'd also sit in on writing workshops to encourage others and show them it wasn't as 'scary' as they thought, being in a workshop about writing stories. She has never learned to read (because nobody ever took the time to help her), but she still took part in many meetings and planning sessions. She is so patient with people and 'speaks' with her eyes and hand gestures, even though the lack of mobility in her hands is very severe. I was one of the many people she taught to understand her, using her own special way of communication. She never got frustrated. She should have had the good education she deserved. I know she would have made a brilliant mainstream teacher of disabled children.

Sandra O'Brien was bringing up four small children while working on her reading and writing problems, and was also writing letters to various funders, being a director, and acting as a volunteer carer for others who attended courses and had physical and other disabilities. Sandra was such a natural at this that she was asked to resign as a director and take up part-time work as a paid carer (legally PWC directors are not allowed to be paid for any work they do). She continued attending courses whilst doing this. Today sees her employed full time as a senior care assistant

(NVQ qualified) at a residential care home for elderly people who are mentally ill, and back at PWC she works as a volunteer director in her spare time. She attends the college in the evenings to work on the courses (such as health and safety) she has to do for her job to keep her skills updated.

Joe Flanagan, who'd come to England from Ireland as a young man, had great difficulty with his reading and writing. Joe, a founder member of the college, was determined to write about his life after finding himself redundant at the age of 55. He found himself so busy helping set up the college over the years he was writing his story, that he is still (almost 22 years later) editing his life story. The story has been published by PWC but Joe is still not satisfied with it and beavers away at it daily. Joe won't give up, and one day he will be happy with what he has written. His commitment shows in the way he has stuck with being a director of the college for all these years. He believes he has to be perfectly satisfied that all is correct in his book before he'll give it up.

I liked and admired these people, and wanted to be a part of their group. They gave me the chance to help others, to sit with groups of people and help them to realize they could do a lot more for themselves and could also help others themselves.

In the past words like 'illiterate' had taken on a different meaning for people at PWC. To them illiterate didn't mean people who couldn't read; it had become a term like 'stupid' or 'thick', and suggested that they 'couldn't think for themselves'. So words like these were banned from their vocabulary and were never spoken or written in their work. I too began to think about words like 'learning disabilities' and 'illiterate'. These were used to describe people who, in olden days, were usually labelled as 'backward', but who were taking on teaching roles within the community. Where were their labels now?

They would successfully raise thousands of pounds from government bodies to run their organization, without filling in the standard application forms but using their own letter writing and meetings with funders. They have also voluntarily given back thousands of pounds and struggled on without funds when funders insisted that things had to be done their way, for example that exams should be introduced, people should move through and away from the college at a much quicker pace, and higher standards should be set.

After 21 years PWC has become a model of good practice in adult basic and community education. Funders and other bodies who in the past dismissed the college now inform other education organizations in the community that their funding is dependent on them working with PWC and taking note of and using PWC's methods in their own work.

PWC is run over two sites and at venues out in the community. The college premises are housed in a partly renovated old Co-Operative Society warehouse and shop. Strangely enough, when it had in its earlier days been a Co-op, the warehouse owners realized that many of its employees couldn't read or write, so a room in a cottage at the back of the building was used to give lessons to these workers. The cottage is now incorporated into the main PWC building and its use has come full circle!

Subject to funding, courses run 3 full days and 3 evenings a week in the college building, which has workrooms, a dining room, kitchen, dormitory style bedrooms, accessible toilets and showers, good access to the building, a lift, and a small office. The cellar and attic areas are yet to be fully redeveloped to contain more bedrooms, workrooms, a new, larger, and fully accessible kitchen, and new reception and dining areas.

The main office, based 12 miles away, has a large outreach planning area, a large meeting room, a kitchen and a small reception area. Besides the volunteer directors, many other volunteers are based here too. Short and long courses in office skills and committee skills are held here, as are the many meetings to allow PWC to run smoothly. Meetings happen almost daily, for planning, evaluation and monitoring, and just plain managing. Other courses are also held at various venues out in the community, for example at the local library, local community centers and church halls.

A day course usually has about 12 participants, a paid workshop leader, a volunteer workshop leader, a 'writing hand', a carer and often some support volunteers. A weekend residential course will have two main workshop leaders and numerous other workshop leaders who do 1–2 hour sessions. These people will often be participants learning to read or write but able to pass on other skills. About 16–20 participants stay the weekend, and often another 10 or more attend daily.

People use public transport to get to college if they are able to access it, and those who can't because of disability or vulnerability have a minibus or a taxi sent for them. People come from all over, from Merseyside to Doncaster (a radius of 100 miles), often traveling for 2 hours or more on our minibus or public transport with 2 hours to get home again.

The FWWCP and PWC are the people who made me what I am today, after years of voluntary work: an employed outreach worker and workshop leader in adult basic and community education; a creative writing tutor, especially for people with disabilities; and a publisher of working class people's writing. My first 'published' book of others' writing was produced using an old fashioned typewriter loaned to me by a friend. I typed up the pages, laid them out and photocopied them whenever I had access to an office – especially an unattended one! I'd provide the paper and slip this through the copier unknown to the staff. 'Smart Publications' was totally non-profit-making!

Many of the FWWCP workshops based in Liverpool joined with others to form the Merseyside Association of Writers' Workshops. With so many writers it was possible to set up a course in publishing skills at Liverpool Community College, one of only two colleges left in the North West of England which taught printing. The course ran for a day a week, starting with around 12 writers. Although the course was originally set up for only 1 year, along with the main student apprentice printers and by becoming involved in a City and Guilds course, I was able to keep the course running longer, and about 50–60 books were published. Most of these were given to family and friends by the authors; those that they sold would just about fund the paper and card for the next book, but not the labor! The first published book I was involved with was *Don't Judge*

This Book by its Cover,[2] published by the Merseyside Association of Writers' Workshops, which contained the work of many local writers.

The course students provided the contents and materials. Our writers were taught how to run the printing machines, lay out pages, and take and develop photographs to make printing plates. The course ran for 5 years, until the college realized what was happening and thought we were making money. In fact, we'd often give away books to enable the writing to get out there so that people could begin to read it, and would want to write for themselves and for future generations about their own lives and their own working class history. It isn't just *their* own history – we need to take responsibility for the way our own memories are recorded for others to have, without anyone else's interpretation.

Many chapters in this book are about occupational apartheid, occupational injustice, and work with marginalized people. My work is with people who have been marginalized, like me, and who might not have imagined that they could have an occupation that they could choose, or that they could use the fact of their marginalization, such as their need for basic writing and reading skills, or access to the arts, to achieve what they wanted by telling their own stories. What can you do with *your* history?

References

1. Frost G, Hoy C (eds). Opening Time. Manchester, UK: Gatehouse; 1985.
2. Merseyside Association of Writers' Workshops. Don't judge this book by its cover. Liverpool, UK: Merseyside Association of Writers' Workshops; 1990.

Useful Addresses

The Federation of Worker Writers and Community Publishers, Burslem School of Art, Queen Street, Stoke-on-Trent, ST6 3EJ, Tel: 01782 822327, Website: www.thefwwcp.org.uk

Pecket Well College, Keighley Road, Hebden Bridge, West Yorkshire, HX2 8DB, Tel: 01422 347665, Fax: 01422 343565, Email: pwc@pecketwell.fsnet.co.uk

SECTION 2

Philosophical and theoretical arguments

SECTION CONTENTS

INTRODUCTION

If in the previous section we have been exploring what might exist outside the borders of occupational therapy, the writers in this section survey the capacities within the profession for making new openings, new transcending opportunities. If, like ancient mariners, occupational therapists have sailed within sight of land, building a picture of holism from safe and assured landmarks, inevitably there comes a point where familiarity ends, a fog descends, and when it lifts a new horizon is revealed. To make sense of the new it is necessary to challenge old assumptions, re-examine, reconsider, and reflect.

There is a tendency for our profession to be inward looking and self-referential, and yet the holistic project of occupational therapy, with its concern for the relationship between human adaptation and the environment, suggests multiple complexities, a drawing of parallels and interfaces with many areas of knowledge, science, and the arts. Our extended three part foray into setting out a basis for confronting occupational apartheid (Ch. 6) offers a tool for appraising political activities of daily living, and the discussion of issues which arise from these is offered as an initial exploration. What emerges from these reflections is a new assertion of the ideological component in occupational therapy, as Townsend and Whiteford affirm, 'the radical, political stance on occupation' (see Ch. 9). The direction this suggests, again and again, is toward a negotiated, participatory, and shared perspective, rather than one that is prescribed, i.e. worked out with rather than done to. This entails reframing the position of occupational therapy and its practitioners in the hierarchical panoply of treatment givers, in other words relocating occupational therapists into territories that accommodate *not* a practice without definition, but rather one in which there can be greater flexibility and agreement about where boundaries should fall, or need to be situated. It requires a positioning of the profession that recognizes its work with the extremities of human experience, and being able to confront rather than collude with the processes of occupational apartheid explored in Section 4.

This implies a practice that becomes more context-dependent, more action oriented, more intuitive and spiritual, because it is closer to the everyday need for participation. This would seem more like common sense than radicalism, but Iwama's chapter (Ch. 10), like Peloquin's exploration of the heart of occupational therapy (Ch. 8), explores how the dust thrown up in the collision of the Western scientific paradigm with the practical and rational aim of providing occupation filters rather than illuminates the purposefulness of activity. Reading his chapter, we are asked to question the assumption that client-centeredness is necessarily directed to maximizing autonomy. To what extent is dependency a purposeful function? How do occupational therapists, with their aim of maximizing independence, negotiate the social needs of people to be dependent on others?

One of the key human requirements that Burgman and King explore in their chapter on child spirituality (Ch. 12) is belonging, which is given meaning through the experience of having one's needs fostered through others and at the same time is a component of resilience. Occupation is therefore based in social interaction and in the experience of social meaning which confirms one's relationship to the world. The implication of this argument is explored in Galheigo's proposal in Chapter 7 that occupational therapy requires a sociocritical standpoint to meet this inclusive demand. If meaningful occupation is related to a sense of social belonging, then both the nature of the society to which individuals are obligated and the basis on which membership is determined are problems for occupational therapists. How acceptable is it for a society to accommodate or refuse the requirements of specific minorities? How should we be working to enable the social integration of people into society, to enable them to conform irrespective of their perceived needs, or should we work to empower them to have their needs recognized? As social participants ourselves, how do we recognize the difference between empowering the expression of social need and the channeling of needs and desires to other social outcomes by corporations, governments, the media, and other institutional and ideological social influences?

In Chapters 14 and 15 Abelenda et al and Egan and Townsend explore how occupational therapy models can be employed in the analysis of these questions and can enable therapists and the people they are working with to make sense of their experiences, unravel the process of occupational apartheid, and determine actions and goals which will overcome the barriers they face in social participation. Fransen (Ch. 13) explores how community-based rehabilitation (CBR) approaches address poverty as the fundamental cause of disability, and the central contributions that can be developed by occupational therapists in working toward occupation-based goals. Her conclusion suggests that the relationship between CBR and occupational therapy offers many mutual benefits and will contribute positively to the evolution of our professional philosophy and practice.

Finally, Michael Iwama (Ch. 10) makes a case for occupational therapists to question the cultural assumptions underlying their professional philosophy, or else find themselves embarrassed in trying to implement aims which do not engage with local realities. At the close of this section (Ch. 16) he gives an introduction to the *kawa*, or river model, which offers an environmentally harmonious counterpoint to the more driven basis of Western occupational therapy approaches.

Chapter 6

Overcoming Occupational Apartheid
A preliminary exploration of the political nature of occupational therapy

Frank Kronenberg, Nick Pollard

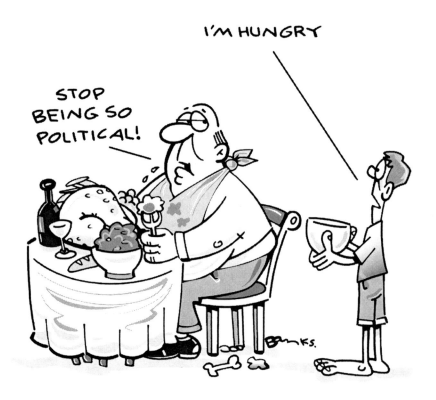

Occupational therapists view humans as occupational beings, and engagement in dignified and meaningful occupations is as fundamental to the experience of health and wellbeing as eating, drinking, and being loved.[1]

Whoever is fond of the comfortable and the fortunate stays out of politics. He does not want anything to change.[2]

(Italian peasant boy)

OVERVIEW

Why must we know about occupational apartheid? The German philosopher Kant said: *'Begriffe ohne Anschauungen sind leer, Anschauungen ohne Begriffe sind tot.'* (Until you give it a name, you will not perceive what you see.)[3] Occupational therapy appears to be perceived as an apolitical profession by its practitioners.[4,5] Through the introduction of the notion of occupational apartheid within the language, discourse, and practice of occupational therapy – a 'louse in the fur' if you like – the authors of this text envision raising critical awareness and understanding about the political nature of occupation (people's dignified and meaningful participation in daily life) and this profession's enabling roles in relation to occupational apartheid.

We use the term 'people experiencing disabling conditions' as a point of departure for describing how personal participation in daily life is limited or denied through broader factors than physical or cognitive disability, to suggest that sociopolitical conditions themselves can be the principal barrier to access, which would be in line with the *International Classification of Functioning, Disability and Health*,[6] 'allowing occupational therapy to be proactively descriptive of all people and not just those with illness or disability'.[7]

Occupational apartheid departs from the Aristotelian assumption that not all people are equal, some are better, more worthy, deserve more than others, and that this is the natural way of the world.[8] Ancient Greek democracy was limited in its inclusiveness. It did not extend across gender or to all social classes in a society which depended heavily on slaves.

Occupational apartheid also departs from the inspiring notion of occupational justice,[9] which includes a Rawlsian[10] sense of justice arising from respect and equality; unlike occupational injustice, which covers a broader range of situations, occupational apartheid demands calls for action, identifying situations with which one cannot ever feel comfortable. Occupational apartheid therefore describes circumstances which go beyond the description of occupational deprivation: 'a state of preclusion from engagement in occupations of necessity and/or meaning due to factors that stand outside the immediate control of the individual',[11] (p. 201) although occupational deprivation may be a contributing factor to or a product of occupational apartheid. Occupational apartheid should not be confused with the politics of apartheid in the former South African regime, but the use of apartheid is deliberate, and in this instance refers to systematic segregation of occupation opportunity.

Our chapter does not pretend to present the only framework for analyzing politics, but it does offer a working concept, a set of key questions and illustrations which can enable readers to explore the political nature of various everyday living situations that occur in occupational therapy practice, research, and education. Preliminary explorations require broader and more in-depth study to increase the scope and to consider alternative views, therefore any conclusions we draw at this stage can be no more than a summing up of progress to date, and we invite other people to contribute to this discussion.

PROLOGUE

The examples below serve as a backdrop to our discussion of occupational apartheid in this chapter.

Example 1

The International Day of Tolerance in Guatemala was part of a process to promote a culture of peace in a country that suffered more than 36 years of horrific internal armed conflict. 'Survivors of the Street' were the youth of the occupational therapy project who performed an impromptu theater piece about life on the streets, using percussion on recycled plastic drums decorated with graffiti, dance, acrobatics, and juggling. A crowd of over 1200 pupils from privileged schools, the minister of education, UNESCO (United Nations Educational, Scientific and Cultural Organization) representatives, and the national press watched and applauded a great presentation. The actors and accompanying project staff were glowing with pride and joy. Suddenly, 2–3 minutes before the end, a woman, who did not identify herself but who was a representative of the former government party, approached the group and tried to cut short the performance. She fumed angrily, spoke about disrespect, took the Guatemalan director of the performance outside, and scolded him for the 'disgraceful presentation'. She did not feel it was appropriate for street children to serve as role models in the celebrations.

All of us were dumbstruck by her attitude. Some of the kids came outside to find out what was going on, and soon figured out that they were the cause of the conflict. Another slap in the face, blowing away the boosted self-esteem and joy they had experienced minutes before (see Ch. 19).

Example 2

In some parts of the United Kingdom there are significant numbers of people from ethnic minority groups, many of whom migrated to find work in the booming economy of the 1960s. Many of these people initially gave up traditional practices in order to fit in with a foreign society. Some aspects of the impact of this migration have had a significant effect on British culture, for example the popularity of Asian foods, and trends adopted from Indian cinema and in popular music, but the majority of white British people still know little about these cultures, which are now an established part of their society.

For an elderly Sikh person, for example, who may be unable to communicate in English, this presents significant problems. Whereas an elderly white person may be able to access assistance with personal care and daily living activities, language and cultural barriers may prevent older Sikhs from obtaining equipment and other resources to meet their needs.

Most hospital based occupational therapy departments contain assessment kitchens, to determine whether a person is able to make their own meals or drinks, but few of these can accommodate the cultural practices of people who cannot use utensils which have held meat. Often occupational therapists performing home visits are unable to access professional translators and family members are pressed to perform this service. Consequently, people are unable to express their needs, or reluctant to disclose issues they consider personal. The purpose of the visit and the job the occupational therapist carries out remains a mystery to the person for whom the intervention is being planned. The occupational therapist may order equipment which is culturally unsuitable, overriding the person with disabilities who has been attempting to explain why they cannot use it.

The consequences are that Asian people with disabilities are more likely to be restricted in or denied the ability to perform personal care and daily living activities according to their social, religious, and cultural needs. A person may have a bath that they cannot use fitted in their house, and then have to finance further alterations which need not have been necessary; another may require toileting aids which would prevent having to perform personal care impurely with the right hand. These issues have a deep impact on the ability of some people to achieve basic independent functioning in comparison to those with similar problems living in the same society, but within the dominant culture.

Example 3

A group of people with early onset of dementia approached a city council official in order to obtain funding for a day center. Early onset of dementia is generally under-recognized and people who have it often do not receive services appropriate to their generation; without a place to go, they can be socially isolated and confined to their homes.

One of the group members, a former council official himself and a former colleague of the man they are addressing, asked his old friend where he spent his holidays that year. Bemused by the request, which seemed to be a product of the dementia, he replied with an account of his walking tour of the Tyrol. 'Now ask me where I'm going,' said the group member. 'Remember the nursing home we put up several years ago? That's where I'm spending my holiday. I've no choice, there's nowhere to go when my wife needs a break from me.'

Example 4

The World Federation of Occupational Therapists (WFOT) approved their first ever position paper on community-based rehabilitation (CBR)[12] at the council meeting in Cape Town, South Africa in 2004. The WFOT is the key international representative for occupational therapists and occupational therapy around the world, and the official international organization for the promotion of occupational therapy. For the first time in its 52 year history, the organization used a newly developed process and took an official stand on an issue of global relevance that transcends what many view as its traditional professional interests.

In this document, the WFOT acknowledges the world-wide existence of an estimated 600 million people with disabilities, predominantly in (but not limited to) 'developing countries', who with their families and communities are restricted in or denied access to dignified and meaningful participation in daily life. The council recognized the need to develop a critical awareness and understanding about these realities, and in response accepted the new and emerging notions of occupational apartheid, occupational deprivation, and occupational justice to guide and inform occupational therapy thinking and action. The WFOT council meeting follows rules that allow for debate and discussion of any item brought before it. The WFOT delegates represent the (then) 57 member countries of the Federation, and at the Cape Town meeting there was an even representation from both 'developed' and 'developing' countries. The final vote of acceptance of the discussion paper followed lively discussion and a healthy debate.

Clearly the profession faces different challenges in different countries, and the debate reflected this. It began with some delegates proposing a motion for an amendment to delete the terms 'occupational apartheid, occupational deprivation, and occupational justice' from the paper, because these terms were felt to be 'too politically charged', based on the premise that the WFOT is a non-political organization. Furthermore, these delegates explained that occupational therapists in their countries were insufficiently familiar with the meanings of this new language.

The leader of this project was invited to comment on the motion. He argued that this 'new language' had been included in the paper after a lot of deliberation, following significant exchanges with the profession internationally, and on the basis of the WFOT's aspiration to be a forward-looking global leader of the profession. Examples were offered of occupational therapy congresses in Europe and Africa where these concepts had been addressed as core themes, indicating 'new directions' in the international discourse of occupational therapy. He strongly recommended that the terms should be retained in the position paper.

Other delegates spoke in favor of the terms, saying that this new language connected with the experiences of daily living of many people in their countries, and described their practice realities. One delegate said: 'We would rather have no position paper than a mutilated one'. A vote was called for on the amended motion, and defeated. A 'middle way' motion, to remove 'occupational deprivation and occupational apartheid' and retain 'occupational justice', as this term was perceived to be less emotive and politically charged, was also defeated. And so the final vote was taken on the original position paper, which was accepted by a clear majority. Clearly democracy works within WFOT.

PART 1 INTRODUCTION TO OCCUPATIONAL APARTHEID

AWARENESS AND ACTIONS

Meaningful human activity begins with awareness,[13,14] which comes about through practice and experience with the world; rather than doing things in response to awareness, we become aware and learn through doing things. Learning and empowerment take place in a social context.[14-16]

In dealing with limits, we become acutely aware of the nature of power as we experience confrontations and learn to assess risks and benefits. As Chomsky[14] says: 'there's an interaction between awareness and action ... awareness is only the beginning, because people can be aware and still not do anything – for instance, maybe they're afraid they'll lose their jobs. And obviously you can't criticize people for worrying about that; they've got kids, they've got to live. That's fair enough. It's hard to struggle for your rights – you usually suffer.'

According to the WHO (World Health Organization),[17] health is determined mainly by factors outside the domain of medical, technical, or public health, such as social, economic, and political conditions. Hunger, ill health, wars, and similar phenomena result from unfair distribution of land, resources, and decision-making power. A key to widespread improvement in health is strong political commitment to equity in meeting all people's basic needs.[18] Thus the healthy person, family, community, or nation is one that is relatively self-reliant – one that can relate to others in a helpful, friendly way, as an equal.[2] This, as Lanthenas remarks, writing in 1792, requires that the person is empowered:

> *The first task of the doctor is … political: the struggle against disease must begin with a war against bad government. Man will be totally and definitively cured only if he is first liberated: Who, then, should denounce tyrants to mankind if not the doctors, who make men their sole study, and who, each day, in the homes of the poor and the rich, among ordinary citizens and among the highest in the land, in cottage and mansion, contemplate the human miseries that have no other origin but tyranny and slavery?* [19]

Occupational therapists and occupational scientists view humans as occupational beings[20,21] and believe that people's engagement in occupations that they themselves find meaningful and useful in their given environment, is as fundamental to experiencing health and wellbeing as eating, drinking, and being loved.[16,22,23] However, a constructively critical look at everyday practice reveals a dissonance between our proclaimed philosophical roots, values, and beliefs – who we say we are and what we stand for, our rhetoric – and what we do, our practice in the real world, in relation to the people we serve (see Ch. 1).

This realization became apparent to the first author while researching the development and implementation of occupational therapy with street children in Mexico[22] and Guatemala[24] (see Ch. 19). Occupational therapy literature has not discussed the development of practice that would facilitate and empower such children and the communities in which they live to effect real changes. This would seem to limit the usefulness of occupational therapy which has not until recently been enabled to challenge the perpetuation of deprivation and marginalization.[16] The lived experience of these projects enlightened the first author's awareness of the need for a critical exploration of the political nature of occupational therapy.[25,26]

His extensive review of general political science and specific occupational therapy and occupational science literature explored the meanings of the terms 'politics' and 'political' in relation to the doing, being, and becoming[27] of our profession. This review found that politics, of its very nature, is a controversial term around which there is little agreement, politics and political as keywords have rarely been discussed in relation to occupational therapy's primary role of 'enabling occupation'.[28]

More recently, Watson[7] (p. 10) has asked whether 'Occupational Therapy [is] ready to move forward and make occupation a political issue, thus ensuring that occupational risks are addressed as a social development issue and not only as a health concern?' Watson describes four international perspectives, which are outlined below.

Watson[7] (pp. 10–11) tells how Hocking and Wilcock describe proposals to develop political activism amongst occupational therapists in New Zealand and Australia. First they propose informing occupational therapy educational curricula from examples of Maori initiatives in dealing with the social and health inequalities these people have experienced since colonization. This proposal is paralleled in some of the education initiatives discussed in Chapter 31, and in one of the WFOT–CBR master project plans to develop an occupational therapy and politics education module.[29] Next, they advocate getting students to work with occupational injustices in their local communities. Finally, they propose that New Zealand and Australian professional associations proactively monitor employment, unemployment, and education and justice policy and legislation.

Whiteford, another Australian whose work is described by Watson,[7] (pp. 11–12) calls for occupational therapists to take the responsibility for making their professional and philosophical ground clear without looking over their shoulder in case other health professions alienate them. While recognizing that this political commitment operates at both the personal and professional levels, Watson argues that occupational therapists have to make themselves visible in order to affect moral and political challenges.[7]

Watson[7] (pp. 13–14) gives an account of Roberts' description of how three measures, i.e. a recent redefinition by the College of Occupational Therapists[30] of occupational therapy as a complex intervention, changes in the professional and academic status of therapists through the development of consultant posts, and an emphasis on evidence-based practice, are enabling occupational therapists to influence policy. Occupation has become a political issue in the UK and therapists' social concerns are not confined to their own nation but reflect the globalization of occupational therapy. Added to this, the *International Classification of Functioning, Disability and Health*[6] together with the *Ottawa Charter for Health Promotion*,[31] offer the profession the means to address the needs of local populations both in the UK and world wide, developing community action and public health strategies through facilitative approaches.

Watson[7] (pp. 14–15) also describes Sadlo's suggestion that occupational science concepts such as occupational deprivation and occupational marginalization have coincided with changes in the College of Occupational Therapists' internal structure to enable it to better represent the profession politically on issues such as employment, housing, transport, mental health, and prisons. Occupational science is now a core part of occupational therapy curricula, but high caseloads are impeding some practitioners in developing approaches to tackle social issues. Watson is optimistic that new graduates from the universities will be equipped to evidence measures to address the occupational roots of problems such as drug use, vandalism, overwork, homelessness, and disillusionment which are widespread in the UK.

There is a clear case, therefore, for occupational therapists to develop measures that enable them to deal with political questions in relation to occupation. To enable the development of understanding and the possibility of future application the first author[4] derived a broader approach from a political scientist, Cees van der Eijk, who regards politics 'as an aspect of human occupation and human relationships that occurs everywhere, in all situations'.[32] This judgement underlines the importance of an informed holism as the basis for empowerment. According to van der Eijk, after Hobbes[33] and Clauswitz,[34] the main characteristics of politics are conflict and cooperation, and specific key questions can help determine and understand the political nature of any given situation.

OCCUPATIONAL APARTHEID: GENESIS OF THE TERM

Occupational apartheid is based on a premise that some people are of different economic and social value and status than others. Although at an abstract level and in rhetoric all people may be considered equal,[35] in everyday reality 'some [people] are more equal than others'.[36]

The term arose through the first author's exploration of the potential for occupational therapy practice with street children in Mexico[22] (see Ch. 19). Street children's occupational and social participation is denied or restricted to survival at the margins of society, where the predominant occupations are derived from crime, drugs, prostitution, and affiliation with gang culture. The profession had no concept that could either explain the origin of the phenomenon of street children or offer a response from a specifically occupational therapy perspective. The first author's research preliminarily described occupational apartheid as 'more or less chronic established environmental (systemic) conditions that deny marginalized people rightful access to participation in occupations that they value as meaningful and useful to them'.[22]

Outside occupational therapy and occupational science literature, Staples and Steinberg used the terminology occupational apartheid in the context of race awareness to describe situations where the range of work-based occupations available to certain ethnic groups are limited by those in power.[37]

Even the earliest Western descriptions of society have discussed inequity in the distribution of money, power, and prestige.[38,39] Macionis and Plummer[40] describe how this inequity in distribution determines the hierarchical nature of social stratification along a number of categories, e.g. social and economic, gender, ethnicity, age, educational attainment, and other factors such as disabilities, language and dialect, and sexuality. They further point out how social stratification is a matter of four basic principles:

1. It is a characteristic of society, not simply a reflection of individual differences.
2. It persists over generations.

3. It is universal but variable.
4. It involves not just inequality but beliefs.[40] (pp. 240–241).

An obvious and crucial example for both Macionis and Plummer's discussion and ours is South Africa's apartheid history. Through the policy of apartheid (which became law in 1948), the dominant white minority population legally denied citizenship, land ownership, and democratic rights to the black majority.

> *Implicitly apartheid had an occupational [i.e. work-related] dimension; black people were discriminated against as a subordinate caste, given only sufficient education to enable them to perform the low-paying jobs deemed inappropriate for whites. By comparison white people earned on average four times more than black people, and virtually every white household was able to afford a black household servant.*[40]
>
> (Plummer, 1998:242) (See also Ch. 32.)

Since the overthrow of apartheid in 1994 the South African government estimates that half of all black people continue to live in conditions described as 'desperate', and over half the population live below the poverty line.[40] The main reason for this is not a lack of resources but lack of opportunity to earn an income,[41] therefore the facilitation of human occupations depends on the political influences operating in the social and economic environment.

Occupational apartheid results from political constraints which may extend to encompass all aspects of daily living and human occupation through legal, economic, social, and religious restrictions, and can be found as a consequence of chronic poverty and inequality in many countries across the globe. Occupational apartheid has also been used to describe 'situations where occupations are classified, paid, valued and enhance life for some, while in the same places and times occupations are taken for granted, exploited and trivialized for others'.[16] Although we recognize this description we emphasize the systematic and even deliberate aspect of most circumstances of occupational apartheid which occur through unresponsive, collusive, or exploitative policy measures maintaining privilege over poverty (see Ch. 1). In other words, there is a reluctance to confront occupational apartheid because the privileged elements of the world's economies have been benefiting from it materially and in terms of local political and social stability; for example, Dundas[42] suggests that counter-terror policies adopted by these economies since the announcement of the international 'war on terror' are negatively affecting overseas development aid.

We therefore seek to draw the distinction between occupational apartheid and occupational injustice. Occupational injustice occurs 'when participation in occupations is barred, confined, restricted, segregated, prohibited, underdeveloped, disrupted, alienated, marginalised, exploited, excluded or otherwise restricted'.[16] Although the terms are complementary; occupational injustices occur *within* a system of occupational apartheid. Townsend and Wilcock[16] point to the problem that the term 'occupation' presents in English, as a classifying term for occupational therapy, and the difficulty of introducing new terms prefaced by 'occupational'. Thus for example, in their workshops on occupational justice, participants have been confused by the breadth of application for 'occupational' in such terms as occupational justice, and have been unable to distinguish it from 'social' justice.

As we will discuss later through the use of 'political Activities of Daily Living (pADL) questions' (see below), what we do is dependent on the social opportunities and resources available to us to facilitate our occupational participation and exercise our occupational rights.[16] The availability of occupational justice is determined by political factors in the occupational environment. Thus opportunities can be created, and restricted or denied, to produce situations of occupational apartheid through the systematic operation of political forces. People do these things to other people, and the problems they present therefore have a just and human solution. As occupational therapists we can choose, as Townsend and Wilcock[16] point out, to comply with occupational injustice and occupational apartheid or advocate for justice. But this is not only an issue of professional responsibility; for us it is an issue of ethical responsibility and global citizenship in which there is not really a choice. As we made clear in Chapter 1, there is no defence in maintaining that we know nothing about it.

The authors' working definition of the term occupational apartheid is given in Box 6.1.

This short, initial definition, which the authors are continuing to refine, describes a phenomenon which requires an active dialogue between occupational therapists and the people they work with to make more politically informed choices about needs, practice, and negotiation of outcomes.

Occupational apartheid is imbedded in economic, social and cultural practices, and therefore enters people's individual and collective states of minds, or attitudinal environments.[6] The problems it engenders are to be confronted and overcome at individual, community, and social levels. Our use of the term occupational apartheid was coined to inform occupational therapy practice, and its conceptual development and refinement will be influenced by a diversity of disciplines such as political science, sociology, anthropology, and in particular the emergent occupational science, which is concerned with the study of humans as occupational beings.[20,21] The social, cultural, and political dimensions of human occupations, their environments, and their interactions, everything we

---

Box 6.1   Working definition of occupational apartheid

Occupational apartheid refers to the segregation of groups of people through the restriction or denial of access to dignified and meaningful participation in occupations of daily life on the basis of race, color, disability, national origin, age, gender, sexual preference, religion, political beliefs, status in society, or other characteristics. Occasioned by political forces, its systematic and pervasive social, cultural, and economic consequences jeopardize health and wellbeing as experienced by individuals, communities, and societies.

do as humans, may potentially become factors in a political process of occupational apartheid. One of the principles with which we therefore question the nature of human occupation is *'Todos somos responsables por todo'* ('Everyone is responsible for everything')[43] (p. 44) (see Ch. 1).

OCCUPATIONAL APARTHEID AND OCCUPATIONAL THERAPY

Because we are social agents, engaged in and concerned with human occupation, this concern with reclaiming social responsibility (but not examining underlying causes) has implications for the ways in which occupational therapists conceive their practice and underpinning philosophy. There is evidence that the profession is developing a more proactive stance around the world, as suggested by the contributors to this book and by Watson and Swartz.[44] As Example 4 in the prologue of this chapter suggests, occupational apartheid, deprivation, and marginalization are global issues. Through our occupational interactions we all contribute to and are all implicated in any outcome. One might say, for example, that the wealthier lifestyles of many people in the northern hemisphere depend upon, and are products of, occupational apartheid amongst impoverished people in the southern hemisphere (see Ch. 1, first principle).

Although when considering the socio-economic and political differences across the globe it has been common practice to refer to 'the developed and the developing world', the globalization of poverty may have brought the southern and northern hemispheres far closer than indicated on a map – perhaps within easy reach of almost everyone's home. Aristotle's state, in which he thought the wealthy were best suited to govern,[8] depended on slavery. Poverty was held to be natural in the midst of wealth. This is why we have not referred to the developing world – in our view problems of development are ubiquitous. There are, none the less, economic and political inequalities between countries, which result from a recent colonial past and its corporate inheritors. This divergence impacts on the occupational choices that are accessible to societies and individuals in helping to instigate the circumstances of occupational apartheid or develop the strategies to overcome it. We refer again to Example 4 from the prologue. Had occupational apartheid, occupational deprivation, and occupational justice not been agreed as issues to be addressed in the WFOT position paper on CBR,[12] then, as one delegate pointed out, the argument would have been 'mutilated'. More than that, it would have been ineffectual; it would in fact have represented a colonialist position which did not recognize the situations of those countries and communities with fewer health resources. In his damning critique of the impact of colonialism on health practices, Fanon[45] explored some of the consequences that arose from culturally inappropriate models of care – which, in his examples, led to racism and complicity in colonial terror. In the new millennium we do not want to repeat these crimes. We argue that our professional concern with human occupation gives us a key position from which to challenge occupational apartheid and change the way in which we discourse the political nature of occupation itself.[22,46]

PART 2 POLITICAL ACTIVITIES OF DAILY LIVING

WHAT WE MEAN BY POLITICS AND POLITICAL

Aristotle[8] thought human beings were naturally political animals. Occupational therapists and occupational scientists view humans as occupational beings.[16,20,21,28] Cardona[47] describes politics as the people's capacity and power to construct their own destiny. Therefore politics is a human occupation, and given the concurrent development of inequalities with civilization, not only occupation but also science has a political aspect. Marcuse[48] points to the potential of science as a liberator that can serve human needs, but points out that the use of science in advancing technology has the effect of increasing human occupations (not only in work but in all aspects of human life) and creating new demands. The technologically advanced societies could make concessions to those which they exploit, but instead they use their technology and economic dominance to protect their advantages.[42,48] Making a point echoing Foucault's[49] description of a disciplinary technology which includes health care as a measure of social control, Marcuse argues that those who have access to the benefits of technology increasingly use it to protect themselves from 'the substratum of the outcasts and outsiders, the exploited and persecuted of other races and other colours, the unemployed and unemployable. They exist outside the democratic process.'[48] As occupational therapists we should recognize that in addition to our position as technicians who assess, monitor, and work to restore or adapt functional capacity in humans, we are also included in the roll-call of agents of social control. If, however, we are to conduct our professional relationships in a person-centered way, we need to empower ourselves as social agents with a capacity for question and critical action.

The choice is between conflict and cooperation, which van der Eijk[32] has identified as the characteristic of 'the political' that occurs everywhere in all sorts of situations and relationships. These terms are descriptive, they do not mean that conflict is 'bad' or that cooperation is 'good', but refer to the aims and actions of individuals and groups. Conflict occurs when individuals or groups work against each other to realize their own goals and interests, while these are mutually incompatible. Conflicts are inevitable and often can't be fully resolved, but to reach a solution for a society as a whole requires cooperation. Cooperation can be viewed as the other side or reverse of conflict, and it can also be viewed as inevitable. In both conflict and cooperation one can distinguish two different aspects: one with respect to content and another with a behavioral or occupational aspect. The content aspect suggests that 'it's about something' – usually indicated by the terms aims and interests. The behavioral or occupational aspect indicates that conflict or cooperation can be perceived in behavior.

Van de Eijk[32] claims that it is impossible to pose and maintain one single, strict definition of 'politics', because the word belongs in the category of so-called 'controversial' terms – a characteristic the term seems to have in common with 'occupation', the core construct of occupational therapy.

Since 'the influence of theoretical principles upon real life is produced more through criticism than through doctrine'[34] (p. 210), in what we hope will be an open, on-going critical dialogue, we propose to consider the multilevel and multistakeholder-serving occupational therapy process of change as a conflict and cooperation dialectic.

According to van de Eijk, descriptions of the concept 'politics' can be classified into two main types, namely the aspect approach and the domain approach to understanding politics. The former implies that politics is an aspect of human occupation and human relationships that can be found everywhere. This is the concern of political Activities of Daily Living (pADL), and the small 'p' aims to distinguish this from the second type, the domain approach (big 'P'), which views 'Politics' merely as a particular, defined sphere of human relationships, indicated by terms such as the state, government, public administration, a political party.[9,32] Other political scientists have described politics as 'shaping the future of a society as a whole, or exercising influence on this shaping'[50] (p. 164) and 'the way in which people change society, and in which other people attempt to prevent these changes'.[51] (p. 55)

Hence, 'politics are concerned with conflicts between groups of people, the development of conflicts, the development of cooperative strategies to influence the outcome of the conflicts in one or another group's desired direction, and the resolution of conflict.'[32] (p. 17) These processes also depend on the choice of political system in which one is interested. However, not all conflict or cooperation has to be political. The only rationale for trying to distinguish political situations from, for example, economic, legal, or cultural issues, is that the nature of the situation largely determines how the given issues occurred, developed, and have become encoded.[32] It is, as Watkins[52] has illustrated, the problematizing of these processes of encoding which dispels myths such as the natural inferiority of classes, races, or gender explaining economic legal or cultural inequalities.

The relationship between this process and that of occupational therapy intervention can be shown from some of the illustrations with which the authors prefaced this chapter. Older Asian people (Example 2) and people with early onset of dementia (Example 3) were unable to obtain services because resources were not available or because a problem had not been perceived. The provision of better translation services or the enabling of a better cultural understanding may have given people the opportunity to discuss their needs. This requires changes in policy which make effective provision. Recognition of the problems resulting from dementia from the stark example given by someone with the illness actually did produce a political response, through the sanctioning of funding to provide a day center. The Guatemalan street children in Example 1 had overcome many difficulties in order to participate in a day of tolerance, but they discovered that what governed the conditions enabling them to take part was not their ability, but the political will to admit them to the world of privilege.

To determine the political nature of a situation one can ask a set of specific questions (see Box 6.2). These key questions, framed as 'pADL questions' by the authors, are interrelated and interdependent, meaning that the answer to one question will have implications for the other questions.

> ### Box 6.2   pADL (political Activities of Daily Living) key questions
>
> 1. What are the characteristics of the conflict and cooperation situation?
> 2. Who are the actors (occupational beings)?
> 3. How do the actors conduct themselves? What are their aims, interests, and motives?
> 4. What are their means?
> 5. What does the political landscape look like?
> 6. What is the broader context wherein conflict and cooperation manifest themselves? [32]

We follow the introduction of these questions with a presentation of occupational therapy practice examples in which these questions are applied as a preliminary reasoning tool towards the following ends:

1. Raising awareness and understanding of and actively facing up to the political nature of people's participation in daily life;

2. Enabling people-centered self-empowerment. Self empowerment is not a Nietzschean process of strengthening individualism at the expense of weaker others,[53] nor is it an inward looking affirmation of the self geared to disempowering collective and political awareness,[54] (pp. 135–173) either of which may weaken the community as a place in which to realize empowering cooperative occupation. Indeed, as Rousseau[55] suggests, a just process of self-empowerment actually requires individuals not to use their innate natural power (such as physical strength), but to derive their power from cooperation with others.

3. Encouraging Occupational justice. Occupational justice has been proposed as the foundation and fundamental purpose of occupational therapy, a profession which exists 'to address injustices'.[16,26,56] In Rousseau's terms, this requires that occupational therapists therefore act by negotiation with the community, since they cannot achieve anything unless the community wishes it to be effective. Although occupational therapists are not legally empowered, they might be described as 'engineers' who facilitate the proposal of the mechanisms by which the community chooses to operate. They are not, then, like Rousseau's lawgiver,[55] but instead provide a catalyst in the process of overcoming systems of occupational apartheid.

A WAY OF LOOKING AT THE POLITICAL NATURE OF SITUATIONS – THE pADL QUESTIONS

What are the characteristics of the conflict and cooperation situation?

First of all, what is the conflict and cooperation situation about? 'Characteristics' are those aspects that can be distinguished in any conceivable concrete situation: e.g. the number of actors and what is at stake for each of them; or the extent to which force is used to realize goals/interests. These are factors which affect the relationships between the actors.

We need to think about conflict and cooperation from a more general and theoretical perspective rather than in the specific situation being examined. Deciding which characteristics are relevant enables an analytical description of the situation. An empirical, accurate, and reliable description is required for the outcomes to be useful.

At first sight very different situations appear to share characteristics: aspects of conflict and cooperation at local level are to be found in national and international issues. They can provide models for explaining the origin and interrelationships of different characteristics to gain a general understanding of political situations. This enables us to make sensible predictions and set realistic outcomes in new investigations. Box 6.3 draws out some practice examples for the reader.

Box 6.3   Illustrations from occupational therapy

As we discussed earlier (p. 8), there is a dissonance between 'who we say we are' and 'what we do', i.e. between the walk and talk of occupational therapy. We espouse client-centered practice[57] but, as Examples 2 and 4 from the prologue illustrate, for whom or on whose behalf are occupational therapists working? As de Souza has asserted in his fifth principle, as described by Freire,[58] 'there is no public ethic without a personal ethic', and as Freire[58] has argued, every professional should reflect on whether the activity carried out in the name of a profession corresponds with real needs or political demand. This distinction is not always obvious because professional ethics are often couched in terms which serve the hegemony that, after all, supports their existence. Therefore we prefer not to refer to the people occupational therapists work with as clients or consumers here, as readers may have noted in Chapter 1. We feel it is appropriate to make the reason for this clear in this chapter on overcoming occupational apartheid. The implication of words like 'client' or 'consumer' is that people have the economic means to buy access to services from occupational therapists, but this distinguishes those who have from those who have not. This free market terminology appears to us to fly in the face of human rights, and is an example where occupational therapy itself may unintentionally contribute to conditions of occupational apartheid. Rather than use the term client-centered, we prefer to adopt the term 'people-centered' from Werner and Bower,[2] Mason,[23] and Turner[59] since this can refer to both individuals and communities irrespective of wealth and means.

Declarations of human rights or of professional responsibilities are written to accommodate so many factors that the result is generalized, rather than specific to their underpinning values. Values have to serve needs without being impossible to deliver, and the limitations on delivery are posed by political, economic, social, and cultural structures. The greater the number of interests being served by a measure, the less representative and the more excluding it will be; one rationale for having political representation is that it is impossible to have a fully participative society if people are to have any other occupation.[60] 'Thus it is that other structures are subservient to politics because it is through political systems that power is expressed. Professionals 'who do their work uncritically, just to preserve their jobs, have not yet grasped [their] political nature'.[58]

Inevitably the true professional is drawn into or becomes acutely aware of the conflicts and contradictions surrounding their role, and must seek to achieve cooperative solutions to resolve them. Watkins[52] describes how in a complex interplay of cultural, social and economic hegemonies there are many ever-changing and situational meanings which make these conflicts difficult to perceive or anticipate accurately but none the less they are there. Nor will the potential for cooperation be immediately obvious: partners may come together to serve different aspects of a purpose which suits their individual interests, which, as Dasgupta[61] suggests, may arise from pressure to serve a multiplicity of individual, social, familial, civil, and other obligations – combining both motives of expediency and altruism. As we saw in Example 1 in the prologue, occupational therapists may have the impression that a project they are involved in will fit into a community event such as the Day of Toleration, but others' views of the extent to which cooperation applies may be limited by their own perspectives, for example the need to protect privileged children from the influences of street children.

Box 6.3 continues

Thus, while conflict may turn into cooperation, cooperation may serve interests which maintain other conflicts. For example, consider the negotiations which take place about the introduction of new therapeutic activities, the development of new staff posts or new facilities, the multiple interests at work in multidisciplinary teams, or the process of applying for funding to undertake research in an occupational therapy department. In such issues occupational therapists are often working from the position of being in a professional minority, and themselves experience occupational injustice from an organizational framework which systematically excludes their involvement.[16]

In these conflict and cooperation situations, occupational therapists maintain their professional objective of being people-centered, through achieving the three pADL aims. In other words, raising awareness and understanding of people's participation in daily life, enabling people-centered self-empowerment, and encouraging occupational justice requires a constructive engagement in the issues of conflict and cooperation around professional practice and the people we work with. Occupational therapists aim to empower the people they work with, but recognize that the therapeutic relationship is time limited. Although it is negotiated toward mutually agreed outcomes, these in turn may produce new situations of conflict and cooperation.

Box 6.4   Illustrations from occupational therapy

Almost 400 years ago, Shakespeare wrote:

All the world's a stage,
And all the men and women merely players:
They have their exits and their entrances;
And one man in his time plays many parts.[63]

(Act II scene vii)

The interface between occupational therapists and the people they work with is not fixed. Their roles can be interchanged – occupational therapists are also health service clients. A people-centered practice, therefore, ultimately appears to serve everyone's needs. Before wholly accepting a stakeholder consensus for society, we should consider the actors' scripts, which are informed by a variety of needs, wants, pressures, and obligations, according to their social position and the rights and responsibilities allowed by their role.[62] In a hospital many hierarchies may be evident, governing the different clinical, administrative, and other supportive functions, in which some actors have a bigger stake in the production than others and wield

more influence. Many actors are involved in several hierarchical structures. An occupational therapist may belong to an occupational therapy service, but work in a multidisciplinary team. It is not uncommon for therapists to have split posts between two teams. Some may be advocates for a particular therapy within their professional group, others will find that to develop their career they have to leave behind clinical work and enter a managerial hierarchy. Thus occupational therapists will be engaged in conflicts and cooperation around, for example, obtaining more posts in multidisciplinary teams or issues of role blurring in generic work demands, in-service training which favors certain professional groups or clinical interests over others; supervision needs; balancing obligations between different aspects of their work, as well as attending to their case-load. This range of dramatis personae and their multiple parts in the play suggests an interplay of obligations which, as Dasgupta[61] says, is governed by rules rather than discretion. This leads to the next pADL question.

Who are the actors?

The actors are those individuals, groups, and organizations who are actively involved in the given situation of conflict and cooperation, including those incidentally affected by the consequences, and those who choose not to do anything. It is important to know the capacity in which actors are participating. All actors occupy multiple roles through the complex interplay of social relationships in which they are engaged, whether they are individuals, groups, or organizations. An organization may serve different purposes to different individuals:[62] it may be the provider of a service, an employer, a litigant, or a consumer, roles that may also be occupied by the individuals who make up the organization. Thus it is necessary to distinguish between individual and collective actors. One of the criteria for exploring this is power (addressed later in this part of the chapter under the heading 'What are their means?'), which may determine such categories as 'elites' and 'ordinary people'.

We are concerned not so much with actors but with the cooperation or conflicts that develop between them. 'Who is the ally, partner, or opponent of whom?' This question recognizes that actors may cooperate in some areas and conflict in others. Allies or partners do not agree about everything, but if they happen to be on your side in other conflicts this may benefit your mutual relationship. It is important to consider how relationships between actors can become a source of power and influence through cooperation in conflict situations. This is illustrated in Box 6.4.

How do the actors conduct themselves? What are their aims, interests, and motives?

Understanding how conflict and cooperation started and developed requires insight into the occupational behavior of the people who are involved. It does not merely concern personal psychological profiles, but a broad understanding of the background to the political behavior of the actors.

It is important to recognize the aims, interests, and motives of the actors to get an idea of what they are trying to achieve (see Ch. 19). *Aims* refers to what the actors consciously strive for, *motives* refers to actors' 'less conscious or less publicly expressed desires', and *interests* refers to what actors strive for consciously in a way which is clear to others.[32] (p. 42) Political science is concerned with aims and motives because political behavior has long been viewed as purposeful, and goal-oriented.[33,64] However, there are also behaviors which do not stem from political aims and motives, but from a reflex-like impulse, from an instinctive reaction, or from personal motives. Besides aims and interests, the actors' reasoning is important for a good understanding of their behavior. This includes the 'logic' which the actors employ with their goal-oriented behavior. These features (aims, motives, interests) contain their perception of the world as well as the 'causal reasoning' which they use.[32,33,64]

In this context, it doesn't matter if this logic is fact or fantasy, complete or incomplete. Just as the occupational therapist employing the Canadian Occupational Performance Measure begins from the client's determination of their own needs, irrespective of any professional observation, goal-oriented behavior is based on how one *thinks* that the world functions. The perceptions and causal argumentations in this subjective logic offer each actor the basis for their own assessment of the situation in terms of risks and the possibilities for the realization, costs, and benefits of goals, just as, in carrying out an activity, the therapist must account for risk and benefit. These estimations and expectations are then the basis for what an actor decides to do. Box 6.5 illustrates these processes.

What are their means?

Van der Eijk[32] says that *means* refers to everything that actors can use to realize their political aims in conflict and cooperation situations in which

Box 6.5   Illustrations from occupational therapy

Iwama (Ch. 10) discusses the implications of Western and Eastern systems of conceptualization for interpreting occupational behaviors as respectively individualistic or group focused. In a global commodity market, where even models of occupational therapy are marketed across cultures, there are many pitfalls for the application of modes of working and assessment materials that do not fit all sizes. Both Iwama, and Townsend and Whiteford (Ch. 9) warn against the misconceptions which arise from the export of occupational therapy concepts combined with the cultural effects of a global power imbalance favoring wealthier countries. Imported models may be more effectively marketed to practitioners, who may favor them over a locally derived and culturally appropriate model. The consequences of forcing square pegs into round holes on an occupational assessment aid may well produce occupational injustices where therapists and the people they are working with alike may be set on tasks which are unachievable, incomprehensible, and inappropriate. The systematic use of inappropriate approaches which subjugate local cultural forms may well result in occupational apartheid, preventing the people we work with from being enabled to articulate their needs[45,65–67] (see Ch 10 and 26). This may also be seen in Example 2, where people have migrated, bringing their cultures to other countries where systems have not adapted to the wider range of needs brought about through diversity. The insufficiency of occupational therapy approaches from the northern hemisphere has led, in Brazil (see Chs 7 and 11), to the development of well established social approaches to occupational therapy to meet the complex needs of a society with many social and economic differences.

The ability to recognize occupational apartheid depends, as we have already discussed, on critical awareness, an issue which is explored further by Townsend and Whiteford in Chapter 9. But even the development of a critical awareness is conditional on resources, and other wants, and depends on the actors' ability to cooperate with others sufficiently well to obtain the means. Some actors lack sufficient insight to recognize the need to take certain parts in order to achieve their aims, or serve their interests and motives. The occupational therapist's role may be to assess these actors' interests and enable them to both recognize them and develop the appropriate roles – to restore a kind of justice through the analysis of reality.[58] Out of this follows the need for an integrated needs and rights-based approach to occupational therapy practice, education, and research.[4,68,69]

In one sense this puts the occupational therapist in the role of the soft policeman, but the question of addressing occupational apartheid demands that occupational therapists are enabled to interrogate both the actors and those around them. Rousseau[55] suggested that those who made laws should be without power in order to be truly independent in thought, perhaps a position many occupational therapists have recognized themselves to be in, but consequently not heeded.[16] Mindful of lawgiving, we refer to the detective story and the questions it asks. This is not merely the solving of a formal intellectual problem; the occupational therapist is required to understand the 'not so very fragrant world' we live in, and thus be 'a complete man and a common man and yet an unusual man [sic]'.[70] As Chandler continues, 'The story is this man's adventure in a search for a hidden truth and it would be no adventure if it did not happen to a man fit for adventure. He has a range of awareness that startles you, but it belongs to him by right, because it belongs to the world he lives in'.[70] (pp. 198–199).

they take part. This key question is concerned with phenomena that deal with power and influence, and other related notions (see Ch. 30).

Power is often viewed as a capacity of actors to determine or change the behaviors or choices of others. The question of how power can be made visible – how it can be investigated empirically – is one of the most important ones in political science. The capacity indicated by the term power is based on the means of power or resources of power. This includes not only means of force and coercion, but also other means such as connections, money and capital, information, or having means of communication at one's disposal.

Influence is the capacity of actors to determine or change the availability of a range of behaviors or choices to other actors.

Box 6.6   Illustrations from occupational therapy

From this knowledge of the world arises a paradox which occupational therapists in a people centered practice need to recognize. One of the key issues is the lack of means of power of people experiencing disabling conditions; their marginalized position outside society is the fulcrum for a creative involvement for mounting challenges to the status quo. To have meaning, activity may be a social contribution but it may also contain a reflective element, as we have already explored. Part of the value is in the capacity it gives for rebellion – not violent revolution or rebellion for its own sake but, as Baldelli[72] (p. 24) remarks the application of 'critical intelligence' to a process of change.

As occupational beings we need to consider the implications of our roles within society. These operate at several levels, as an anecdote from Sennett and Cobb illustrates: 'I got three kids now, right, I got to put money away for their schooling and all, like I don't want to let them down, I mean I won't be holding up my end if I don't work.'[73] Thus, if as Baldelli[72] suggests, one might demonstrate one's critical intelligence by taking oneself out of oppressive and exploitative structures, one is still faced with other moral obligations to family and other interests, and with individual promises and commitments one may have made. The exploitative nature of society and of occupational apartheid ensures that if a person is unable to sustain commitments because of a reduction in ability, very often they, rather than those in power, receive the blame from those closest to them. Thus power operates to influence and contain behaviors and choices so that broader questions are not asked about where, why, and by whom the decisions are made that determine the limited range of choices available to other actors. Occupational apartheid not only denies or restricts occupational opportunities, but provides a means of power for others.

In a profession centered on occupation, a profession of educated middle class individuals who have learned about universal truths about the human nature of and need for occupation, it is easy to lose sight of this problem and to assume that occupational therapists hold the key to a truth that the client is unable to assimilate, and use manipulations that the client cannot perceive (see Examples 2 and 3 above), where assumptions about culture and diagnosis impact on the service users' interests. This is a false position, for the illusion that one group holds the truth and another does not have the capacity to realize it is another manifestation of occupational apartheid based on a restriction of opportunity and means. To see how this is, we need to look at the political landscape.

It does not follow that having these means at one's disposal will result in the same power in every conflict and cooperation situation. The availability of power and influence to actors depends on the domain in which they are operating and the mutual dependencies arising from the aims, motives, and interests that develop between actors over different fields of conflict and cooperation.

Asking the question 'What are their means?' gives insight into the actors' means of power and the power that these means yield. The political system is concerned with questions about the structure of power that characterizes the system as a whole. What matters is not whether some actors have a lot of power and others less, but what the pattern of power relations looks like. For example, is there one small group that has most power in all fields, or are there more groups that each have a lot of power, but in different fields? How equally or unequally is power distributed over different groups within society? Pollard and Walsh[71] discussed the problems of status that have restricted the professional power of occupational therapists due to the gendered nature of the profession through much of its development. This leads to difficulties both in representing the profession's interests in a male medicine-dominated health system hierarchy, and also for unqualified occupational therapy support workers trying to develop their skills and have their abilities recognized by their departmental colleagues. Box 6.6 elaborates further on these power relationships.

What does the political landscape look like?

Conflict and cooperation take place in a political system.[32] How they arise and develop is partly dependent on the organization of the system, which includes among other things institutions and rules. Political institutions are usually more or less established forms for the organization of behavior. They include 'concrete' and 'procedural' institutions.

Examples of *concrete institutions* are the House of Commons in the United Kingdom, The House of Representatives in the US, the United Nations, but also other institutions such as national occupational therapy associations and educational programs, and regional (Council of Occupational Therapists for the European Countries, Occupational Therapy Africa Regional Group, Confederación Latinoamericana de Terapeutas Ocupacionales) and world (WFOT, WHO, UNICEF, etc.) governing bodies. These institutions manifest themselves by performing certain tasks or aims, having people who do the work, an office and address where they are established, and so on.

Examples of *procedural institutions* are regular and free democratic elections, annual general meetings, WFOT council meetings, etc. These manifest themselves through stable patterns and procedures of occupational performance, e.g. procedural reasoning, protocols, and guidelines.

Concrete institutions are largely the embodiment of procedures for behavior, and are often formal institutions, with more or less established tasks and responsibilities for certain matters, defined for example, in a constitution. In many democratic political parties, the party congress is the institution that determines the political direction of the party and takes important decisions. In the WFOT this role is undertaken by the bi-annual Council meeting (see Example 4).

Many political scientists take a more empirical stand; finding out who really determines the political course of the party is a question for research, and one must be wary of constitutional and procedural details that do not describe the actual mode of operation used by those actors with influence or power. Concrete political institutions can be actors themselves (their tasks are, after all, in the terrain of politics), therefore they *must* be taken into account in the examination of conflict and cooperation: we must ask which institutions are really involved, and which are able to become involved – given their aims and methods of working – and what consequences this could have for the power relations that determine the regulation of a political system as a whole. Besides institutions, the political landscape also includes 'rules', codes for what is and what is not allowed or appropriate in the conduct of political conflict and cooperation. Rules should not here be confused with any legal principle, but instead refer to method.[34,64] In the arena of politics, rules are often vague and there is no external referee, yet rules present an important source of conflict and cooperation. For a better understanding of conflict and cooperation, a knowledge of these rules, and awareness of how they are continuously subject to changes and reinterpretations is essential. This is explored further in Box 6.7.

Box 6.7   Illustrations from occupational therapy

The Canadian Model of Occupational Performance (CMOP)[28] divides the environment into physical, cultural, social, and institutional elements. The institutional element includes policies, decision-making processes, procedures, accessibility, and other organizational practices. It includes economic, legal, and political components. Of the various occupational therapy models and approaches, CMOP most explicitly addresses these environments, and in its most recent refinement appears to offer a means of asking the question: what does the political landscape look like?

Example 4 described the process that led to the approval of the WFOT position paper on CBR by the Council meeting.[56,74] The WFOT endorsement of the terms occupational apartheid, occupational deprivation, and occupational injustice gives occupational therapists both a means of influence and a means of power to act to overcome occupational apartheid, where we could not act previously as we had no name for the problem and therefore no official mandate, a dilemma also identified in Chapter 19. This example demonstrates the way that rules were operated within WFOT procedural and concrete institutions in order to formalize and operationalize its support of occupational therapists advancing the principles of CBR. The position paper was the point of departure for the formulation of the WFOT master project plan on CBR. This plan also includes the development of an educational module on 'Occupational Therapy and Cooperative Politics', which aims to raise awareness of the political nature of occupational therapy and its core construct, occupation (dignified and meaningful participation in daily life), within and beyond the field of CBR.[29]

What is the broader context wherein conflict and cooperation manifest themselves?

According to van der Eijk[32] (pp. 45–46), in the arena of conflict and cooperation, political occurrences and processes are not isolated from the context of the world; they don't take place in a vacuum. Politics and context influence each other mutually, without one being the exclusive result of the other. Developments in politics must be principally understood from the logic of political interactions and process. The reverse is equally valid.

Relative autonomy refers to the relationship between politics and *context*, in which both to a certain extent have their own existence, while they still mutually influence each other. Some parts of the context hardly ever, especially not in the short term, lend themselves to conscious change through human intervention, e.g. because they result from geographical, climatic, and physical features. Here the relative autonomy is very wide. These contextual features provide a source of means from a political perspective, because organization is required at certain periods, for example to maintain flood defences or deal with natural disasters. On the other hand, they are a source of permanence since they make up preconditions wherein human existence, including its political dimension, takes place.

Relative autonomy between politics and context must not be confused with personal autonomy, which other authors apply to citizenship as the basis of individual participation in society.[75] This distinction is necessary because other parts of the context are the products of human occupation and are therefore, in principle, open to deliberate influencing by political actors. Important aspects of the context of politics – which themselves are mostly also viewed as relatively autonomous – are the economy, the sphere of the law, society, culture and language, the field of mass communication. For each of them the following question can be posed: under what circumstances is their relative autonomy in relation to politics stronger or weaker? This demonstrates that the level of autonomy of aspects of the context in relation to politics is different from place to place over the course of time. Box 6.8 relates this to the situation of occupational therapists.

Box 6.8	Illustrations from occupational therapy

Pollard and Walsh[71] have argued that a number of contextual factors have impacted on the potential power of occupational therapists to develop a more independent position within mental health systems in the UK. They list the following factors: high turnover in posts, coupled with the attractiveness of the flexibility produced by a demand for occupational therapists exceeded by supply, contributing to a lack of professional development because of interrupted careers; the concern of the profession with basic life activities that are perceived socially as low status, and the perception that in gaining professional status women occupational therapists are distancing themselves from concerns with domestic occupational therapy activities; and the secondary status of a female profession in relation to male partners' employment needs, producing disruptions in career patterns for women therapists. Consequently, occupational therapists have historically been compromised in developing research interests and gaining professional promotion, while at the same time, because of the difficulties in gaining status, they have remained invisible to other health professions who are often unaware of what they do. As some of the contributors to Watson and Swartz[44] have suggested, this perspective may be changing, but occupational therapists who wish to tackle occupational apartheid also need to face up to some of the restrictions and denials that compromise their own access to self-determination.

PART 3 BEING AND BECOMING FIRM AND RESOLUTE

DISCUSSION

Occupational apartheid has already proved a controversial term, and we acknowledge that even amongst the contributors to this book it is not one which everyone is comfortable or in agreement with. It has been described, for example, as an 'emotional sledgehammer', and as language which is 'too politically charged'; South African colleagues have found it difficult to accept a term which combines the core of their profession with a word which represents 'a historical evil', which they fought and have left behind.

We acknowledge and respect these difficulties, particularly when we are introducing this language into a profession which, as suggested by Example 4, and by Sadlo (in Watson[7]) has hardly counted itself as one with political objectives. However, the disabling realities to which occupational apartheid refers and which are experienced by very large numbers of human beings predominantly in (but not limited to) 'developing countries', are malignant and require appropriate terms.

To use phrases which are less controversial does not serve people experiencing such disabling conditions as those which result from the combination of poverty, disability, deprivation of rights, and other inequalities. Certainly these conditions are examples of occupational injustice and occupational deprivation, but these terms do not suggest that such phenomena are the consequences of political and economic decisions, in other words, that there is a systematic relationship between the phenomenon and the causes. Occupational apartheid is a term which confronts these realities, and demands the unravelling of the complex and often mysterious processes which produce them. Furthermore, as Hocking, Wilcock, Whiteford, Roberts and Sadlo appear to suggest in Watson,[7] (pp. 10–15) having analyzed the process, action is necessary. Often an awareness of the phenomenon requires participatory action in order to begin the process of analysis, and a sustained program of collaboration in order to effect substantial change. 'A sense of stake-holding does not fall from heaven. If it is acquired at all it is acquired with great difficulty and considerable social cost.'[75] (p. 112)

Example 3 described the political actions of a group of people with early onset of dementia, a group that requires early health intervention to delay the progress of the illness. This means that they need a prompt diagnosis in order to obtain treatments and plan occupational outcomes for themselves effectively to maximize the potential of a time limited life in dignity and meaning. To be empowered in this, the person with early onset of dementia needs to be told exactly what their situation means. Delaying the message loses them vital time.[76] Similarly, although we realize that many people will struggle to recognize occupational apartheid, particularly in social contexts of relative economic prosperity, the longer it takes to address the global issues to which it refers, the more lives will continue to be blighted or even negated of meaning through the systems which thrive upon it. If occupational apartheid is not named, then the realities that are experienced by vast numbers of people every day around the world do not exist in the sense that they are not seen. It is, as Fanon says,[45] (p. 251) 'time to change our ways … The new day which is already at hand must find us firm, prudent and resolute.'

Townsend and Wilcock[16] refer to trivialization of occupations as a result of occupational apartheid. Again, this is something we would like to highlight, especially as the idea that occupations can be 'trivialized'[16] (p. 77) suggests a paradoxical relationship with meaningful occupation. This occupational absurdity is an underpinning condition of occupational apartheid in which occupational meaning is negated through the nature of an occupation, producing an effect of occupational alienation.[16] Two examples are described in the following paragraphs.

The first example is from the experience of the second author, who was told by both staff and patients at an asylum where he used to work that as recently as the 1980s a group of people with chronic mental illnesses were daily sent to occupational therapy in order to knit squares. The completed squares were passed to another group of people in the same room who unravelled the squares back into balls of wool. These exercises were offered to give them an occupation. It may not have occurred to the people who first devised this activity that it was absurd, but it seemed so to some of those engaged in it and certainly to those who had to supervise it.

Lafargue[77] provides the second example in his description of the lives of French textile factory workers. Their jobs were dangerous, involved long hours, and produced poor quality cloth which was dumped on the market because it was no longer fashionable. To produce these goods they worked so long they had no leisure time, and got into poor health. Production of a cheap commodity was therefore linked to occupational imbalance'[78] a situation where the availability of enriching and meaningful life experiences is compromised. Although Lafargue was writing about conditions in a previous century, similar conditions continue in many contemporary societies, for example in the production of fashion items, toys, and electronic components.[79] These are often the basis for new economies, yet there is a paradox for the individuals concerned, who will not realize the benefits of participating in the new wealth because they do not have the leisure or sufficient wages to enjoy it, or their damaged health will not allow them to, and they lack the resources to campaign for better conditions. For them this occupation is only beneficial in the sense of offering a choice between perpetuating their poor working conditions or starving. This is an absurdity.

In neither of these examples are the occupations 'enriching'[16] rather, they have lost their connection with meaning. The first is an example of work for work's sake; the second is an illustration of the skewed consequences of the profit motive which render the product and the work unnecessary. There is no point in making things which are immediately dumped or destroyed, unless you are enabled at least to enjoy the process of making them. However, both the asylum inmates and the factory workers had no choice but to engage in absurd occupations. Of course they could have stopped work, but the regime of the asylum may have prevented access to any other activities, and in the case of the factory workers, they would have had to find new work. If their work in the factory paid them at subsistence level, then they were merely working to exist, and were deprived of the benefits of meaningful occupation. Occupational apartheid deprives people of experiencing meaning through occupations.

Occupational absurdity results from engagement in those occupations which not only alienate those performing them but actually contribute to the perpetuation of occupational apartheid, or which are positively harmful personally and in a broader social sense. Occupational apartheid is itself an occupational absurdity.

In situations of extreme adversity such as armed conflicts, poverty, and chronic illness people have developed mechanisms which enable them to face and obtain a distance from their circumstances. These devices enable them to put their situations into perspective and speculate about the possibilities of resolving them.

Absurdity is deliberately used to describe these situations because often those people experiencing these conditions are deprived of most of the resources they need to overcome them and develop occupations which are meaningful and enriching, including, means of developing awareness (see beginning of this chapter). Recognition of occupational absurdity and alienation, however, can lead to means they can generate themselves, weapons of mass construction, deconstruction, and reconstruction. These critical, paradoxical weapons are ubiquitous, e.g. humor,[80] the arts, philosophy, and have a long history of use in many cultural traditions, particularly in the question of obtaining meaning and questioning social and even political practices. Occupational therapy processes and technologies are also, as many of the contributors to this book suggest, capable of this work.

Even so, in the informal discussions with many colleagues around the world that have contributed to the development of this chapter, strong feelings of anxiety have been expressed about developing a critical political position within the occupational therapy profession, and similarly about the use of humor and even the arts to advance serious points. We agree that used carelessly, such weapons of mass construction, deconstruction, and reconstruction can easily misfire, but their use is well established and respected, with examples from Jesus,[81] Buddha Drukpa Kunley (the 'Crazy Wise' Tibetan teacher)[82] and Taoist philosophers,[83] all of whom have posed reflective questions akin to the pADL questions we have outlined above. The critical awareness such teachers enable people to develop is eminently portable and applicable to many situations; indeed, a questioning of practices and rules is at the core of what Fish and Coles[84] have termed 'professional artistry', consideration of which is intended to enable health professionals to account for their decisions and actions. Rigor is vital in such questioning, as we have suggested in our discussion on the need to 'face up' to occupational apartheid. As Fish has commented, the practitioner has to deal with 'a critical professional audience (including the practitioner and immediate colleagues) and the public'.[85] (p. 130) It was indeed, Fanon's[45] incisive use of the paradoxical and absurd in his depictions of medical case dilemmas which so forcefully made his case against the abuses of colonial medicine, and illustrated how the ethics of care were undermined under a colonial regime.

Fish[85] assumes that unlike practitioners, artists rarely meet the audience for their work, but this does not take account of participative and political uses of the arts by the people occupational therapists work with. Questioning approaches, such as the pADL examples above, are not solely for the use of health professions; people with experience of disabling conditions are already developing them and deriving strength from them. Recent examples of this approach can be found in Mad Pride, a UK-based mental health survivors' organization who have reconstructed the word 'Mad' with a capital letter to politicize the inequalities experienced by people with mental illness. Mad Pride, which borrows its tactics from Gay Pride, and Survivors' Poetry, another United Kingdom-based organization of over 2500 poets who have survived mental distress,[86] use the arts to promote a positive image of mental illness. Such critical weapons[87] can be guided by a set of values provided by the concept of occupational justice (see Ch. 9) and the concepts outlined in part 2 of this chapter in the pADL questions, and in the principles set out in Chapter 1. By themselves they are not enough, unless they are connected to outcomes through action. Occupational therapists can develop links with such activist groups to help empower the people they work with in challenging occupational apartheid (see Ch. 21).

CONCLUSION

At this point, let us return to David Werner's foreword: 'Through a cycle of analysis, reflection, and action, Freire's methodology aimed to enable concerned and disadvantaged people to discover their self-confidence and work together to 'change the world.' *Occupational Therapy without Borders* shares a similar vision: its scope extends from the personal to the global.' Coming out of the closet as political beings can not be done if we are not more transparent about where we're coming from, what our aims, motives, and interests are, and what we both can and want to offer to the processes in which we engage. The discussion of ideas such as partnerships, emancipatory approaches, enabling, and empowering those who are not participating due to disabling conditions, implies choosing to support those whom the system has marginalized, in order to work for occupational justice.[16]

However, the relative autonomy of the broader context is that we are employed and managed by institutions that were created and funded by that same system which produces marginalization. For whom or on whose behalf do we work? We have identified the need to use pADL questions to explore this question critically, and we urge all readers to engage in an on-going open dialogue about the political nature of who we say we are, as articulated in our philosophy, principles, values, beliefs, and aspirations in doing, being, and becoming.

There have been and there are voices within the occupational therapy community that encourage us to embrace a business paradigm, saying 'if we don't, we might not be around in the future to talk about it.'[88] Acknowledging that the health, social care, and education arenas in many affluent countries in the world seem to accommodate market driven practices, we agree that it is important to understand this macro process related to globalization that is taking place, and to determine our position in this scheme.

We argue that occupational therapy's means are our principles, values, and beliefs. These define who we are and what we do. They are our critical weapons of mass construction, deconstruction, and reconstruction, with which we defend our identity, integrity, and dignity. If we lose these, those we aspire to serve, who really legitimize our existence and are our means to power, have more to lose. So whatever choices we make as occupational therapists, individually and collectively, they are political and so are their implications and consequences.

We recognize that we are presenting part of a complicated picture, and asking readers to take on this complexity in order to be able to apply its content appropriately. It is a participatory action process, which also requires collaboration with people who experience disabling conditions, with occupational scientists, and with others in the development of new weapons of mass construction, deconstruction, and reconstruction, not only to overcome occupational apartheid, but also to address other conditions that deny or restrict dignified participation in meaningful occupation. The outcomes and the realizations of what is involved cannot yet be evaluated. This chapter is itself an initial foray, a manifesto in which the authors proclaim the direction of their future work. We welcome the opportunity to engage with our readers in the scrutiny and further development of these concepts and their application in practice.

Our deepest fear is not that we are inadequate,
Our deepest fear is that we are powerful beyond measure.
It is our own light, not our darkness that most frightens us.

We ask ourselves, 'who am I to be brilliant, gorgeous, talented and fabulous?'
Actually, who are you not to be? Your playing small does not deserve the
world.
There's nothing enlightened about shrinking so that other people won't feel
insecure around you.
It's not just in some of us; it's in everyone.
And as we let our own light shine, we unconsciously give other people
permission to do the same.
As we are liberated from our fear, our presence automatically liberates others.

Nelson Mandela, quoted in Russell[89]

Acknowledgements

We would very much like to thank the following for their inspiration, constructive criticism, and assistance in the production of this chapter: Cees van der Eijk, Dennis Jubb, Manvir Manku, and our colleagues Reg Urbanowski, Michael Iwama, Sandra Galheigo, Marion Fourie, Marilyn Pattison, and Kit Sinclair.

References

1. Kronenberg F. Occupational therapy without borders. Paper presented at the 30th National Congress of the Occupational Therapy Association of South Africa, Cape Town, May 2004.
2. Werner D, Bower B. Helping health workers learn: a book of methods, aids, and ideas for instructors at the village level. Berkeley, California: The Hesperian Foundation; 2001.
3. Kant E. *Kritik der reinen Vernunft, Einleitung zu einer Idee einer transzendentalen Logik*. Hamburg: Philosophische Bibliothek, Taschenbuch; 1998.
4. Kronenberg F. In search of the political nature of occupational therapy. MSc OT paper. Linköping University, Linköping, Sweden. 2003.
5. Griffin S. Occupational therapists and the concept of power: a review of the literature, Austr Occup Ther J 2001; 48 (June): 24–34.
6. World Health Organization. International classification of functioning, disability and health. Geneva: WHO; 2001.
7. Watson R. New horizons in occupational therapy. In: Watson R, Swartz L, eds. Transformation through occupation. London: Whurr; 2004: 3–18.
8. Aristotle. The politics. Harmondsworth: Penguin; 1962.
9. Townsend E, Wilcock A. Occupational justice. In: Christiansen C, Townsend E, eds. Introduction to occupation: the art and science of living. Thorofare, NJ: Prentice Hall; 2003.
10. Rawls J. A theory of justice. Oxford: Oxford University Press, 1973.
11. Whiteford G. Occupational deprivation: global challenge in the new millennium. Br J Occup Ther 2000; 63(5): 200–204.
12. World Federation of Occupational Therapists. Position paper on community based rehabilitation. WFOT. Forrestfield, Western Australia. April 2004. Online. Available: www.wfot.org.
13. Freire P. Education for critical consciousness. New York: Continuum Press; 1983.
14. Chomsky N. Understanding power: the indispensable Chomsky. New York: The New Press; 2002.
15. Freire P. Pedagogy of the oppressed. Harmondsworth: Penguin; 1973.
16. Townsend L, Wilcock A A. Occupational justice and client centred practice: a dialogue. Can J Occup Ther 2004; 71(2) 75–87.
17. World Health Organization. Primary health care: report on the International Conference on Primary Health Care, Alma Ata. Geneva: WHO; 1978.
18. Werner D, Sanders D. Questioning the solution: the politics of primary health care and child survival. Palo Alto, California: Healthwrights; 1997. Online. Available: http://www.politicsofhealth.org/
19. Foucault M. Birth of the clinic. Routledge; London: 1986.
20. Yerxa EJ. Occupational science: a new source of power for participants in occupational therapy. Journal of Occupational Science 1993; 1: 3–10.
21. Wilcock AA. A theory of the human need for occupation. Journal of Occupational Science 1993; 1: 17–24.

22. Kronenberg F. Street children: being and becoming. Research study. Heerlen, The Netherlands: Hogeschool Limburg; 1999.

23. Mason M. Incurably human. London: wORKing Press, 2002.

24. Kronenberg F. Juggling with survivors of the street: occupational therapy and clowns in Guatemala City. Paper presented at the 13th WFOT congress. Stockholm. 2002.

25. Kronenberg F. Occupational therapy without borders: occupational justice education. Paper presented at 9th annual meeting of the European Network of Occupational Therapy in Higher Education. Prague. 2003.

26. Kronenberg F. Understanding and facing up to the political nature of occupational therapy. Paper presented at the 7th European Congress of Occupational Therapy. Athens. September 2004.

27. Wilcock AA. Reflections on doing, being and becoming. Can J Occup Ther 1999; 65(5): 248–256.

28. Canadian Association of Occupational Therapists. Enabling occupation: an occupational therapy perspective. Ottawa: CAOT; 2002.

29. WFOT–CBR project team. Master project plan. WFOT; 2004. Online. Available: www.wfot.org

30. Creek J. Occupational therapy as a complex intervention. London: College of Occupational Therapists; 2003.

31. World Health Organization. Health and welfare, Canada. The Ottawa Charter for Health Promotion. Ottawa: Canadian Public Health Organization; 1986.

32. van der Eijk C. *De kern van politiek*. Amsterdam: Het Spinhuis; 2001.

33. Hobbes T. Leviathan. Oxford: Oxford University Press; 1996.

34. von Clauswitz C. On war. Harmondsworth: Pelican, 1968.

35. United Nations. United Nations General Assembly: Universal Declaration of Human Rights. New York: United Nations; 1948. Online. Available: http://www.un.org/rights/50/decla.htm and www.hrweb.org

36. Orwell G. Animal farm. Harmondsworth: Penguin; 1951.

37. Steinberg S. 'Race relations': the problem with the wrong name. New Politics 2001; 8(2). Online. Available: http://www.google.co.uk/ search?q=cache:F7SSV6fXPSQJ:www.wpunj.edu/ ~newpol/issue30/steinb30.htm+STeinberg+ %22occupational+apartheid%22&hl=en?

38. Engels F. The origin of the family, private property and the state. Foreign Languages Press, Peking: 1978.

39. Rousseau JJ. A discourse on inequality. Harmondsworth: Penguin; 1984.

40. Macionis JJ, Plummer K. Sociology: a global introduction. London: Prentice Hall Europe; 1997.

41. Watson R, Fourie M. International and African influences on occupational therapy. In: Watson R, Swartz L, eds. Transformation through occupation. London: Whurr; 2004.

42. Dundas C. From the war on poverty to the war on terror? The shifting priorities of ODA. Available: http://www.bond.org.uk/networker/march04/ odasecurity.htm.

43. Molinas Moldinado MM, Monroy Peralta JG. *Sistematizacion de experiencias: una invitacion para la accion una propuesta para instituciones y/o programas que trabajan con el sector de la infancia*. Guatemala City: Childhope; 1999.

44. Watson R, Swartz L. Transformation through occupation. London: Whurr; 2004.

45. Fanon F. The wretched of the earth. Harmondsworth: Penguin; 1967.

46. Urbanowski R, Kronenberg F, Pollard N, Simo Algado S. The politics of occupation. Paper presented at the 2nd Canadian Occupational Science Symposium. Toronto, May 2004.

47. Cardona CE. *¿Qué es y para qué sirve la política? Educación para la Paz*. Documento interno. Edición 1. Guatemala: Oficina Pastoral Social Arzobispado de Guatemala OPSAG; 2001.

48. Marcuse H. One dimensional man. London: Routledge; 1991.

49. Foucault M. Discipline and punish. Harmondsworth: Penguin; 1991.

50. Kuypers G. *Grondbegrippen van politiek*. Antwerpen/Utrecht: Het Spectrum; 1973.

51. Poldervaart S, Reinalda B. *Vrouwenstudies, politicologie en de omschrijving van politiek*. In: Fennema M, van der Wouden R, eds. *Het politicologen-debat: wat is Politiek?* Amsterdam: Van Gennep; 1982: 35–56.

52. Watkins E. Throwaways: work culture and consumer education. Stanford: University Press; 1993.

53. Nietzsche F. On the genealogy of morals. In: Kaufman W, ed. *On the genealogy of morals* and *Ecce homo*. New York: Vintage Books; 1989: 15–311.

54. Dorfman A. The infantilization of the adult reader. In: Dorfman A. The Empire's old clothes. London: Pluto; 1983: 135–173.

55. Rausseau JJ. The social contract. Harmondsworth: Penguin; 1968.

56. Kronenberg F. WFOT discussion paper on Community Based Rehabilitation. Forrestfield, Western Australia: WFOT; April 2003. Online. Available: www.wfot.org

57. Sumsion T. Overview of client centred practice. In: Sumsion T, ed. Client centred practice in occupational therapy. Edinburgh: Churchill Livingstone; 1999: 1–14.

58. Freire P. The politics of education: culture, power and liberation. South Hadley, MA: Bergin & Garvin; 1985.

59. Turner A. Patient? Client? Service User? – What's in a name? Br J Occup Ther 2002; 65(8): 355.

60. Lucas JR. Democracy and participation. Harmondsworth: Pelican; 1976.

61. Dasgupta P. An inquiry into well-Being and destitution. Oxford: Oxford University Press; 1993.

62. Goffman E. Interaction ritual. Harmondsworth: Penguin; 1972.

63. Shakespeare W. As You Like It. In: The Complete Works. Omega Books; Ware: 1986: 622.

64. Machiavelli N. The Prince. Harmondsworth: Penguin; 1996.

65. Dorfman A. The Empire's old clothes. Pluto Press, London: 1983.

66. Kymlicka W. Multicultural citizenship. Oxford: Clarendon Press; 1995.

67. Iwama M. The issue is…toward culturally relevant epistemologies in occupational therapy. Am J Occup Ther 2003; 57(5): 582–588.

68. Canadian International Development Agency. Action plan for 2001. Quebec: CIDA; 2001.

69. Townsend E. Occupational justice: ethical, moral and civic principles for an inclusive world. Keynote presentation at the Annual Conference of the European Network of Occupational Therapy Educators. Prague, Czech Republic. October 2003.

70. Chandler R. The simple art of murder in *Pearls are a Nuisance*. Harmondsworth: Penguin; 1964: 181–199.

71. Pollard N, Walsh S. Occupational therapy, gender and mental health, an inclusive perspective? Br J Occup Ther 2000; 63(9): 425–431.

72. Baldelli G. Social anarchism. Harmondsworth: Penguin; 1972.

73. Sennett R, Cobb J. The hidden injuries of class. London: Faber and Faber; 1993.

74. WHO. Report of International Consultation to Review Community Based Rehabilitation in Helsinki. Geneva: World Health Organization; December 2003. Online. Available: www.who.int.ncd/disability

75. Clarke PB. Deep citizenship. London: Pliuto Press; 1996.

76. Harris PB. The subjective experience of early onset dementia: voices of the persons. 55th Gerontological Society of America Annual Meeting. Boston. 26 November 2002. Online. Available: http://www.dasninternational.org/archive/subj_exp_eoad.pdf

77. Lafargue P. *Le droit a la paresse*. Pantin: Temps de Cerises 1996.

78. Wilcock AA. An occupational perspective of health. Thorofane, NJ: Slack; 1998.

79. Frost S. Labour standards in China: the business and investment challenge. Hong Kong: Association for Sustainable and Responsible Investment in Asia; 2002. Online. Available: http://www.asria.org/publications/lib/LabourStandardsInChinaReport.pdf

80. Fernandez JD. *Hacia una pedagogía del humor*. Revista Ñaque: Teatro, Expresión, Educación 1999; 3(9): 1–9.

81. Wilson AN. Jesus. London: Flamingo; 1993.

82. Dowman K. The divine madman. The sublime life and songs of Drukpa Kunley. Middletown, CA: The Dawn Horse Press; 1998.

83. Watts A. Tao, the watercourse way. Harmondsworth: Pelican; 1979.

84. Fish D, Coles C. Developing professional judgement in health care. Oxford: Butterworth Heinemann; 1998.

85. Fish D. Appreciating practice in the caring professions. Oxford: Butterworth Heinemann; 1998.

86. Survivors' Poetry. Online. Available: http://66.102.11.104/search?q=cache:gfP841WuaZUJ:groups.msn.com/survivorspoetry+survivors+poetry&hl=en

87. Mad Pride. Online. Available: www.madpride.org.uk/about.htm+Mad+Pride&hl=en

88. Jacobs K. Recreating occupational therapy. Paper presented at the 5th European Congress of Occupational Therapy. Paris. 2000.

89. Russell M. Living in remote rural Australia. In: Voices of the unheard – testimonies from the People's Health Assembly. Dhaka, Bangladesh: People's Health Movement; May 2002: 47.

Chapter **7**

Occupational therapy and the social field
Clarifying concepts and ideas

Sandra Maria Galheigo

OVERVIEW

This chapter aims to introduce the reader to the discussion of the role of occupational therapy in the social field. The author proposes a theory of occupational therapy in the social field from a critical standpoint, based on her long-term Brazilian experience, both as an academic and a practitioner. To build up the argument and to clarify concepts currently used, broad sociological concepts such as marginalization, exclusion, disaffiliation, and apartheid are presented. Their meanings are scrutinized and their imbedment in major theoretical frameworks is portrayed. Emancipation, empowerment, the construction of subjectivity, and citizenship are presented as essential elements that organize the discourse, cement the principles, and inspire occupational therapy action from a critical view. In conclusion, considerations for action in the social field are offered, including the need to think about action on both a local and a global basis, from singular and collective perspectives.

THINKING ABOUT OCCUPATIONAL THERAPY FIELDS

Is there such a thing as a 'social' occupational therapy? Will this be a new, reductionist approach to organizing information and attending to people's needs? What is the best way to promote debate and produce knowledge and practice, with regard to a population that has been largely excluded from social welfare? What theoretical standpoint should occupational therapists adopt? Will it be necessary to take sides? Should sociologists, health and social workers, and occupational therapists necessarily be partisans, in addition to their primary role as scientists and practitioners? To begin with, what is the best way to refer to those in need anyway: excluded, marginalized, vulnerable, survivors, deviant, under apartheid, disadvantaged, disaffiliated? As social constructs, these descriptions harbor implicit meanings that may give place to different interpretations (or misinterpretations) of the phenomenon of inequality. Is all this questioning an issue only for the Third World, or is it, despite the variations, at the core of a contemporary global debate concerning social affairs? Are occupational therapists world-wide interested in this, and ready to play a role different from the one they have been used to playing in rehabilitation? Is their role in the social field professional or political? Is it possible (or even essential) to have it both ways?

These are questions that have been the focus of occupational therapy debate in research, practice, and teaching in Brazil since the late 1970s. Besides its traditional role in rehabilitation, occupational therapy has increasingly developed a significant experience with the population below the poverty line, which is in a doubly vulnerable condition with regard to both emotional bonds and social support. Based on this three decade experience, this chapter addresses the issue of the role of occupational therapy in the social field in the contemporary world. As a consequence, it aims to answer the questions above from a critical standpoint, in which social reality is seen as deriving from the interplay between structure and social practices. In this framework, social phenomena also need to be carefully thought about, bearing in mind the objective and subjective aspects of social reality.

CLARIFYING CONCEPTS: MARGINALITY, EXCLUSION, AND DISAFFILIATION

Since its origins, occupational therapy has subscribed to humanistic principles and practices. The concern with human action, from the most basic activities of self-care to the most creative and productive accomplishments in social life, has oriented its humanitarian approach. Consequently, it is legitimate to assume that there is still a significant role to be played by occupational therapists in matters related to social affairs.

Whether there should be a so-called social field in occupational therapy or whether the theoretical framework should be given by a universal model is still a point of controversy. However, this contention is not limited to the social domain but encompasses a broader debate in occupational therapy. The argument in favor of a specific discourse and practice for a social occupational therapy is that, in the social field, the core rehabilitation concepts of normality and functionality are of no use. Instead, they should give way to concepts such as equality, accessibility, and inclusion. This argument also implies that occupational therapists should commit themselves to the cause in favor of people's human rights, transcending an immediate professional role or academic interest. As a matter of fact, a critical standpoint provides the foundations for such an argument, as will be explained later in the chapter.

Focusing on a particular field makes it possible to unveil the meanings of terms, notions, and concepts that have been socially and historically constructed, and have varied throughout time and space. Their clarification is important in the shaping of coherent and effective policies and methods of action.

Despite everyday usage of some of these terms, concepts such as marginality, deviance, inclusion/exclusion, equal opportunity, apartheid, vulnerability, and disaffiliation have their meanings imbedded in some major theoretical frameworks. Using them interchangeably may lead to inconsistencies in the comprehension of arguments and implementation of actions. Examining briefly the three most substantial concepts – marginality, exclusion and disaffiliation – may clarify their further analysis.

Marginality is a concept that has been used for a wide range of social conditions relating to urban poverty. Robert Park[1] first used the concept of marginal man in the 1920s in his study of the behavior of migrant communities in Chicago. The marginal man, according to Park, was marked by instability since he lived in two different cultural realities and felt a stranger in both of them. However, whatever negative features one might see in this character, Park envisaged in the marginal man the chance to understand better the processes of civilization and progress. Consequently, at this point, the concept was associated with social change and non-conformity, a meaning still present today.

In Latin America, the diverse usage of the notion of marginality points to a common explanation: marginality means lack of integration.[2] However, there is a divergence about its causality, as shown by the two major streams of thought that emerged in the period: the functionalist approach (associated with the theory of modernization) and the Marxist approach (associated with the theory of dependence). The structural–functionalist analysis assumes that because society is a systemic organization and works on a consensual basis, marginality takes place when one of its members does not adapt to its rules. Marginality and the lack of integration here are reduced to the adaptation, or failure to adapt, of a person to a given social structure.[2] In contrast, according to the Marxist standpoint, marginality is a result of the social relations of production, specific to the capitalist accumulation. Marginality is thus understood as a social conflict resulting from the marginal incorporation of the population in the labor market and is used to refer to dependent economies (i.e. typical of peripheral countries).

From the 1950s to the 1980s in Latin America, the notion of marginality came to be attributed to various circumstances related to urban poverty, poor living conditions in the slums, lack of access to the benefits of the urban, industrial society, and the unstable position of the production process.[3] Also, it came to be seen as a way of transgressing the social order, which led to the stigmatization of the term in Brazil by the association of the term 'marginal' with 'troublemaker'.

Exclusion is a notion which Foucault[4] started to use, without particular emphasis, to refer to the so-called 'Great Confinement'. At that time, those whose common feature was their incapacity for productive work, such as the insane, the disabled, the poor and the deviant, were confined in the *Hôpital Général* in Paris. According to Foucault, this was the seed for the establishment of public asylums by the end of the nineteenth century. Therefore, the term exclusion was primarily associated with the ideas of banishment, confinement, and social control. Later, René Lenoir,[5] another French author, used the term to allude to the subjective dimension of being poor in twentieth century France, particularly in the 1970s and 1980s. Also, exclusion was used to refer to the instability of working relations and personal bonds in the contemporary world.

At the turn of the millennium, the process of exclusion may represent the collapse of the ideas of inclusion and the universality of human rights; a disintegration process by which an astonishing number of people come to be unquestioningly accepted as disposable, and become segregated either culturally, spatially, ethnically, or economically. The term exclusion is thus related to the opposite concepts of equality and citizenship, and expresses the disruption of social bonds, either material or symbolic. It may refer to different processes and groups, modes and causalities, and it cannot be used to signify a specific phenomenon in a particular society. The term exclusion exceeds the condition of unstable integration in the labor market and suggests a wide set of circumstances, which may affect identity, social cohesion, and the sense of belonging.[3]

Escorel,[3] following Hannah Arendt's works, argues that social exclusion may reduce social groups to the condition of *animal laborans*, i.e. people whose main concern is exclusively the maintenance of their survival. These people are expropriated, and therefore excluded, from their condition of *homo faber* (which involves the human capacity of doing, creating, and building the living world) and *bios politikos* (which involves the drive for interaction and participation in public life).

The extensive and diffuse uses of the notion of exclusion have also been reason for criticism. First, if one takes diversity and plurality in contemporary societies as an example, one has to be careful not to mistake exclusion for difference, since not all difference leads to exclusion. Second, the concept of exclusion cannot be applied indiscriminately to all social systems, without considering each one's cultural attributes. Although one should think in global terms as far as universal human rights are concerned, one should take into account local realities, customs, beliefs, and peculiarities in social stratification and social structure.

Exclusion is also considered an inadequate notion to be applied in circumstances where, rather than inequality or discrimination, there is a strict dividing line, restricting social mobility and religious and ethnic relations, and creating two disconnected worlds. In this case, the terms *apartheid* or *social apartheid* are preferable, since they stress difference and define better a fragmented territory, a social fracture. The idea of social apartheid implies the existence of two separate and opposing worlds, each one with its internal solidarity principles and social dynamics.[3,6,7]

Robert Castel[8] points out that exclusion has become an all-encompassing term for all global miseries. He argues that the excluded person is actually a *désaffilié*, whose path is made up of a series of disruptions in the balance of the previous living conditions. *Désaffiliation*, a French neologism freely translated here as disaffiliation is a concept created by Robert Castel to approach, in a more adequate way, the 'new social question', i.e. the result of the rise of unemployment and the growing vulnerability of working conditions in the 1990s in France. Castel[9] chooses to approach it as an outcome of the intersection of two axes: the axis of integration/non-integration in work and the axis of belonging/not belonging to a family sociability. The multiple combinations of these factors will define one's condition, which may deteriorate from *integration*, when there are satisfactory professional and family guarantees, to *vulnerability*, when there is some fragility both in work and family life, to *disaffiliation*, when a rupture occurs in both. By the end of the process of disaffiliation, a process of weakening and rupture of social bonds, economic loss becomes complete deprivation and relational fragility becomes isolation.[3,10] This extreme condition is, for example, the one faced by homeless people, street children, and refugees around the world.

As shown above, the concepts of marginality, exclusion, social apartheid, and disaffiliation are attached to particular theoretical frameworks and their origins are inscribed in specific social domains. Making them clear contributes to a better approach to the object, or rather the subject, of social occupational therapy, i.e. the marginalized, the excluded, and the disaffiliated. Lack of integration may be seen from different standpoints and occupational therapists will always have to evaluate which one is most appropriate to the reality they are dealing with. They have also to decide whether to root their actions in broad sociological concepts, such as the ones presented above, or go after concepts specific to occupational therapy, such as occupational justice and occupational apartheid (see Chs 6 and 9).[11,12]

Occupational therapists have to be careful not to be invasive in local affairs and should be prepared to read the peculiarities of local tensions and conflicts, recognize prejudice and discrimination, and be aware of the way power relations are established. Occupational therapists should make use of cultural relativism, which takes into account the beliefs and customs of other peoples within the context of their own culture rather than the therapist's. They also have to keep in mind the cherished universal human rights, such as the right to life, dignity, and self-determination. Other concerns occupational therapists should have are to avoid patronizing people and using their professional power to disregard people's inclinations.

It is important to stress that although the concepts described above are useful as a point of departure, they still focus on the failure, the absence, or the lack of something, i.e. on negative features. Other key concepts should be pursued in order to focus on more positive aspects, such as empowerment, emancipation, the construction of subjectivity, collective action, and citizenship, which are the aims of occupational therapy in the social field. As these ideas are inscribed in a critical standpoint it will first be necessary to present the foundation upon which occupational therapy in the social field should be laid.

OCCUPATIONAL THERAPY FROM A CRITICAL STANDPOINT

What are the aims of occupational therapy in the social field? The answers usually vary around the theme of integration. Some of the usual answers are: to integrate people into society, to re-adapt people, to promote inclusion. These answers, however, do not convey a precise meaning. On the contrary, they are ambiguous and may corroborate a functionalist view of society, which continues to be hegemonic in some fields of knowledge and in educational, social, and health practices.

The functionalist standpoint is based on the belief that society has a functional organization based on harmony and consensus. According to this view, society and its organizations are meant to be kept in order and equilibrium. Social change and social conflict are considered secondary phenomena and a menace to the proper function of social institutions.

As a consequence, people and families who do not live according to what is established as normal or adequate, end up being considered dysfunctional, troublesome, or deviant. The role of the professional, in this view, is to help these people to work out their own difficulties and re-enter or re-adapt to society and social life, as if they had intentionally left mainstream social life behind or had disregarded some previously established social contract.

This standpoint – in Janowitz's[13] words, the 'social psychology of conformity' – became dominant in sociological theory and analysis and came to influence a whole generation of professionals who worked with social problems. Because of this influence, the casework approach became the main strategy used to treat a variety of social problems in very different social, economic, and political contexts, such as Western societies or the peripheral countries under their influence.

The conservatism of the order theories has been much criticized by conflict theorists, who argue that order theories fail to explain social change properly. Since order theories put the emphasis on stability and order, social change is considered a temporary event, a sort of deviance that will soon be eliminated. Following the same path, social conflict is regarded as harmful and aberrant. Social problems are therefore reduced to psychological matters limited to individual behavior. No political context is used to explain the origins of certain social conditions.

Social practices based on functionalist premises are considered, by critical standards, methods of social control that disregard history and politics,[14] procedures that conform people to their existing social conditions, no matter how appalling they are.

The critical standpoint, in contrast, understands social exclusion as part of the capitalist way of life and social conflict as part of the dynamics of social relations. Consequently, excluded people cannot 're-enter society' because they have never left it. Their main problem, actually, is being excluded from access to basic social rights, and from participation in social and political life.

The critical view stresses that there is no point in blaming the victim. In addition, this view is not limited to the reality of specific countries or particular regions of the world. Although exclusion is more apparent in the peripheral countries, in contrast to the relatively stable conditions of those at the core of the economic system, the rise of neo-liberalism, the decline of systems of social protection, and changes in contemporary work patterns have had an impact on living standards and quality of life across the whole world. These problems have to be dealt with globally, although one must admit that the peripheral countries have borne the major burden.

Actually, for occupational therapists to embrace a critical standpoint they must first understand clearly the importance of encouraging people's consciousness regarding their role as social actors. Also, occupational therapists should acknowledge the importance of helping people to empower themselves in order to take their history into their own hands.[15] However, adopting a critical standpoint implies putting this view into practice in all the spheres of action, i.e. with the users of occupational therapy services, within multi professional teams, in the education of future practitioners, and in professional associations at local, national, and international levels.

For this to happen, emancipation and empowerment need constantly to be fostered. It goes without saying that these concepts should be used within a critical framework.[16,17] Marxism sees freedom as self-determination, a result of the removal of obstacles to human emancipation.[18] Emancipation is understood here in terms of going beyond the customs and conditions of hierarchical domination. It implies the reduction of inequality, oppression, and exploitation and seeks a better redistribution of power and resources. In this way, it is a concept that follows the ethics of justice, equality, and participation. Empowerment and re-appropriation are meant to be the processes through which people experience opportunities to make decisions and contemplate new courses of action, and through which they take notice of new demands as well as new life opportunities. In doing so, these processes foster non-conformity and self-determination on a collective basis. Also, they imply a move toward making people aware of their right to have rights. Actually, this is what the concept of citizenship is all about. The struggle for the extension of human rights has to become part of daily social life and the outcome of organized collective action.

Nevertheless, occupational therapists should be careful not to overestimate the collective and political issues and deny the person who is part of the whole process. In order to favor the idea that a subject is someone who has rights, occupational therapists should first consider the existence of the previous personal experience of the subject, seeing them as a person who has dreams and desires, who makes use of free expression, who enjoys thinking, doing, and creating. As Winnicott[19] says, a subject is the outcome of the interaction of objectivity and subjectivity, i.e. someone who experiences life as the melding of subjectivity and objective observation. This interaction takes place in an intermediary area between the inner reality of the individual and the shared reality of the external world.

Consequently, subjectivity may be defined as a complex outcome of the interaction of the subject (with biological and psychological attributes) with family and the territory, under the influence of cultural bonds, social stratification, power relations, and the media.[20]

Subjectivity expresses itself through human praxis. Occupation, activity, human action, and praxis are concepts that refer to the human capacity to make an imprint in social life. Used sometimes interchangeably, these concepts are still a matter of controversy in occupational therapy. Societies (with their own cultures) and languages (with their varied senses) do not always acknowledge the term occupation as the one which best conveys the proper meaning when describing human beings' capacity to make use of intentionality and planning to transform the world.

Subjectivity is a complex interaction that brings about a singularity that can only truly exist when conformity, oppression, alienation, and a mass-produced identity are denied. This is the axis around which occupational therapy in the social field may think about itself: wherever the subject and the collective converge. In other words, occupational therapy makes possible the expression of human action entwined with the manifestation of culture and collective action.

Labor, despite its exploitations, makes possible the manifestation of the creative potential of human beings, the appropriation and the production of daily life, the fabrication of solidarity, and the exchange of labor force into income and goods necessary for life maintenance. The denial of labor as an organizing phenomenon of social relations has had a disrupting impact on society, as we know, mainly for those people excluded from its benefits. The picture gets worse when the state ceases to fulfill its function as provider of basic social policies. As a result, the lack of proper policies in education, health, housing, and relief programs aggravates even more the life conditions of people whose disadvantaged position worsens progressively.

The most familiar target of social disruption is the family, which becomes increasingly unable to cope with basic daily life functions, because it is denied its rights of access to resources and opportunities that would enable it to carry out its responsibilities of holding, developing and maintaining its members. Some institutions have severely criticized the performance of the family and have sought to substitute its functions. The dominant law and order perspective still persists in proposals that involve individualizing, criminalizing, and medicalizing social problems. However, in opposition to this, more initiatives should be taken, through wealth redistribution, the reduction of social inequality, the strengthening of social bonds, and the fostering of solidarity, to discriminate positively in favor of people, their families, and communities.

The failure of the social support network, be it the family, as the provider of basic care, the social fabric, as the promoter of solidarity, or the State, as the one responsible for basic social policies and, ideally, the safekeeper of social justice, has engendered a huge demand for social programs. Among these there are relief programs, which might guarantee subsistence and survival, protection policies, which can assist the vulnerable groups, and human rights defence programs, which can protect people from being abused either by their families, by institutions, or by the State, and can guarantee human rights.

Occupational therapists may contribute to changes in the conditions described above in many ways. They should participate in these programs and, equally, support any other initiative that aims to provide options for people to empower themselves. However, as mentioned previously, these actions should not be based on conventional medical ideas of functionality and normality, i.e. on the well-known health–disease paradigm. Likewise, these actions should not restrict themselves to a single frame of reference. Inasmuch as the problem reports to a complex situation, one should not approach it from a single point of view, a unidimensional perspective. On the contrary, different aspects should be considered.

Summing up, a critical approach should begin with a comprehension of the macrostructure that defines the ethical, social, cultural, economic, and political boundaries. This helps the development of an understanding of the reality experienced by the people involved and of the history and context of people's lives as socially constructed processes. A critical approach may also contribute to a better understanding of the ideological limits social life imposes on the transformation of the social reality and people's emancipation.

In addition, one has to consider the impact of contemporary life on the construction of self-identity and on the way reality is socially constructed. In parallel, it is important to understand social reality from the point of view of those involved. For occupational therapists, it is crucial to study and better comprehend the dynamics of day-to-day social life. The everyday life, either on a personal or a social basis, gives structure, form, and meaning to what people do, and to what people are. It is also essential to get to know how people experience their daily lives and what representations they make of their own condition. Only then can meaning be properly accessed.[21-25]

This broad sociological perspective should keep pace with an understanding of the subjective aspects of people's doings, which are manifested through the dynamics of their inner and outer reality. Also to be considered are the establishment of emotional bonds, and the study of the impact of negligence, deprivation, and abuse in the constitution of the self. Nevertheless, while threading through all these different ideas, occupational therapists need to make use of their own views on everyday life affairs, on people's doings and their lifestyle contexts. After all, the uniqueness of the subject manifests itself in daily practice determined by the cultural imprint and the means of production of a particular society.

CONSIDERATIONS FOR OCCUPATIONAL THERAPY PRACTICE IN THE SOCIAL FIELD

Occupational therapy practice in the social field, as described above, depends on the social reality as to where its efforts will be focused. The first step should be to gather information and examine local needs and the local support networks. It is important to have a clear picture of the reality in order to avoid duplication of services and waste of effort. The second step is to encourage local initiatives, whether developed by local governmental or non-governmental organizations. The idea is to work on a network basis, connecting the various initiatives and resources that local governmental and non-governmental action can provide. For this, it is important to get people in the community involved in the planning and implementation of programs. Working in proximity to people's daily lives always guarantees better results than the traditional top-down approach. Emancipation and the construction of a consciousness around the right to have rights must be the focus of community care. As already stated, broad notions of health protection and health promotion should replace previous curative models that were based on the idea of treating dysfunctional people, and sought to adjust, or rather, conform them to their deprived condition.

Organizations, social activists, and professionals, when working with excluded people, have manifold actions to undertake. Confronting social exclusion means working for social inclusiveness, i.e. for social justice. As a consequence, occupational therapists must address the problem in the wide perspective, rather than focusing exclusively on the person. The role of *social articulator* is one of the first roles occupational therapists should develop in working with vulnerable populations. This means occupational therapists should focus on building up inclusive environments. As social articulators, occupational therapists should contribute to the strengthening of family and community ties, since an inclusive approach means developing the sense of connectedness and belonging of this population. Helping people to develop ties of affection and solidarity are the first steps to be taken in overcoming the resistance to engagement manifested by those who are vulnerable. It is also essential to listen to their stories and opinions, recognize their resilience, and learn the strategies they develop to endure and survive the difficult circumstances of their lives.

Collective action should be encouraged, such as using community organizations to engage with people's primary needs, or engaging in cultural activities such as popular celebrations, bazaars, and festivals. It is important for the community to assess its own needs, and to learn how it can demand the vouchsafing of its social rights, and know where in the social network its members may find any assistance they need. Also, it is important to revive the sense of communal feeling that is provided symbolically in cultural events.

Occupational therapists should also think about other specific roles in this context. When they conceive their action they should both contribute to the preservation of social and cultural bonds, and at the same time bear in mind contemporary issues that may affect people's judgement. To begin with, it is important to consider the disadvantaged conditions that poor people face. Illiteracy, poor reading skills, and poor access to cultural and social goods are known to impoverish communication and life experience.

This is aggravated by the role played by corporations and the media, who keep producing meanings and colonizing desire, influencing people's needs, experiences, and lifestyles.[26] This leads to the consumption of the dominant ideology in an uncritical and an ahistorical way that encourages people to accept the reproduction of facts and ideas without further consideration. Such attitudes contribute to emptying out the value of occupation in its different manifestations. Expectations in life become detached from real, existing conditions. Consumerism and the worship of image are represented by the ideal of a successful being, and this becomes the object of desire in the social imagination.

The feeling of not achieving a desired lifestyle is immediately associated with the identity of a loser. The experience of being below the poverty line, i.e. not having means for life maintenance, becomes confused with the lack of satisfaction of the ever-present needs created by the consumer society.

Both converge on the identity of the outsider. Violence occupies the privileged space of speech and becomes one of the ways of communicating and mediating dissatisfaction and conflict. Violence also becomes one of the few opportunities people have to exercise power and self-determination.

Group activities are essential for favoring the development of identity and belonging that is so much needed. Occupational therapists should focus on strengthening people's perception of their abilities, a perception sometimes made fragile by low self-esteem. People should be offered opportunities to learn how to express their feelings and communicate with others in a more effective way, and to rescue or preserve their cultural roots, improving their sense of belonging. Occupational therapy action should admit the possibility of encouraging people to experiment and broaden their understanding of occupation in order to establish more satisfactory emotional and social bonds. Understanding the reasons for one's social exclusion is part of the process of feeling included. People should not believe that their life condition is their own fault. Instead, discussing the social and political life of their country gives them the opportunity to acknowledge themselves as social actors, entitled to human rights.

Depending on the seriousness of the living conditions of vulnerable people, fostering basic relationships on dual-term basis may be necessary. In these cases it is essential to get in touch with the people and institutions that are involved in these people's lives, such as family, friends, school, and street mates. The main principle for dealing with vulnerability is to look at it in comprehensive terms, learning about and respecting personal motives but always keeping in touch with the broad scenario. In the end, social problems need social answers and collective initiatives.

In conclusion, working with people who live in vulnerable conditions within a fragile social support network is a challenge, given the dramatic conditions they experience in daily life. Familial and social violence, difficulty in accessing welfare, and the harsh experiences of intolerance and social inequality are causes of mental suffering that may be expressed in a number of different ways, such as irritability, aggression, emotional frailty, apathy, rebelliousness, or indifference. People's living conditions are structurally determined and cannot be sorted out simply by therapeutic intervention. However, occupational therapists are in the privileged position of being involved in the development and implementation of projects among people who have very limited life perspectives; and we are able to strengthen and empower them, both as individuals and collectively, to search for and find more constructive and less socially violent ways of addressing their situations.

References

1. Park R. Human migration and the marginal man. AJS 1928; 33:881–893.
2. Quijano A. *Notas sobre o conceito de marginalidade social*. In: Pereira L, ed. *Populações 'marginais'*. São Paulo: Duas Cidades; 1978:11–71.
3. Escorel S. *Vidas ao léu: trajetórias de exclusão social*. Rio de Janeiro: Fiocruz; 1999.
4. Foucault M. *História da loucura na idade clássica*. São Paulo: Perspectiva; 1978.
5. Lenoir R. *Les exclus*. Paris: Seuil; 1974.

6. Buarque C. *O que é apartação: o apartheid social no Brasil.* São Paulo: Brasiliense; 1993.

7. Nascimento EP. *A exclusão social na França e no Brasil: situações (aparentemente) invertidas, resultados (quase) similares?* In: Diniz E, Lopes JSL, Prandi R, eds. *O Brasil no rastro da crise: partidos, sindicatos, movimentos sociais, Estado e cidadania no curso dos anos noventa.* São Paulo: Hucitec/Anpocs/Ipea; 1994:289–303.

8. Castel R. *As armadilhas da exclusão.* In: Belfiore-Wanderley M, Bógus L, Yazbek MC, eds. *Desigualdade e a questão social.* São Paulo: EDUC; 1999:15–48.

9. Castel R. *De l'indigence à l'exclusion, la désaffiliation: précarité du travail et vunérabilité relationelle.* In: Donzelot J, ed. *Face à l'exclusion – le modèle français.* Paris: Esprit; 1991:137–168.

10. Castel R. *Les métamorphoses de la question sociale: une chronique du salariat.* Paris: Fayard; 1995.

11. Townsend EA, Wilcock AA. Occupational justice. In: Christiansen C, Townsend E. Introduction to occupation. Thorofare, NJ: Prentice Hall; 2003:243–273.

12. Kronenberg F. Street children: being and becoming. Research study. Heerlen, The Netherlands: Hogeschool Limburg; 1999.

13. Janowitz M. Sociological theory and social control. AJS 1981; 81:82–108.

14. Cohen S, Scull A. Social control in history and sociology. In: Cohen S, Scull A, eds. Social control and the state: historical and comparative essays. Oxford: Martin Robertson; 1983.

15. Francisco B. *Terapia ocupacional.* 2nd edn. rev. Campinas: Papirus; 2001.

16. Freire P. *Pedagogia do oprimido.* 23rd edn. Rio de Janeiro: Paz e Terra; 1996.

17. Freire P. *Educação como prática de liberdade.* 22nd edn. Rio de Janeiro: Paz e Terra; 1996.

18. Bottomore T, ed. A dictionary of Marxist thought. 2nd edn. Oxford: Blackwell, 1991:172.

19. Winnicott DW. *O brincar e a realidade.* Rio de Janeiro: Imago; 1975.

20. Neto JC. *Mutações da esfera pública.* In: Baptista D, Soria M, Silveira ML, et al, eds. *Cidadania e subjetividade: novos contornos, múltiplos sujeitos.* São Paulo: Imaginário; 1997:73–121.

21. Geertz C. *A interpretação das culturas.* Rio de Janeiro: Zahar; 1978.

22. Berger P, Luckmann T. *A construção social da realidade.* 8th edn. Petropolis: Vozes; 1990.

23. Goffman E. The presentation of self in everyday life. Harmondsworth: Penguin; 1969.

24. Lefebvre H. Everyday life in the modern world. London: Allen Lane; 1971.

25. Minayo MC. *O Desafio do conhecimento: pesquisa qualitativa em saúde.* 6th edn. São Paulo, Rio de Janeiro: Hucitec–ABRASCO; 1999.

26. Steinberg S, Kincheloe J. *Cultura infantil: a construção corporativa da infância.* Rio de Janeiro: Civilização Brasileira; 2001.

Chapter **8**

The art of occupational therapy
Engaging hearts in practice

Suzanne M. Peloquin

OVERVIEW

In this chapter, I discuss the unique art of occupational therapy, both in principle and as it occurs in practice. I begin with professional artistry's association with the human spirit, its meaning in occupational therapy, and its distinctions from and confluence with science. My discussion then turns to powerful stories from earlier times as well as from more recent global arenas, to exemplify four elements of the artistry of practice: the capacity to establish rapport, the enactment of empathy, the act of getting others to know and use their potential, and the act of helping others to become participants in a community of others.

My discussion of artistry reflects an understanding of the construct drawn from my cultural context. My personal and professional development within the United States shapes my vantage point. Although I start from that admittedly provincial point, I press past its confines to show the manner in which traditional constructs such as the art of practice can expand to include a global vision. I hope that readers will conclude that discussions of the old theme of artistry have much resonance with discussions of more current themes of inclusion, political advocacy, and social justice.

INTRODUCTION

When it comes to discussions of survival and the capacity of the human spirit to overcome adversity, the artistry of occupational therapy practice seems vital to consider, both in principle and in practice. Artistry is common to most professional practices, even those better known as scientific, and it is artistry that is closely linked with a profession's expressive and compassionate functions, those associated with its spirit. There are unique dimensions to the art of occupational therapy practice, a helping profession within which persons collaborate toward an empowerment drawn from meaningful occupation. This chapter examines the unique art of occupational therapy both in principle and in practice.

THE PROFESSION'S SPIRIT

It seems important to share the meaning of my association of the art of practice with the profession's *spirit*, particularly given the theme of spirit that courses through this book. When colloquially one says, 'That person has spirit,' an image emerges of someone with a positive blend of energy, courage, and resilience. The spirit of any professional group, while similar in terms of its evocation of vitality, is more often identified as its *ethos*. Shaped from its inception by leaders who have given it life and sustained its voice, the ethos of occupational therapy is one of *caring about persons and their occupational natures*.[1] It is thus for the sake of persons and their occupational natures that practitioners manifest energy, courage, and resilience in the enactment of their art and science.

I have argued elsewhere that it is time to reclaim the profession's ethos and to *inspire* practice, i.e. to liven and animate it relative to its caring functions. We need to 'make something happen, to build something from the inside out.'[2] (p. 457) That image of edification has bearing on the work of this chapter: expanding a common view of the profession's art.

A HERITAGE OF CONCERN FOR THE HUMAN SPIRIT

The profession has a long history of concern for the human spirit, with strong associations made early by founders of the Society for the Promotion of Occupational Therapy.[3] Barton,[4] for example, cited the human spirit when characterizing occupational therapy as a making – not of a product, but of a person stronger physically, mentally, and spiritually than before. Kidner too,[5] (p. 385) spoke of a spiritual making:

> *May you realize in increasing measure the value of certain spiritual things which are the real making of life, but which we call by many common names. Kindness, humanity, decency, honor, good faith – to give these up under any circumstances whatever would be a loss greater than any defeat, or even death itself.*

More recently, I enfranchised the concept of making, suggesting that practitioners look past the details of what they do with others to see the depth of their work as a participation in the making of lives and worlds.[3] Colloquialisms reveal the deeper meaning and the creative making in such mundane activities as grooming (making oneself presentable), cooking (making a meal), or working (making a living). The human spirit manifest in such making is clear.

Many occupational therapy practitioners engage with others in such making. The expression of human spirit that can occur through occupation is well portrayed in this poem by Petersen:[6] (p. 61)

There is a shouting SPIRIT deep inside me:

TAKE CLAY, it cries,
TAKE PEN AND INK,
TAKE FLOUR AND WATER,
TAKE A SCRUB BRUSH. TAKE A YELLOW CRAYON.
TAKE ANOTHER'S HAND – AND WITH ALL THESE SAY YOU,
*   SAY LOVING.*

So much of who I am is subtly spoken in my making.

Many occupational therapy practitioners also animate the human spirit in health delivery systems. Whether they practice in hospitals or schools, prisons or community programs, halfway houses or shelters, practitioners hear comments that note their singularity in livening the settings within which they work. Through the use of empowering occupations, our therapy programs transform settings. Baum[7] (p. 515) said that we bring care to systems because we 'harness will and give the individual control through activity. That is human. That is care.' Our role in helping individuals to connect with occupations through which they can take control is both powerful and unique.

This millennium calls practitioners to extend the caring ethos of occupational therapy, its spirit, beyond traditional boundaries. The ethos needs reclamation in delivery systems that have grown depersonalized. It begs unfolding within groups untouched by its benefits. In a world grown small because of easier travel and widespread media coverage, those who are poor, disenfranchised, socially isolated, and marginally cared for beckon to us as they have never done before. When Herbert Hall[8] (p. 164) spoke of the mission of the Society for the Promotion of Occupational Therapy, he might have been noting the challenge for occupational therapy today as 'a human reclamation service touching vitally on matters of vast social and economic consequences'.

Such reclamation work, done for the sake of persons and their occupational natures, might warrant spirited actions often associated with bold artistry. These include brave-hearted acts such as those proposed by Davies;[9] engender a restlessness throughout the system; disturb complacency; and insist that rules be broken when there is good and sufficient reason. The spirit of our founders calls to our own. We can parallel today their wholehearted responses to early twentieth century needs.

THE MEANING OF THE ART OF PRACTICE

I turn now to a common understanding of the art of practice, one manifestation of our spirit. In 1972, the American Occupational Therapy Association (AOTA) described occupational therapy practice as 'the art and science of directing man's participation in selected tasks ...'.[10] (p. 204) Later, Mosey[11] analyzed the art of practice, indicating that it was not a desire to help others, not the skilled application of scientific knowledge, and not the act of being a sympathetic or systematic listener. She described the art instead, as 'the capacity to establish rapport, to empathize, and to guide others to know and make use of their potential as participants in a community.[11] (p. 4) I see the therapeutic relationship in occupational therapy as an expression of its artistry whenever it realizes an early vision of practitioners who reach for hearts as well as hands.[1,12] The vision captures well our ethos of caring.

RELATIONSHIP OF THE ART TO THE SCIENCE

Much over the years has led to a dichotomization of art and science in health care, with artistry's emotional aspects disregarded in favor of the more rational dimensions of science, a disregard that has made holistic functions more difficult. A thorough discussion of the philosophical streams and historical/political events that have contributed to this dichotomy and invited dominance by a model of technical rationality[13] goes beyond the scope of this chapter. Brief mention of the effects of such forces on practice contexts seems important, however, because some of these are dispiriting. Some squelch the profession's artistry.

Societal beliefs and professional requests that health care should be more accountable, effective, and productive have been linked with a trend toward depersonalization.[14,15] Long-neglected but sound management principles have been applauded as responsible practice. Sound methods based on evidence and best protocols drawn from knowledge have also gained respect. Unfortunately a problem-solving mentality, along with a for-profit ethos (work for the sake of financial gain and solvency), so dominate many delivery systems that practitioners deem care and relationship, constructs rich with artistry, to be at risk.[16,17,18]

The perceived dichotomy between art and science seems excessive. Science is commonly seen as a rigorous quest for knowledge and truth and is best known for its use of objectivity and analysis. Art, on the other hand, is thought to be an imaginative quest for beauty and meaning and a use of synthesis and self-expression. Emerging models within science, among them qualitative and constructivist approaches to knowing, seem more holistic and artistic. Conversely, highly technical forms of art built on mathematical calculations resemble reductionistic forms of science. Conceptual distinctions between art and science are still writ large for many, pressing them to choose one over the other. If distinct and complementary, art and science are more kindred practices than we acknowledge, and it is for this reason that occupational therapy practitioners can move fluidly between them to achieve an integrative excellence while enacting a caring ethos.

Much within the literature of the arts and sciences affirms their common features, a hardly surprising fact when one considers their common human origin. Koestler[19] noted that the finest creative work, whether in art or science, emerges when an individual is fully engaged, reasoning and feeling as a unified self. The artist Arnheim[20] argued that both productive thinking and creative action occur in art and science. Gilmour[21] noted that artists are as much concerned with truth as are scientists. Finding scientific characteristics in art's methods, Goodman[22] suggested that a picture is much like a crucial experiment that adds to human knowledge. Good science, said Bruner,[23] builds on wild metaphors that can be very personal. Good science, he said, demands passion, intuition, and imagination alongside its objective stance and rigorous analysis. Debates over the preferential value of art and science, based on their differences, fail to include the radical similarities through which both art and science can manifest the human spirit.

When occupational therapy defines itself as an art *and* a science, it characterizes itself as a practice that is both creative and productive in its work among thinking and feeling selves. The definition of practice as an integrated art and science suggests a profession constituted of people who are concerned with engaging with other people in occupation. It affirms a practitioner's commitment to a search for meaning and truth, to the disposition to be both personal and objective, to the use of imaginative synthesis and analysis, to the enfranchisement of feeling and thinking capacities. And that integrative ethos is one that reflects what Collins and Porras[24] named 'the genius of the AND'. When one hears stories of excellent occupational therapy practice, the art and the science within them seem truly confluent.[1]

The best of practitioners can only analytically tease out that which distinguishes artistry from science in what they do. In reality the two occur at once and as one. I believe that only when the best of artistry and science coexist can practitioners extend the profession's ethos more broadly into the world.

ILLUSTRATIONS OF ELEMENTS IN THE ART OF PRACTICE

Because this discussion turns more on the unique dimensions of the art of practice, I will turn now to consider more deeply those elements of the art named critical by Mosey:[11]

1. The capacity to establish rapport
2. The enactment of empathy
3. The act of guiding others to know and make use of their potential, and
4. The act of helping others to become participants in a community.

For a real understanding of the art of practice, one must consider its manifestations in reality alongside its characteristics, in principle. I have thus culled illustrative stories from the biography of Ora Ruggles, *The Healing Heart*,[12] to exemplify her artistry. Ruggles was a pioneer occupational therapist who practiced in the early part of the twentieth century; her early title was that of wartime reconstruction aide.

In many ways, conditions in the United States during the time of Ruggles's early practice reflected an unrest like that felt more globally at the start of this millennium. Hospital treatment was thought inadequate in meeting personal needs; war killed and isolated many; industrial work was thought dehumanizing; new technologies produced maiming accidents; contagious diseases could not be held in check; city leaders struggled with poverty and sanitation; large numbers of immigrants challenged social services with the volume and uniqueness of their needs.[25] The stories of a therapist practicing in such a time seem highly relevant to this discussion.

The stories of Ora Ruggles also seem apt to consider because they describe her work among individuals often marginalized because of economic status, social position, or visibly disabling and/or contagious conditions. Additionally, the stories come from a less modern time when economic frugality, low technology, and reason seasoned with intuition dominated occupational therapy practice.

Because my aim is to expand traditional views of the art of practice, I end the illustration of each aspect of the art of practice with either a late twentieth century story that exemplifies artistry practiced in a less traditional realm or with a modern story that calls for artistry in a compelling way.

The capacity to establish rapport

Ruggles found a variety of ways through which to establish rapport with her patients, as this brief collection of stories will show. The term *rapport*, coming from the French, means a relationship or connection that is characterized by harmony, accord, or affinity. One form of Ruggles's making of harmonious connections was through her use of the environment. Shortly after Ruggles arrived at the Kula Sanatorium established in Hawaii for patients with tuberculosis, she was given a stark room with tables and chairs. When a few patients first came to the room and moved close to the windows, Ruggles sensed that they craved the warmth and color of the world outside. She quickly got permission to redecorate the workshop with simple and inexpensive materials. She and her patients made colorful drapes; they painted warm murals of Chinese, Japanese, Hawaiian, and Korean scenes, reflecting well the diversity of the group. They made bright cushions for the floor. One older woman, much cheered by the changes, brought others to chat in surroundings that were much livelier than the wards below. The room conveyed a warmth that drew them to Ruggles and to occupation. Transcending the probability of contagion and any perceived differences in culture that she might have reframed as boundaries, Ruggles established rapport.

The term rapport, remember, means a relationship characterized by harmony, accord, or affinity. Such rapport often begins with a practitioner's attempts at making it, even when cultural conventions challenge such attempts. A more current story that has salience within the context of a broader establishment of rapport unfolds within Tenberken and Kronenberg's account in this book (see Ch. 3).

Sabriye Tenberken openly tells her story of being born with sight and later becoming visually impaired and ultimately blind.[26] That story earned her the trust of Tibetan parents, Chinese authorities, European funders, and her partner, with whom she started, developed, and runs the first rehabilitation and training center for the blind in Lhasa, Tibet. Within that school she encouraged the process of mutual storytelling to create a strong rapport among blind children and adults from many parts of the country.

As they learned to read and write in Braille, individuals from widely divergent places found an affinity and told their stories in such a way that they realized their own potential while helping others to shed cultural biases against blindness. Through their story about the power of stories, Tenberken and Kronenberg show us an artistry in establishing rapport, an artistry that was nested within everyday engagements.

Enactment of empathy

In its fullness, empathy calls for a practitioner's being there for another, to appreciate that person's thoughts and perspectives, and to apprehend that person's feelings.[27] Because the manner of *being with* in occupational therapy is a unique enactment of *doing with*, and because the trappings of occupation are imbedded within the helping relationship, portrayals of its enactment are important to share.

Ruggles's empathy toward a child named Ruby illustrates a turning of the soul that Katz[28] said is central to empathy in that it represents a sound grasp of the views and the feelings of another. When Ruggles met Ruby for the first time, she saw a rather unattractive 12-year-old who retaliated against the taunts of other children by destroying their work. Hoping to understand better this child's interests, Ruggles asked Ruby if she might like sewing. The child said, 'Why? So I can grow up and be an old maid and sit at home with my sewing? Is that what you do?'[12] (p. 215) Although Ruggles's inner urge was to feel anger, she checked that impulse and thought, 'This girl dislikes people because she can see that they dislike her. I must alter my attitude. I must change my hate to love. I must show Ruby that I love her.'[12] (p. 215) This turning of soul pressed Ruggles to ask what Ruby hoped to be when she grew up. In a small voice, Ruby said that she hoped to work in a beauty parlor. As Ruggles saw this child anew in light of her yearning for beauty, she softened. She taught Ruby to shampoo and set her hair, and she arranged for her to spend time in a beauty shop. Ruggles noticed a change over time. As Ruby connected with others, her inner beauty emerged. The turning of soul that had happened first in Ruggles led to a soul turning in Ruby.

A salient contemporary story that illustrates such a turning of soul is present within Fujimoto and Iwama's discussion in Chapter 26. Within this discussion of occupational injustices against children with severe disabilities in Japanese society, the stories of Satoko, Ayumi, and Yukimi are poignant calls for empathy. Despite what Fujimoto and Iwama name a valuable interdependence in Japanese culture, they also note a cultural press for sameness so strong that children with unique needs are often excluded. Many occupations are withheld because inclusion might warrant efforts at accommodating one child's needs that transcend those made on behalf of the typical child.

Fujimoto and Iwama share the image of a father having to be present and tending to the needs of his child during every moment of the school day. They tell of a child being made to sit at poolside in the hot sun watching her friends swim, denied her great joy of swimming because of extra preparations associated with her disability. They tell of children dying of despondency from such exclusion. These stories call for the soul turning of empathy. Fujimoto and Iwama ask all practitioners to turn to those who are marginalized and to extend to them the principles of social justice. These writers call to the empathy that is part of our artistry. They call each of us to generate restlessness within systems grown either uncaring or complacent.

Guiding others to know and make use of their potential

The art of occupational therapy is not a coercive process of doing *to* another but more of a collaborative and guiding process of doing *with*. That collaboration has as one primary aim an individual's recognition and realization of personal potential. The story of Kilgore illustrates the artistry of this process quite well. Kilgore was a soldier who worried Ruggles because he was often angry and impulsive. Ruggles spoke to a physician who told Ruggles that Kilgore, once a cowboy, was filled with rage and revulsion over the wartime brutality in which he had engaged. Ruggles thought about Kilgore and then consulted with the foreman of the hospital blacksmith shop. She found Kilgore and showed him a design for spurs, asking if he would help her start a metalwork class; he agreed. Within the hour he was in the shop. He mastered the work quickly, and his drinking, gambling, and angry outbursts soon stopped.

After discharge, Kilgore started an ironwork plant that grew to be the largest in the Southwest. He wrote this to Ora Ruggles, years later:[12] (p. 91)

> *I've been doing a lot of thinking lately Ruggie. It started out last week when some of the boys around town asked me to run for mayor. It makes me realize again, Ruggie, how much I owe you. I wonder what the boys who asked me to run for mayor would think if they knew an army doctor once scribbled on my medical record, 'This man is a menace to society.'*

In Chapter 23 Ramugondo tells a salient contemporary story about the efforts of occupational therapy practitioners who guided impoverished mothers of children with human immunodeficiency virus (HIV) and/or acquired immunodeficiency syndrome (AIDS) to know and use their potential to play with their children. As an occupational component of a support group, these mothers also made playthings. The toys were sold to a foundation that supplied them to children's homes in other impoverished regions.

This story captures the imaginative artistry of occupational therapy. How fine that 'child's play' could extend from one caring circle to others who also found and used its potential. These mothers, empowered by their own capacity, engaged in a creative act that empowered others.

Guiding others toward participation in a community

Always attentive to the various groups within which her patients sought to belong and participate, Ruggles structured activities to facilitate that participation. The story of Leo illustrates this artistry on several levels. Poverty troubled many patients at Olive View Sanatorium, especially those with families. Ruggles ran a shop in the hospital where patients sold their crafts to defray expenses. After Leo arrived, he was sent to bed with a high fever. He was restless and troubled because he had a wife and four children to support. His small farm was mortgaged, and his family needed $15.25 a month to keep the farm. Leo's physician thought him too sick with a high temperature to work with Ruggles. Although she accepted that judgement initially, Ruggles spoke once again to the doctor as Leo's condition worsened. She was convinced that Leo's deterioration was more mental than physical, so she proposed to work with Leo at his bedside but to stop if his temperature rose.

Ruggles told Leo that he could earn $20 a month selling leatherwork. Although his first efforts were crude, he soon produced fine items. His first earnings amounted to $22.65 and the physician's pronouncement that he was well enough to work outside the ward. Leo became an assistant to Ruggles, helping other patients as soon as he secured his $15.25. Ruggles's work was credited with saving his farm, his pride, and his life. His leatherwork allowed him to participate in the support of his family and in a helping process among peers in the hospital.

Thibeault[29] describes a more recent occupational therapy venture in Sierra Leone among African bush wives. The project exemplifies an artful guidance of others toward participation in a community. Abducted in their pre-school years and taken into slavery by rebel troops, these young bush wives had been raped repeatedly. After a period of psychosocial healing, the women were guided to consider vocational possibilities.

The women decided to establish a fish-salting cooperative. They were challenged by the granting agency, which recommended smoking the fish instead, to produce a more marketable item. Aware of the limits already imposed on their community by deforestation, the women were guided to negotiate successfully their more implementable and environmentally sensitive choice – salting fish. The women's participation in a community of wage earners was one level of their engagement, but a deeper level of belonging occurred in their sensitive accommodation of their needs to the larger needs of their community. The therapeutic guidance that supported such negotiation was real artistry.

SUSTAINING THE ART OF PRACTICE: RECLAIMING THE VISION

Clearly the art of practice, as illustrated in all of these stories, requires a commitment to the occupational therapy ethos and a courage, energy, and resilience for meeting the commitment. One source of the necessary inspiration for those hoping to emulate such practice is the vision of 'reaching for heart as well as hands,' that appeared early in the biography of Ora Ruggles and reappeared at its end.[12] On the first occasion, this vision structured one of the many stories that make the book compelling. Here is the story. During the First World War and thus early in her career, Ruggles was unusually quiet as she entered the army barracks at Fort McPherson. Her friends asked what she was thinking. She said that she had made a great discovery, one that she could not get over because it was so simple yet so effective. When pressed to share, she said, 'It is not enough to give a patient something to do with his hands. You must reach for the heart as well as the hands. It's the heart that really does the healing.' After several silent moments, a colleague said, 'That is a tremendous discovery, Ruggie. I think we'll all benefit from it.'[12] (p. 69)

Her colleagues were correct, and the wisdom of this early vision resonates well among practitioners today who hold the art of practice dear. Most who consider this early vision can 'see' a vivid affirmation of caring. The phrase 'reaching for hearts' depicts at least a practitioner's earnest striving to care. And, certainly, images of the heart are so widely used as icons denoting love that their meaning is certain. The phrase 'reaching for hands' depicts a practitioner's earnest striving for competence. The vision also captures a commitment to the art and science of practice. Practitioners so inspired may carry that same vision past traditional practice realms.

While writing this chapter, I discovered the work of practitioners world-wide who have led bold initiatives for the sake of persons and their occupational natures. Anne Lang-Etienne, for example, carried into the late twentieth century a global vision of reaching for hearts and hands. Thibeault[29] (p. 197) described Lang-Etienne as 'a spirit that moved and shaped a generation of occupational therapists.' Lang-Etienne's dream, 'a penetrating vision that soared beyond convention,' affirms the profession's artistry. Listen to Thibeault, who reframed Anne's dissidence so that we can see its artistry:

> *Anne dreamed of a dissident profession that would resist social pressure and challenge commonly held views. She dreamt of a profession dedicated not only to the functional but to the essential. Through focusing more on mindfulness and less on conformity, she hoped for renewed awareness and maturity that would revitalize our collective engagement.... She envisioned the contribution of occupational therapy to socially or environmentally devastated communities with collective healing as our aim.... She was convinced that the values intrinsic to occupational therapy, if expressed more forcefully in the public sphere, could provide appropriate solutions to some pervasive ills.[29] (pp. 199–201)*

Ora Ruggles and Anne Lang-Etienne both heard a call to reach past the confines of common practice with energy, compassion, and resilience; they helped others to make new lives and worlds for themselves. They invited us to also move beyond conventional boundaries to meet the spirits of survivors. The artistry in such ventures consists of finding bold ways to establish rapport, to engage empathically, and to guide others to use their potential within communities. Such outward reaching is a building of the profession, from the inside out. And it is 'a human reclamation service touching vitally on matters of vast social and economic consequence.'[8] (p. 164)

References

1. Peloquin SM. Reclaiming the vision of reaching for heart as well as hands. Am J Occup Ther 2002; 56(5):517–525.
2. Peloquin SM. Now that we have managed care, shall we inspire it? Am J Occup Ther 1996; 50(6):455–459.
3. Peloquin SM. The spiritual depth of occupation: making worlds and making lives. Am J Occup Ther 1997; 51(3):167–168.
4. Barton GE. 1920. What occupational therapy may mean to nursing. Trained Nurse and Hospital Review 64:304–310.

5. Kidner TB. Address to graduates. Arch Occup Ther 1929; 8:379–385.

6. Petersen J. A book of yes. Niles, IL: Argus; 1976.

7. Baum CM. Eleanor Clarke Slagle lecture – Occupational therapists put care in the health system. Am J Occup Ther 1980; 34:505–516.

8. Hall HJ. Editorial – American Occupational Therapy Association. Arch Occup Ther 1922; 1:163–165.

9. Davies GK. Teaching and learning. What are the questions? Teaching Education 1991; 4(1):57–61.

10. American Occupational Therapy Council on Standards. Occupational therapy; its definition and functions. Am J Occup Ther 1972; 26:204–205.

11. Mosey AC. Occupational therapy: configuration of a profession. New York: Raven; 1981.

12. Carlova J, Ruggles O. The healing heart. New York: Julian Messner; 1946.

13. Schön DA. The reflective practitioner: How professionals think in action. New York: Basic Books; 1983.

14. Breines E. The end of OT? We have a choice. Adv for Occup Ther Pract 1999; 15(9):6.

15. Peloquin SM. The depersonalization of patients. Am J Occup Ther 1993; 47:830–837.

16. Howard BH. How high do we jump? The effect of reimbursement on occupational therapy. Am J Occup Ther 1991; 45:875–881.

17. Joe B, Hettinger J. Hand therapy in the grip of managed care. OT Week 1995, July 27; 9(30):18–20.

18. Kerr T. Managed care blues. Adv for Occ Ther Pract 1999, May 3; 15(9):11, 61.

19. Koestler A. The act of creation. New York: Macmillan; 1964.

20. Arnheim R. Visual thinking. Berkeley: University of California Press; 1969.

21. Gilmour J. Picturing the world. Albany: State University of New York Press; 1986.

22. Goodman N. Languages of art: an approach to a theory of symbols. Indianapolis: Hackett; 1976.

23. Bruner J. Actual minds, possible worlds. Cambridge: Harvard University Press; 1986.

24. Collins JC, Porras J. Built to last: successful habits of visionary companies. New York: Harper Collins; 1994.

25. Peloquin SM. Occupational therapy service: individual and collective understanding of the founders, part 1. Am J Occup Ther 1991; 45(4):352–359.

26. Tenberken S. My path leads to Tibet: the inspiring story of how one young blind woman brought hope to the blind children of Tibet. New York: Arcade; 2003.

27. Peloquin SM. The fullness of empathy: reflections and illustrations. Am J Occup Ther 1995; 49(1):24–31.

28. Katz RL. Empathy: its nature and uses. London: Free Press of Glencoe; 1963.

29. Thibeault R. In praise of dissidence: Anne Lang-Etienne. Can J Occup Ther 2002; 69(4):197–203.

Chapter **9**

A participatory occupational justice framework
Population-based processes of practice

Elizabeth Townsend, Gail Whiteford

OVERVIEW

Proposed in this chapter is a participatory occupational justice framework for use with populations who are restricted from participation in everyday life. The framework is applicable to economically wealthy as well as poor nations. The chapter offers literature, processes, and reflective questions for population-based practice in occupational therapy and other professions. Three related concepts provide the cornerstones of the chapter: occupation, client-centered enabling, and justice. The authors, from Canada and Australia, believe that justice is an implicit social vision in occupational therapy. Six processes are proposed that invite thoughtful experimentation rather than the use of prescriptive techniques. The participatory framework emphasizes population and specific client participation throughout. The significance of this chapter is its emphasis on a justice of inclusion in ordinary, daily life – in situations that are right in front of our eyes. The processes offered are a practical means of identifying and addressing injustices; not through rhetoric, but by determining what people need and want to do. Analyses of occupational injustices will differ across the globe, yet they are available for us all to see through our cultural lenses on real, daily life.

INTRODUCTION

Canada and Australia are two of the world's wealthiest nations. As citizens of these two nations, we propose a participatory occupational justice framework for use wherever populations of certain ability/disability, age, social class, or other features are excluded from opportunities to be meaningfully occupied. The significance of this chapter is its synthesis of vision, theory, and practice grounded in justice. We do not offer a single definition of occupational justice, given that occupations and justice are culturally defined concepts that will differ world-wide. Instead, to advance

Figure 9.1 Three pillars of occupational therapy knowledge.

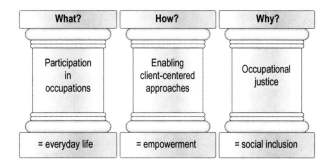

the dialogue on occupational justice,[1] we offer literature, processes, and reflective questions for population-based practice. The six processes of practice proposed in this chapter are not new in themselves – they have been field tested for centuries, if one considers the immense amount of work by populations to develop more inclusive participation in the occupations typical of places ranging from schools and workplaces to health services and homes.

As illustrated in Figure 9.1, to highlight *what* concerns us, we will focus on participation in the occupations of daily life. To explain *how* client-centered occupational therapy works with populations, we will propose personal and systems-enabling approaches. To consider *why* occupational therapists are enabling participation in occupations, we will raise questions about justice. If occupation, enabling, and justice are pillars of occupational therapy knowledge, justice is the pillar that names an invisible social vision. It is likely that every occupational therapy practice includes elements of the six processes, and likely that occupational justice could be made more explicit by using the six proposed processes to:

1. focus on occupations, client-centered enabling, and justice
2. draw on social critique and program development
3. adapt the stages and actions of the Canadian Occupational Performance Process (OPP)[2,3] and
4. incorporate concepts of participation restrictions in the World Health Organization's *International Classification of Functioning* (ICF), *disability and health.*[4]

Orienting language and ideas

In English or translated into other languages, the profession's *occupational* perspective would typically be understood narrowly as pertaining to work,[5] or aggressively as pertaining to military occupation. We, the authors of this chapter, join those who take a radical, political stance on occupation. We allocate value and respect to a broad view of occupations, not confined to economically defined categories.[2,6–11]

Occupational therapists' *enabling* perspective orients us to participatory, empowerment-oriented approaches – what the profession describes as client-centered practice.[12–15] The emphasis is on collaborating, listening, animating, facilitating, coaching, enabling, developing, partnering and other empowerment-directed processes for working *with* individuals and populations.[16–18] Enabling encompasses an array of holistic, contextual, participatory practices. These are dialectically opposite to paternalistic, reductionistic, standardized, care-giving practices that do things *to* or *for* others without their participation and decision making. In the sense that enabling processes favor participation over autocratic, hierarchical relationships, an enabling perspective is ideological and politically aligned with notions of participatory citizenship. There are acknowledged tensions in using enabling, client-centered approaches in hierarchical systems.[17,19–21] Nevertheless, enabling approaches compel professionals to make practice relevant, effective, and publicly accountable.

Linking occupation and justice generates the *occupational justice* perspective first described by Wilcock and Townsend.[22] Occupational justice speaks to issues of difference and social inclusion, taking individual and group differences in occupational participation into account.[22,23] As Fujimoto says, occupational injustices are right in front of our eyes (H Fujimoto, personal communication). The authors' conception of occupational justice is congruent with the ICF[4] concept of participation restrictions. In naming occupational justice as a pillar of occupational therapy knowledge, the profession extends the ICF meaning of participation restriction. Occupational injustices exist when, for example, participation is barred, confined, segregated, prohibited, undeveloped, disrupted, alienated, marginalized, exploited, or otherwise devalued. In Chapter 6 Kronenberg and Pollard describe these injustices as occupational apartheid.[24] Townsend and Wilcock have used the term occupational apartheid with reference to times and places where occupations are classified, paid, valued, and life enhancing for some, while in the same times and places occupations are taken for granted, exploited, and trivialized for others.[1]

Considering power and the political nature of professional practice

The more we, as authors, have explored what a participatory occupational justice framework means, the more we have sought out research on how power, privilege, and political action work in professions. In reflecting on power, we will raise questions about negotiating power when professionals engage in the processes of structuring programs, as well as in the processes of implementing and evaluating them. We will use literature on the politics of power.[25–30] In considering a justice of difference and social inclusion in this chapter, our conception of occupational justice is aligned with postmodernism's interests in diversity and its critiques of universal theories.[31,32]

Despite the commercial origin of the word client, we use this term to link the work of enabling occupational justice to occupational therapists' 'client-centered practice'.[12–15] In practice, occupational therapists may want to refer to active participants in programs by the names participants want to use, such as residents, workers, community members and so on. Client-centered practice is certainly problematic given managerial priorities and hierarchical services characterized by professional dominance.[21,33,34] Our approach emphasizes the ideal of client-centered practice – that is, practice where day-by-day actions are driven by a vision of changing systems to serve better those who experience occupational injustices.

A PARTICIPATORY OCCUPATIONAL JUSTICE FRAMEWORK

The proposed participatory occupational justice framework reflects occupational therapists' ongoing naming and framing of practice,[35] and is subject to our own as well as others' critiques. The framework (see Figure 9.2) is depicted as six non-linear, interrelated processes. Four of the processes address the environment and social change through attention to resources, naming of population injustices, and negotiation with client organizations or advocates on a justice framework and the program. Two processes are condensed from the Canadian OPP for working with individual clients, based on the Canadian Model of Occupational Performance (CMOP),[2,3] and described more fully in Chapter 15 by Egan and Townsend. Here, we describe a single process to identify client-specific occupational performance strengths, resources and challenges that encompasses the OPP stages one, three, four, and seven and involves evaluation before, during, and after client-specific services. The rationale for integrating these OPP stages is that evaluations over various stages flow together in real practice, and may be funded separately from planning or intervention. The process to 'plan, implement and evaluate client-specific services' synthesizes OPP stages five to seven, to identify targeted outcomes and plan services, to implement programs using occupations as the medium of occupational therapy, and to evaluate client-specific services. In summarizing each process, below and in Table 9.1, we offer illustrations from Whiteford's work with persons in a refugee camp in Australia, and Townsend's work with persons with severe, persistent mental illness in Canada.

Analyze and coordinate resources

The process of analyzing and coordinating resources requires self-reflection as well as empirical analysis of human and financial resources. Resources may be analyzed before or after other processes in the proposed occupational justice framework. We name resources in a separate process to stretch our awareness beyond the individual, group, family, or local community conditions typically identified for specific clients in the Canadian OPP.[2,3] As illustrated in Table 9.1, after determining the population of concern, this process involves asking questions such as: 'What forum, method,

Figure 9.2 Occupational justice processes.

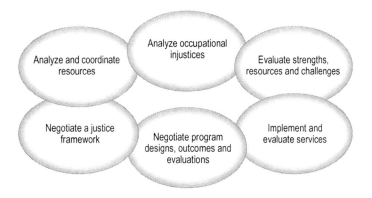

Table 9.1   A participatory occupational justice framework

Processes of practice (Non-linear, interrelated)	Participatory, population-based practice
Analyze and coordinate resources (OPP Stage 4 adapted to structure program/service[a])	● What population(s) is of central concern? ● What forum, method, or database will identify potential population, non-professional, and professional resources? ● What coordination is possible (e.g. collaboration, hierarchy, managed, informal, consensus, majority, leadership and participation modes)? ● What government, corporate, or philanthropic financial resources are available? ● As a human resource, what can I offer? What can I learn? ● How will resources be documented and evaluated?
Negotiate a justice framework (OPP Stage 2 adapted to structure program/service)	● What conflicting and congruent beliefs, values, cultural, and power issues need attention? ● What education, mediation, or arrangements are needed to show respect for the worth, dignity, and rights of all involved?
Analyze occupational injustices[b] (OPP Stage 1 adapted to structure program/service)	● How does the population experience justice or injustice when they participate in occupations? ● What occupational performance and/or environmental issues impact collective experiences of (in)justice? ● What qualitative, quantitative and analytic data exist? ● What qualitative, quantitative, and critical appraisal methods are available to identify and document occupational injustice issues?
Negotiate program designs, outcomes and evaluations[c] (OPP Stages 5 & 7 adapted to structure program/service)	● What occupational justice outcomes will be targeted? ● What programs/services are needed and possible – goals, objectives, locations, times, action-based, occupational, participatory approaches, funding options? ● What education on occupational injustices is needed for the population, for non-professionals, and for professionals? ● Who will advocate for human and financial resources? ● What evaluation and documentation is needed to demonstrate program/service accountability to the population, to professionals, and to funders?
Evaluate client-specific strengths, resources, and challenges[d] (OPP Stages 1, 3, & 4 adapted for client-specific evaluation)	● What qualitative, quantitative, and critical analysis methods are available? What education is needed? ● What is the profile of client-specific occupational justice issues, strengths and resources? ● What client-specific occupational performance, spiritual, and environmental issues, strengths, resources and challenges need top priority? ● How will strengths, resources, and challenges be documented for comparison pre, during and post services?
Plan, implement and evaluate client-specific services (OPP Stages 2, 5, 6 & 7 adapted)	● What client-specific services would target the greatest forces that collectively limit occupational justice, while also addressing client-specific issues? ● What is the most relevant, effective and efficient plan and evaluation strategy for client-specific goals and objectives? ● How is the client involved in occupations as the participatory medium of change? ● What enabling approaches address client empowerment? ● How will the impact of services be monitored throughout from client, professional, management, and other perspectives?

[a] Processes of practice adapted from the Canadian Occupational Performance Process (OPP), CAOT, 1997, 2002;[2] and Fearing & Clark, 2001.[3]

[b] Occupational justice issues may be about accessibility, choice, classification, identity, habits, meaning, opportunities, rituals, support, performance, potential, resources, and more. From an occupational perspective, justice would be about enabling or limiting participation in occupations with an impact on health and citizen empowerment.

[c] A participatory design and evaluation could include qualitative methods such as client narratives, and self-reflection, as well as quantitative methods. In a participatory, occupational justice framework, surveys and measures would be completed by educating communities/ populations or individuals to self-monitor their performance, engage in peer evaluation, or otherwise participate in gathering data. Non-professional as well as professional perspectives would be incorporated into the design and evaluation.

[d] The designated client or representatives may participate through verbal interaction, written documents, third party reports, non-verbal expression in photographs and other objects, talking circles, focus groups, etc.

or database will identify potential population, non-professional, and professional resources?'

Using the example of occupational therapy as a human resource, we might start by asking: 'What is occupational therapy's contribution as a human resource? What do occupational therapists need to learn and what do we have the opportunity to learn in population-based practice that makes occupational justice an explicit foundation of occupational therapy? How might we coordinate our work with efforts by the population, lay persons, governments, businesses, and other professionals?'

Occupational therapy is an extremely scarce labor force. Starting in the nineteenth century, the professionalization of this work located occupational therapists, the vast majority of whom are women in Canada and Australia, in a subordinate position within the medical hierarchy and medical funding.[36–39] Table 9.2 provides the most recent World Federation

Table 9.2 Numbers of occupational therapists (OTs) who are members of national associations

Country	Number of OTs	Country	Number of OTs
Argentina	171[a]	Luxembourg	76
Australia	3500	Malaysia	na
Austria	765	Malta	35
Bangladesh	na	Mauritius	na
Belgium	725[a]	Mexico	na
Bermuda	20	Namibia	na
Brazil	890	Netherlands	3312[a]
Canada	7050[a]	New Zealand	903[a]
Caribbean	na	Nigeria	na
Chile	250	Norway	2734[a]
Columbia	na	Pakistan	na
Cyprus	na	Philippines	246[a]
Czech Republic	na	Portugal	ca 250
Denmark	6198[a]	Republic of Korea	505[a]
Greece	231[a]	Singapore	158[a]
Finland	1424[a]	Slovenia	na
France	978[a]	South Africa	1287[a]
Germany	ca 11 000	Spain	540
Hong Kong	ca 800	Sri Lanka	18
Iceland	134[a]	Sweden	9302[a]
India	1912[a]	Switzerland	1718[a]
Indonesia	na	ROC (Taiwan)	744[a]
Ireland	na	Tanzania	na
Israel	1000	Uganda	na
Italy	110[a]	UK	14 482
Japan	20 226[a]	USA	35 692[a]
Jordan	na	Venezuela	500
Kenya	260[a]	Zimbabwe	na
Latvia	na		

[a] 2004 statistics.
na = not available.
ca = approximate numbers.
Source: World Federation of Occupational Therapists (WFOT) database (2004), email correspondence with WFOT Executive 28 January 2004, and 10 March 2004. Presented are numbers of members of the national occupational therapy associations where the WFOT recognizes that occupational therapy education programs meet WFOT minimum national standards.

of Occupational Therapists' database on the world supply of occupational therapists. Using these and population data, one can compare ratios of occupational therapists per 100 000 population in 2000. While today's figures may be higher, it is clear that occupational therapy remains a numerically small profession, and ratios, and thus access to occupational therapy services, vary enormously around the world.

Occupational therapists work on the profound but mundane occupations of real life. Moreover, we aim to use collaborative, enabling approaches with populations who may have even less power than ourselves.[40–44] This situation poses a major human resource challenge for the profession to combine leadership and partnership models that give us identity, visibility, and a voice, with collaborative models for enabling others' empowerment to develop their own identity, visibility, and voice. In Box 9.1 we describe our experiences, as academic occupational therapists, of analyzing occupational therapy resources for developing student learning and research contributions.

Negotiate a justice framework

As Table 9.3 summarizes, the concept of occupational justice expresses ethical, moral, and civic concerns that participation in daily life should contribute to rather than undermine health, empowerment, and quality of life. The contrast is made here with social justice concerns. Typically, social justice addresses processes of dispute resolution, the distribution of goods and services, the restoration of property, or punishment for acts that transgress social norms. Contested in occupational justice are differing social and economic values for occupations, and the implementation of social inclusion.

Box 9.1   Analyze resources

Whiteford

I interview people who have been defined as refugees in order to understand their experiences. To expose both the profession and the refugees to possible collaborations, I use my academic position to introduce students to local refugee populations in Australia, and I have published analyses of occupational deprivation. The occupational therapy labor force available for expanding on this work with refugee populations in and beyond Australia is unknown, and few people even consider the place of occupational therapy in working with people living in refugee camps. Financial resources are available to enterprising occupational therapists. I need to take care to build occupational therapy education and research with persons in refugee camps into the curriculum. There is huge world interest in understanding how to control or dismantle refugee camps, but no occupational critique of what these camps do to entire populations who will require time and resources to heal.

Townsend

I have built on my community mental health clinic experience through ethnographic research with day and community mental health programs. The occupational therapy labor force available for working with populations with severe, persistent mental illnesses has declined since the beginning of the twentieth century to less than 20% of occupational therapists in Canada. From my academic standpoint, I need to take care that the occupational therapy curriculum includes academic and fieldwork experiences in mental health teams in community as well as hospital settings. I need to ensure that students experience teams that are broader than just psychiatric professionals, and that include consumer, family, community, management, fundraising, and professional members. Financial resources appear to welcome occupational therapists who focus on real life occupational issues, but we need to develop skills in social critique and in the qualitative as well as quantitative evaluation of occupational opportunities and barriers for this population.

Table 9.3   Concepts of justice

	Social: procedural	Social: distributive	Social: restorative	Occupational: difference
Concerns	Processes of dispute resolution	Having or acquisition	Repair or renewal	Health, empowerment, and quality of life
Contested terrain	Equality of voice, unequal human and financial resources	Measurement and comparison of assets and deficiencies of social groups	Credibility of perpetrators and victims, measurement of damage and fair compensation of goods or rights	Social versus economic value of occupations, competing needs for opportunities and resources
Aims	Equal voice and procedural rights	Equal rights to and equal responsibility for goods, services, privileges	Restoration of perpetrators, restitution to victims	Enablement of different opportunities and resources, taking differences into account in social structures
Issues of power	Individual defendants and prosecutors to be heard without bias	All social groups to have equal advantages for participation in daily life	Individual defendants to be exonerated, individual or class victims to be compensated	Different opportunities and resources to enable full citizen participation by all individuals, families and social groups
Actions for justice	Equal procedural processes	Equal distribution or allocation	Confession of guilt, compensation to victims	Enablement of difference for social inclusion

Negotiation is an important process for discovering commonalities and differences in participants' implicit or explicit justice frameworks. In this politically sensitive process, the negotiation hinges on naming potential areas of conflict and cooperation. Occupational therapists might help in negotiating a justice framework by asking open-ended questions (see Table 9.1), such as: 'What are the beliefs, values, frameworks, contexts, and power issues in the situation?'

To negotiate a framework for justice, one would first need to understand the diverse views of occupation or daily life and justice that prevail amongst the various human resources who are prepared to act on an injustice. A population-based practice would link global visions of justice[45-51] with local, culturally-attuned frameworks that address human, financial, geographic, political, and other forces that create inequitable participation restrictions. Occupational therapists' biomechanical, psychosocial, neurodevelopmental, cognitive–perceptual, and other professional frames of reference would be blended with the frameworks of beliefs and values of the population. Justice or other professional frameworks should not be imposed or used implicitly without negotiation on how to use them with the population and with others involved in the team. The negotiation is an ongoing process of relationship building, as we discuss in Box 9.2.

Analyze occupational injustices

A population-based practice would analyze social and economic determinants of occupation, with a focus on the environment.[52-54] Internationally, the environment is targeted in naming participation restrictions as the

---

Box 9.2 Negotiate a justice framework

Whiteford

I developed a relationship with leaders and others in the camp through my interviews. The aim was to discover their beliefs and values about life and justice. My method was to observe people respectfully, and invite them to tell stories about the routines, values, service approaches, and economics of camp life. I learned that they value and believe in justice as a daily experience, their emphasis being on the occupations that they pictured would enhance child development, create a cleaner, more stable home life, and provide opportunities for doing something productive, ideally with pay. They wanted to shape new occupational opportunities as participants, not as dependents on a foreign government. As an interviewer, my aim was to negotiate a justice framework with these people by giving voice to their stories.

Townsend

After a 10-year research relationship, I wanted to publish a paper that would give voice to consumers involved in participatory action research (PAR) in the Mental Health Action Research Connection (MHARC). My aim was to display respect while offering experience in the world of professional research. I needed to work within MHARC's justice framework, accepting that persons with a persistent, severe mental illness need opportunities to participate in economically and socially valued occupations, such as research. My professional framework to enable skill acquisition and social critique needed to be explicit and adapted to the MHARC framework.

---

category most related to social handicap in the ICF,[4] or to social determinants in literature on population health.[55]

Critical questions for discussion (see Table 9.1) are, for example: 'How does the population experience justice or injustice when they participate in occupations? What injustices occur when people are alienated from what they do, or are so imbalanced that they have too much or too little to do? What injustices are perpetrated through deprivation of occupations, or persistent dependence in daily life occupations? What injustices are promoted when some people live a life that they view as useless, either from an individualistic perspective, or from a communal perspective. If a community does not value, for instance, the occupational participation of someone with a disability, how can that person belong fully as a citizen? Is there an occupational apartheid, with some community members participating in the occupations they define as meaningful or useful, while others in the same geographic, social, cultural, and political context lack such opportunities?'

Social indicators, sometimes identified through environmental scans, provide important data to analyze population-based occupational injustices as a background for considering the client-specific issues described below. The first step is to determine boundaries in order to delimit the amount of data to be synthesized in examining social indicators. Here, data are limited to Canada and Australia, and further limited to objectifying statistics on homelessness, employment, and disability. To understand fully whether or not these data represent injustices, one would need to expand quantitative and qualitative data collection, for instance by gathering narratives about participation in occupations, as we illustrate in Box 9.3.

Box 9.3 Analyze occupational injustices

Whiteford

My interviews with persons living in refugee camps prompted me to seek data on homelessness, disability, and employment. The refugees are homeless and largely unemployed, having left their homes to live in confined spaces as displaced persons in an unfamiliar environment. Statistics on homelessness and unemployment tell us the number of people with no fixed address or registered employment. Some refugees may have medically diagnosed physical, mental, or learning disabilities, but many more than these seem to live a life of disability in that they are severely restricted from participating in a variety of occupations in and beyond the refugee camp. These daily life struggles with homelessness, unemployment, and medical or non-medical disabilities are excluded from national census data. My interviews are, thus, an academic means of enabling persons who live as refugees to give voice to the meanings of homelessness, unemployment, and disability for those who have left a homeland and remain cloistered in a new land.[56,57] In the following vignette, M, a refugee and sole parent, talked to me about the occupational challenges and injustices of resettlement:

What I felt was that although they gave me some volunteer people to look after me and help me out, it wasn't necessary to have this many people around and most of the ladies were older than me and I found their way of thinking different to mine. They had different routines than what I had and I felt that they didn't really match, they were used to a different way of life. It would have been better if there was one family looking after another family; as it was in my case, there were older ladies; one came to my place and she would sit down for 3 or 4 hours but we couldn't communicate, we couldn't talk. Then someone else would come with something else.... The trouble was we had to walk a long distance from the flat to the school and because I was also studying [English] I'd sit until the older girl came home from school, but then maybe the little one would go to sleep – there was no routine. It would be nice to have somebody like a family member that I could leave the children with when maybe I could find a part time job, some sort of work, though now they're too young to be left as well ... it's totally different at home ... what would be good would be to have the conditions we live in here with the child rearing practices we have at home. It's different there. You know there could be ten villages and you know people from the tenth village and when somebody comes for a visit everybody knows them and it's like a big family ... the neighborhoods were a lot safer back home, you didn't have to walk everywhere with your kids, the people in the neighborhood know each other and help each other, but here you don't ... everybody needs friends and family around and it's particularly hard here in holiday time and the kids are home and its difficult because there's no family to go to, no family circle.

Townsend

My ethnographic studies with people with severe, persistent mental illnesses required me to consider their experiences in relation to common assumptions about homelessness, unemployment, and disability, and the statistics on such experiences. General data provide a starting place for observing and interviewing people about how they fit or do not fit statistics. I have focused my energies on publishing as an academic method of enabling people living with a severe, persistent mental illness to be heard publicly, for example in a shared publication with a member of the Mental Health Action Research Connection (MHARC).[21] To critique the statistics (to know what they actually represent and leave out), I have also consulted the stories of people living with a mental illness.[20,58] The story of Meg in *I Always Wanted to be a Tap Dancer*[59] (a collection of women with disabilities talking about their lives) tells about the injustices Meg experienced in being denied her occupational dream of being a tap-dancer:

Having once had a mental illness, everything you do in the future becomes suspect. I sat through a committee meeting where the issue of mature age people returning to study was being debated. One committee member spoke scathingly about 'fruitcakes' who come to study as therapy.... I never really decided to make the choice to be open about my experiences, they are part of me and my qualifications just as much as my university qualifications and my employment experience. When I applied for my position ... I was asked: Why did I start the Manic Depressive self help group ... so I told them. I am grateful for the tolerance and understanding that has been extended to me in my job. But why should I be grateful? ... I do my job well, yet I am always conscious of needing to prove that I am as good as anyone else or that I have to make up for the years I lost to illness, and most importantly, never appearing to be mad or high or nervous in any way.[59] (p. 112)

To analyze occupational injustices, one combines micro, meso, and macro data on occupational participation. Micro data (measurements, stories, documents) on individual or group occupational performance can be used with meso data on community, family, or friendship (reports, stories, etc.), and with macro data (often statistical tables, policies, laws, regulations, etc.) on cultural, social, geographic, economic, political, or other conditions. An example of linking meso and micro data in occupational therapy research is offered by Iwarsson et al[60] who studied the relationship between participation in daily life occupations and mortality rates. To date, Townsend and Wilcock[1] have considered four cases of occupational injustice: occupational alienation, occupational deprivation, occupational marginalization, and occupational imbalance. Whiteford[57] has offered five illustrations of occupational deprivation, distinguished from temporary occupational disruptions: geographic isolation, problem conditions of employment, incarceration, sex-role stereotyping, and refugeeism.

Negotiate targeted outcomes and design the program and evaluation

Developing successfully funded program proposals is not easy in a climate of competition for resources. Nevertheless, occupational therapists who work with population representatives create a powerful partnership for generating innovation and resources. Reflective questions for program design might start with: 'What occupational justice outcomes will be targeted?' (see Table 9.1)

To develop an evidence-based approach, the partnership would consider diverse forms of qualitative, critical, and quantitative evidence, not limited to scientifically controlled experiments. Attention to occupational justice issues may arouse interest if the proposal is action-based, involving people as participants in various occupations. Look, for example, at the interest aroused by Simó Algado et al[61] who engaged child survivors of the war in Kosovo in healing processes using creative occupations, such as becoming street clowns and artists. Population proposals may succeed best if objectives and concepts relate not only to practical matters in daily life, but also to the spiritual beliefs that can potentially bring a community or population together, as they did with Kosovo children.

If a program already exists, the planning group would examine how the program actually addresses occupational justice issues. One could survey participants and ask what outcomes they believe would make the most difference in their lives. Or one could visit and observe them to determine and document their occupational possibilities and barriers. Managers could examine, critique, and re-formulate the data being used to demonstrate program accountability for addressing occupational injustices. To guide continuing education, professionals could examine their knowledge, skills, and competence to work using an occupational justice framework. In Box 9.4, we talk about including education in the process of negotiating targeted outcomes, and developing program plans and evaluations in our occupational therapy curricula.

Box 9.4   Negotiate targeted outcomes and design the program and evaluation

Whiteford and Townsend

We educate students in program design and evaluation by making this a prominent part of the entry-level and post-professional occupational therapy curricula. We ensure that fieldwork education includes experiences in program design and evaluation, as well as experiences working directly with individual or group clients. We strongly encourage faculty to include assignments that give students experiences in working with population representatives who have experienced occupational injustices. For instance, we foster the use of language to talk about occupational dreams and occupational justice, naming these as learning topics and curriculum foundations. We attempt to create a learning environment where students discuss and rank program priorities with reference to their analyses of resources, justice frameworks, and injustices, and their analyses of occupation, enabling, and justice. To plan programs with this population, we encourage faculty to guide students in learning how to use population data on housing options and barriers, and on employment support services and limitations.

We encourage critical reflection in faculty, students, and ourselves in overseeing university programs that prepare students, for instance, in critiquing how people become medically/psychiatrically diagnosed with a diagnostic and statistical manual (DSM) mental disorder, or become classified under immigration criteria as a refugee. We attempt to create an academic environment that builds students' courage to emphasize enabling in processes of listening to each other openly and respectfully, knowing that enabling individual and social change is difficult to do. We seek ways to give back – for instance in the form of program designs and materials – to agencies that give their time and knowledge to our students. Throughout the learning process, we recognize that we are responsible as occupational therapists for educating others who are not familiar with occupational analysis and the therapeutic use of occupations. Whatever we have done to date to raise occupational justice-oriented, population-based practice to prominence in occupational therapy education and research, there is so much more to do – especially since occupational therapy is an extremely scarce human resource.

Evaluate client-specific strengths, resources and challenges

To make occupational justice more explicit in evaluation processes, we might ask ourselves: 'What qualitative, quantitative, and critical analysis methods are available and respected? What are client-specific occupational justice issues, strengths, and resources? What enabling processes have been used to support population, community, policy or other changes?' In Guatemala, for instance, Simó Algado and Gregori, who lived and worked with Mayan refugees, recognized that Mayan spiritual strengths were a resource for healing.[62] They invited their clients – the population of refugees – to participate in defining what stories and data could be collected, and they implicitly considered three related outcomes: clients' occupational participation, client and environmental enablement processes, and the advancement of justice through greater citizenship participation and inclusion. Changes in occupational participation were that more people became involved, positive energy grew, and the range of occupations of the group expanded. The changes in participation occurred as the Mayan people took greater control of their own occupations related to community building. Evaluation of enabling processes was carried out as people told stories about their experiences in re-settling their community. Stories of justice and injustice in everyday occupations were interwoven within a population-based, community development approach. These seem to have been invisibly blended with occupational therapy frameworks for psychosocial, biomechanical, and other practice.

In Box 9.5 we describe our own experiences of the evaluation process.

Box 9.5   Evaluate client-specific strengths, resources and challenges

Whiteford

The refugee camp itself is the client. I will be trying to enable other occupational therapists to work with this population as an outreach of mental health, child development, housing, employment, or other existing, funded programs. There may be funding for occupational therapists to propose a contract with this population. In such a contract, I would encourage the occupational therapist to work with residents as participants in identifying, prioritizing, and analyzing the occupational performance issues of various age groups within the camp. The selected persons might be educated to analyze occupations, so that they begin to look at their own lives from an occupational justice perspective. For instance, working together as members of a team of lay and professional workers, the occupational therapist and refugee spokespersons might consider which people are deprived of something to do. They might ask what people do if they have a disability, or are very old. Where explanations are clearly offered, the occupational therapist might use quantitative measures for individual performance, educating individual refugees, possibly through a translator, in the purpose and potential use of information gained through measurement. Evaluation tools would include narrative and observation of daily life participation, use of creative media, or story telling, as in the vignette below, in which V talks about his experience in a UN camp:

In our camp there were 40 000 people. There was no water, no way of washing, it was very bad, some people were sick, some died. There was no food, no eating. People returned on buses [from the conflict areas], they had been mutilated by knives, guns. The program was run in Kosovo by the United Nations; people were working day and night for the aid of drink and everything, there was no sleeping. We were all in there together, my mother and father, they're old people. Some people couldn't make it in to eat, the old or sick people, so we helped them, very important to help – all living together, one family. For me, I was up every
morning at 5 a.m. trying to find out which country we would be going to.

Townsend

I encourage occupational therapy students and practitioners to gather data by using the Canadian Occupational Performance Measure (COPM), selected because of its participatory format. Other forms of participatory evaluation may include client surveys to identify the outcomes of occupational therapy from a client versus a professional or management perspective. Mental health clubhouse members' participation in evaluation may be accomplished by enabling them to evaluate the clubhouse: for example, occupational therapy students were involved in observing how clubhouse members learned to develop evaluation research as an occupation required to sustain a mental health clubhouse.[21] Faculty and students are encouraged to talk about how clients – who may prefer to be called mental health survivors – may participate in their own evaluations through verbal interaction, creative media such as painting, third party reports, photographs and other means of evaluating occupational experiences. Client representatives may inform the evaluation process through talking circles, focus groups, or even email, as in Galipeault's comments to Townsend below:

When health professionals examine components of my life or that of others, they have to context their examination in a broad framework that encompasses all of the factors or determinants that affect health/ mental health. These factors have to be viewed and considered, not through a needs assessment, but through an assets charting approach that considers capabilities and strengths. The mental health system has failed me and others because the entire system is built on addressing needs. Consumer/survivors are often viewed as a needy group. People's endless amount of needs cannot and will never be satisfied."

(Pierre Galipeault, owner/manager of The Empowerment Connection, personal communication 2002).

Plan, implement and evaluate client-specific services

The process of planning, implementing, and evaluating client-specific services has been described extensively in occupational therapy literature. We emphasize here three important markers associated with a participatory occupational justice framework: client participation throughout decision making; enabling action and experience using occupations as the medium of client empowerment; and continuous evaluation of client progress toward greater occupational justice. A reflective, participatory approach

---

Box 9.6   Plan, implement, and evaluate client–specific services

Whiteford and Townsend
As working and research relationships evolve with a population, specific theoretical approaches may be renegotiated, and occupational justice issues may be redefined based on the experiences in this process. Program revisions may occur on a large or small scale. Specific programs with individuals, families, groups, or specific agencies will be adjusted as time and resources allow, and goals and outcomes are renegotiated. Alternatively, the plan may involve linking to other services or situations where work on occupational justice issues can be continued. The evidence of program success or failure would be related to negotiated program outcomes, defined in terms of changes in participation, or critiques of enabling approaches. Markers of success would be documented and reviewed by everyone involved. Occupational outcomes would ideally be the signature of occupational therapy participation in population-based practice.

---

would raise questions as in Table 9.1, such as: 'What is the most effective and efficient plan and evaluation strategy for client-specific goals and objectives?' In Box 9.6 we offer only an abbreviated orientation of client-specific services since this process has been described extensively in occupational therapy and other texts, as well as in Chapter 15, by Egan and Townsend.

REFLECTIONS AND CONCLUSIONS

We have proposed six non-linear, interrelated, participatory occupational justice processes for thoughtful experimentation, rather than as techniques to be adopted. One key point in the discussion has been a persistent focus on using occupations as both the process of therapy, and as outcomes defined in terms of occupational performance, occupational wellbeing, and justice. A second key point has been a commitment to participatory, enabling processes that include population representatives or clients, depending on funding and opportunities for partnership. Our questions arise from a participatory framework which includes population representatives or referred clients. The proposed framework emphasizes participation in negotiating a justice framework, and in the naming of goals and methods of client-specific service delivery. The third key point has been to name social inclusion and citizenship as the ultimate and desirable occupational outcomes associated with teams that include occupational therapy.

The six processes are a practical means of identifying injustices, not through rhetoric, but by determining what people need and want to do, then acting with others to enable social change. Analyses of occupational injustices will differ across the globe, yet they are available for us all to see through the cultural lenses we use to perceive real, daily life. Our description of an occupational justice framework is new – but nothing is really new. The processes are based on our own professional experiences, our teaching and research, and the ancient experiences of those who have enabled vulnerable or marginalized populations not only to survive but also to thrive.

What might occupational therapists contribute to society with a more explicit focus on occupations, collaborative processes of enabling, and occupational justice? What might change in the world if occupational therapists and others address occupational injustices in wealthy nations such as Canada and Australia, and around the globe?

Dedication

To those whose efforts day by day reduce occupational injustices in the world.

Acknowledgements

We acknowledge Dr Ann Wilcock of Deakin University, Victoria, Australia, who has been instrumental in formulating the concept of occupational justice. We also acknowledge the populations whose lives of occupational injustice are an embarrassment to the world.

References

1. Townsend E, Wilcock AA. Occupational justice and client-centred practice: a dialogue-in-progress. Can J Occup Ther. 2004; 71(2):75–87.
2. Canadian Association of Occupational Therapists. Enabling occupation: an occupational therapy perspective. Revised edn. Ottawa, ON: CAOT Publications ACE; 2002.
3. Fearing V, Clark J. Individuals in context: a practical guide to client-centred practice. Thorofare, NJ: Slack; 2001.
4. World Health Organization. International classification of functioning, disability and health (ICF). Geneva: World Health Organization; 2001.
5. Jarman J. What is occupation: interdisciplinary perspectives on defining and classifying human activity. In: Christiansen C, Townsend E, eds. Introduction to occupation: the art and science of living. Upper Saddle River, NJ: Prentice-Hall; 2004:47–62.
6. Yerxa EJ, Clark F, Frank G, et al. Occupational science: the foundation for new models of practice. In: Johnson JA, Yerxa EJ, eds. New York: The Haworth Press; 1990: 1–17.
7. Wilcock AA. A journey from prescription to self health, vol. 2. London: British Association and College of Occupational Therapists; 2002.
8. McColl MA. Theoretical basis of occupational therapy. 2nd edn. Thorofare, NJ: Slack; 2003.
9. Law M, Baum CM, Baptiste S, eds. Occupation-based practice: fostering performance and participation. Thorofare, NJ: Slack; 2002.
10. Kielhofner G. Model of human occupation: theory and application. 3rd edn. Baltimore, MD: Lippincott Williams & Wilkins; 2002.
11. Christiansen C, Townsend E. Introduction to occupation: the art and science of everyday living. Upper Saddle River, NJ: Prentice Hall; 2004.
12. Canadian Association of Occupational Therapists. Occupational therapy guidelines for client-centred practice. Toronto, ON: CAOT Publications ACE; 1991.
13. Department of National Health and Welfare. Guidelines for the client-centred practice of occupational therapy, H39–33/1983E. Ottawa, ON: Department of National Health and Welfare; 1983. (Out of print)
14. Department of National Health and Welfare. Intervention guidelines for the client-centred practice of occupational therapy, H39-100/1986E. Ottawa, ON: Department of National Health and Welfare; 1986. (Out of print)
15. Canadian Association of Occupational Therapists. Occupational therapy guidelines for client-centred mental health practice. Toronto, ON: CAOT Publications; 1993.
16. Townsend E, Landry JE. Enabling participation through occupations. In: Christiansen C, Baum C, eds. Enabling function and well-being. 3rd edn. Thorofare, NJ: Slack; 2004.
17. Polatajko H. National perspective – the evolution of our occupational perspective: the journey from diversion through therapeutic use to enablement. Can J Occup Ther 2001; 68:203–207.
18. Dunst CJ, Trivette CM. An enablement and empowerment perspective of case management. Topics in Early Childhood Special Education 1989; 8:87–102.
19. Byrne C. Facilitating empowerment groups: Dismantling professional boundaries. Issues in Mental Health Nursing 1999; 20(1):55–71.

20. Deegan P. Recovery and empowerment for people with psychiatric disabilities. Soc Work Health Care 1997; 25(3):11–24.

21. Townsend E, Ripley D, Langille L. Professional tensions in client-centred practice. Am J Occup Ther 2003; 57:17–28.

22. Wilcock AA, Townsend E. Occupational justice: occupational terminology interactive dialogue. Journal of Occupational Science 2000; 7(2):84–86.

23. Townsend E, Wilcock AA. Occupational Justice. In: Christiansen C, Townsend E, eds. An introduction to occupation: the art and science of living. Upper Saddle River, NJ: Prentice Hall; 2004: 243–273.

24. Kronenberg F. The political nature of occupational therapy. Linkoping, Sweden: University of Linkoping; 2003.

25. Rebeiro K. Reconciling philosophy with daily practice: future challenges to occupational therapy's client-centred practice. Occupational Therapy Now 2000; March/April: 4.

26. Pogge TW. On the site of distributive justice: reflections on Cohen and Murphy. Philosophy & Public Affairs 2000; 29(2):137–169.

27. Ludwig FM. The unpackaging of routine in older women. Am J Occup Ther 1998; 52(3):168–175.

28. Habermas J. The philosophical discourse of modernity: twelve lectures, translated by Frederick Lawrence. Cambridge, MA: MIT Press; 1995.

29. Mattingly CF. What is clinical reasoning? Am J Occup Ther 1991; 45:979–986.

30. Kuhn TS. The structure of scientific revolutions. Chicago: University of Chicago Press; 1989.

31. Atkinson P, Coffey A, Delamont S. Ethnography: post, past, present. Journal of Contemporary Ethnography 1999; 28(5):460–471.

32. Rolfe G. Postmodernism for healthcare workers in 13 easy steps. Nurse Education Today 2001; 21(1):38–47.

33. Campbell M, Copeland B, Tate B. Taking the standpoint of people with disabilities in research: experiences with participation. Can J Rehab 1998; 12(2):95–104.

34. Cervaro RM, Wilson AL. Beyond learner-centred practice: adult education, power and society. Canadian Journal for the Study of Adult Education 1999; 13:27–38.

35. Polatajko HJ. Muriel Driver Memorial Lecture. Naming and framing occupational therapy: a lecture dedicated to the life of Nancy B. Can J Occup Ther 1992; 59:189–200.

36. Frank G. Opening feminist histories of occupational therapy. Am J Occup Ther 1992; 46:989–999.

37. Griffin S. Occupational therapists and the concept of power: a review of the literature. Australian Occupational Therapy Journal 2001; 48(1):24–34.

38. Maxwell JD, Maxwell MP. Inner fraternity and outer sorority: social structure and the professionalization of occupational therapy. In: Wipper A, ed. The sociology of work: papers in honour of Osward Hall. Carleton Library series number 129. Ottawa, ON: Carleton University Press; 1983.

39. Yerxa EJ. Some implications of occupational therapy's history for its epistemology, values, and relation to medicine. Am J Occup Ther 1992; 46:79–83.

40. Townsend E. Power and justice in enabling occupation. Can J Occup Ther 2003; 70:74–87.

41. Pierce D. Occupation by design: dimensions, therapeutic power, and creative process. Am J Occup Ther 2001; 55(3):249–259.

42. Kinsella EA. Reflections on reflective practice. Can J Occup Ther 2001; 68(3):195–198.

43. Forwell SJ, Whiteford G, Dyck I. Cultural competence in New Zealand and Canada: occupational therapy students' reflections on class and fieldwork curriculum. Can J Occup Ther 2001; 68:90–103.

44. Simmons D, Crepeau EB, White BP. The predictive power of narrative data in occupational therapy. Am J Occup Ther 2000; 54:471–476.

45. O'Neill O. Agents of Justice. Metaphilosophy 2001; 32(1&2):180–195.

46. Johnstone M-J. Stigma, social justice and the rights of the mentally ill: challenging the status quo. Aust N Z J Ment Health Nurs 2001; 10(4):200–209.

47. Balcazar FE, Keys CB, Suarez-Balcazar Y. Empowering Latinos with disabilities to address issues of independent living and disability rights: a capacity-building approach. Journal of Prevention and Intervention in the Community 2001; 21(2):53–70.

48. Ignatieff M. The rights revolution. Toronto, ON: House of Anansi; 2000.

49. Woodhead M. Combatting child labour: listen to what the children say. Childhood: A Global Journal of Child Research 1999; 6(1):27–49.

50. Clements L. The human rights act – a new equity or a new opiate: reinventing justice or repackaging state control? Journal of Law and Society 1999; 26(1):72–85.

51. Jensen SB. Mental health under war conditions during the 1991–1995 war in the former Yugoslavia. In: World Health Stat Q 1996; 49(3–4): 213–217.

52. Law M. Muriel Driver Memorial Lecture. The environment: a focus for occupational therapy. Can J Occup Ther 1991; 58:171–180.

53. Rebeiro K. Enabling occupation: the importance of an affirming environment. Can J Occup Ther 2001; 68(2):80–89.

54. O'Brien P, Dyck I, Caron S, Mortenson P. Environmental analysis: insights from sociological and geographic perspectives. Can J Occup Ther 2002; 69:229–238.

55. Daniels N, Kennedy BP, Kawachi I. Why justice is good for our health: the social determinants of health inequalities. Daedalus 1999; 128(4):215–251.

56. Whiteford G. Occupational deprivation: global challenge in the new millennium. B J Occup Ther 2000; 64(5):200–210.

57. Whiteford G. When people cannot participate: occupational deprivation. In: Christiansen CH, Townsend EA, eds. Introduction to occupation: the art and science of living. Upper Saddle Creek, NJ: Prentice Hall; 2004: 221–242.

58. Sozomenou A, Mitchell P, Fitzgerald MH, et al. Mental health consumer participation in a culturally diverse society. 2nd edn. Sydney: Australian Transcultural Mental Health Network; 2000.

59. Smith M. Meg's story. In: Lawrence A, ed. I always wanted to be a tap-dancer. Paramatta, NSW, Australia: New South Wales Women's Advisory Council; 1989: 100–124.

60. Iwarsson S, Isacsson A, Persson D, Schersten B. Occupation and survival. Am J Occup Ther 1998; 52:65–70.

61. Simó Algado S, Mehta N, Kronenberg F, et al. Occupational therapy intervention with children survivors. Can J Occup Ther 2002; 69(4):205–217.

62. Simó Algado S, Gregori JMR, Egan M. Spirituality in a refugee camp. Can J Occup Ther 1997; 64(3):138–145.

Chapter **10**

Situated meaning
An issue of culture, inclusion, and occupational therapy

Michael K. Iwama

OVERVIEW

This chapter focuses on raising awareness of some of the issues that arise when occupational therapists take their practice into new or different contexts and cultures. In order for therapeutic interventions to be effective, they must take into account the realities and shared meanings of the people on whom they are targeted. The chapter highlights some of the assumptions underlying Western occupational therapy practice and frameworks, and shows that these are not necessarily helpful in an Eastern context. By focusing specifically on Japan and Japanese culture and worldview, the author shows that for occupational therapy to be effective and useful, it must adapt and change in response to the culture in which it finds itself being practiced. In order to insure that their practice empowers people rather than oppresses them, occupational therapists are invited to recognize the cultural construction of occupational therapy itself, and to allow the cultural insiders of client groups to understand and dictate the terms by which occupational therapy should be introduced.

INTRODUCTION

Culture can mean different things to different people. Popular notions of culture often include aspects of race and ethnicity, and what has been referred to as 'high culture': fashion, food, music and dance, representative literary works and art forms. A less restrictive view of culture, and the one borrowed for this discussion, is given by social geographer Isabel Dyck, who has a background in occupational therapy. She explains culture as a shared system of meanings that 'involve ideas, concepts and knowledge, and include the beliefs, values and norms that shape standards and rules of behavior as people go about their everyday lives.'[1]

Culture, in this understanding of it, has often been treated as a secondary concern when explaining occupational therapy in our professional discourse. Our assumptions about the nature of human agency, its components, organization, and meanings, are taken as universal qualities which transcend cultural boundaries and seem resistant to attempts at refuting or altering them. After all, what could possibly be wrong with a therapeutic approach driven by an ideology that seeks to empower individuals to improve or actualize themselves through rational, purposeful action? Few Westerners would take issue with a profession that seeks to assist people to be and become[2] through the use of their hands energized by mind and will.[3] Especially for those who share common experiences and worldviews with the profession's leaders, who articulate the profession's values and philosophies, and construct the models that describe and guide our work, the empirical necessity of critically examining and testing the applicability of occupational therapy for others has yet to emerge as a pressing concern. Like a square peg being forced through a round hole, the fit of ideas emerging from one set of cultural contexts into the other is not always a good one. All too often, it is the recipient hole that is forced to yield to the shape of the intruding peg.

Failure of occupational therapy to meet the requirements for wellbeing of the culturally diverse people it encounters, is often constructed as a problem of the individual rather than attributed to some inadequate aspect of occupational therapy. In our clinical practice, we gain glimpses of this issue when clients have difficulty complying with our best intentions to assist them. Whether it is the elderly gentleman who wonders why he is being admonished to perform daily living tasks independently, or a young woman who seems lost when asked to respond to inquiries structured by the Canadian Occupational Performance Measure (COPM),[4] we tend to situate the problem at the interface between client and therapist, rather than in some set of philosophical or value patterns imbedded in the ideology or the structure of the therapy itself. If not deduced to be a language or communication problem, it might be framed as a problem with the client's particular culture that has fallen short of the requirements of occupational therapy. We might even draw the pejorative conclusion that the client is 'difficult' or 'non-compliant', thinking it incredible that anyone might be at odds with the rightness of the therapeutic process or the ideology that drives it. Rarely do we raise the possibility that the problem might actually lie within occupational therapy itself, in the cultural elements imbedded in its perspectives on ontology and epistemology, and in the frameworks that explain and guide its interventions.

It is a perplexing question and one that needs to be visited as occupational therapy pioneers its way into new contexts of practice. The implications and consequences of implementing therapeutic interventions that are out of sync with local people's realities and shared meanings are profound. An occupational therapy out of cultural context could result in a movement that therapists and clients alike cannot understand, thereby robbing the profession of its meaning and potential to contribute something positive to society. At worst, occupational therapy could be an agent of oppression, colonizing and perhaps further marginalizing people by requiring them to acquire competencies that are maladaptive and run counter to their basic value patterns.

To elucidate this issue, we examine culture from a perspective of cultural relativism, a view that fundamental notions of what is considered true, morally correct, and what constitutes knowledge (or reality) itself,[5] are socially constructed and vary cross-culturally. It will be argued that humans are social beings and through their shared experiences ascribe unique meanings to phenomena, and that reality does not necessarily exist independently of the knower.[6] Occupational therapy and its supporting ideologies (for example the assumption that humans are occupational beings), which are construed as cross-cultural universals, are scrutinized and rejected here. In order to bring occupational therapy safely, equitably, and beneficently into the lives of other peoples, whether they be marginalized here or in some other location, culture in occupational therapy needs to be understood in its own terms from the other's vantage-point.

THE CULTURE OF OCCUPATIONAL THERAPY

If culture is at least partially explained by the ideas, concepts, and knowledge, and includes the beliefs, values and norms, that shape standards and rules of behavior as people go about their everyday lives,[1] then an examination of the concepts deemed fundamental to explanations of occupational therapy should afford a view of the culture that is imbedded in current constructions of occupational therapy. Few would take issue with the notion that the occupation in occupational therapy is defined thus: 'the domain of concern and the therapeutic medium of occupational therapy. … Occupation is explained to be everything that people do to occupy themselves, and can include groups of activities and tasks of everyday life, named, organized, and given value and meaning by individuals and a culture.'[4] However, in the realm of Western social experience, occupation appears to be imbued with more profound meanings. Meanings that go as far as defining the construction of one's 'self' become essential to a society that places fundamental emphasis on the individual as a reflective, rationally minded, independent entity. The construct of 'occupation' subsumes many of the common assumptions that many Westerners hold to be true of their world and how being and individual identity are inextricably tied to what we 'do'. Charles Christiansen viewed 'occupation as the principal means through which people develop and express their personal identities.'[7] He added that 'competence in performance of tasks and occupations contributes to identity shaping and … the realization of an acceptable identity contributes to coherence and wellbeing.'[7] For theory, Christiansen drew primarily from Mead's work on symbolic interactionism[8] and from Piaget – even infants come to know the world through the action of 'doing'.[9]

The construction of occupation in occupational therapy is supported by basic streams of modern social thought and social theory, particularly involving, but not limited to, the concepts of agency, praxis, and reflexivity. That the core tenets of occupational therapy often abide within the explanations offered by modern social science has helped to reify them, at least in the West. With such tacit perspectives toward self, society, and the environs, it may be difficult for Western people to imagine occupation as holding particular, culture-bound meanings, shaped and influenced by prevailing social and cultural contexts.

Celebrated notions of 'self' and identity have come to inhabit our ideas of wellbeing and healthy states of being in occupational therapy. Wilcock has coined what has arguably become the defining slogan for occupational therapists: 'doing, being, and becoming'.[2] Westerners would probably agree that fundamental elements of our being, and what we aspire to become, are primarily shaped and determined by what we do. Suffering insult to one's ability to 'do' due to some unfortunate event or circumstance represents an essential problem and an appropriate rationale for occupational therapy intervention.

WESTERN INDIVIDUALISM; THE FOUNDATIONS OF WESTERN OCCUPATIONAL THERAPY THEORY

We may all be observed to do and perform activities similarly, but the personal and societal meanings we ascribe to and imbue our own activities with are profoundly particular and unique. Where and how do these cultural patterns originate and how are they sustained, even through this age of information and globalization? From my vantage-point of having been born and raised in East Asia and later acculturated in Western social con-

Figure 10.1 East Asian version of the cosmological myth.

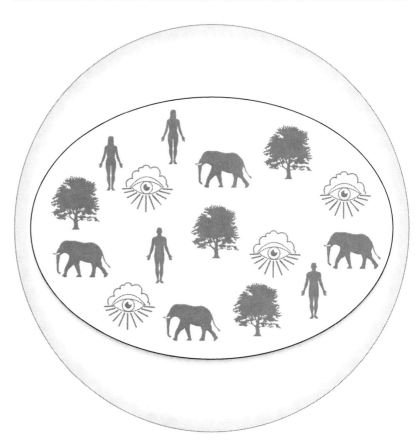

texts, I believe that some of the more profound views on cultural divergence can be better appreciated through narratives of cosmologies and particular worldviews.

The remarkable difference between the East Asian cosmological myth or worldview (see Fig. 10.1) and the Western variation of it (see Fig. 10.2) can be seen in the radical transcendence in the Western view of an all-powerful God, thereby separating the elements of nature, self, society, and deity from their imagined singular, tightly bound unity in the East Asian view into graded entities on a continuum. The transcendence of a single omnipotent deity in Western cosmology [10,11] can be viewed as correlating symbolically with the individual's transcendence over others (society) and nature (environment). This transcendence effects a separation or distinction of self from the social and material environments. We derive from it a sense of individual destiny to act on and occupy our environs, having been bestowed dominion over these elements by God. This sense of individual destiny coincides with the unequivocal social assumption of autonomy and independence evident in Western life. In occupational therapy, independence in daily skills is a universally held and celebrated performance outcome. A requirement to depend on others is perceived negatively, as a state of being requiring amelioration.

Figure 10.2 Western variation of the cosmological myth.

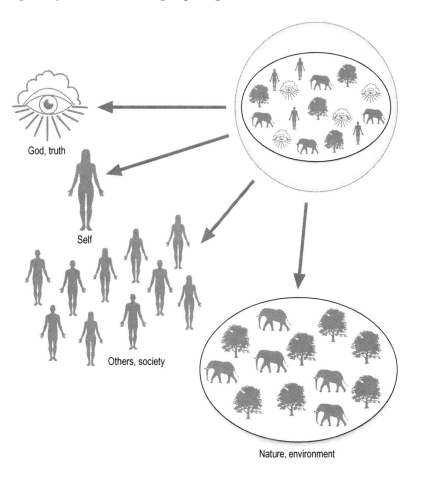

God, truth

Self

Others, society

Nature, environment

Whether or not cosmological myths and particular worldviews have any bearing on a given social group's value and belief systems, certain traits or conceptualizations have often been used in the literature to describe Western individualism. Some of these concepts describe the modal Western individual as being analytic,[12,13,14] monotheistic,[15,10] materialistic,[12] and rationalistic.[16]

Concepts that describe a particular attitude toward doing, such as unilateral determinism,[17] self-efficacy,[18] and personal causation,[19,13] reflect a construal of individualistic intention and construction of 'self' in relation to environment. In Western spheres of experience, the occupation of one's environs through purposeful action is often viewed as a right and an imperative. It assumes, as Lebra postulated, that, for the Westerner, the prime mover[17] for one's actions lies within the individual, with the ultimate objective being to gain competence and independence by establishing control over one's circumstances. In this attitude toward human agency, responsibility for success and failure tends to fall on the individual rather than on the surrounding social context.

Western individualism on a micro level is congruent with monotheism, the tendency to support a 'closed system cosmology' where limits are coterminous with a single truth or omnipotent deity,[10] on a macro level. The congruence between a closed system theology and a closed system *personology*, where phenomena are viewed to be accountable to a single set of laws or moral standards, is evident in virtually all modes and explanations of Western life. Modern science, with all of its positivistic and empirical principles thought to originate from such a worldview, reifies a universe rationally constructed in a logical sequence, reducible to a single basic truth. The orderly division and categorization of reality is not only pertinent to physically 'real' things but presumed also to constitute the structure of immaterial things such as thoughts, ideas, and memories.[12] Thus the Western individual is construed to be especially analytic, preferring a view of reality as an aggregation of parts that fit together in some ultimately logical pattern. Western theorists and researchers have thus sought to 'objectify' the world in a particular way, seeking to reduce the complexities of human thought and action into more linear, logical depictions.

The tendency to construct the world in an analytical, particulate manner, which is congruent with a particulate view of self, society, and nature, represents an important tenet of occupational therapy philosophy. That problematic tenet is the objectification of 'external' objects as existing separately from the observer. The view of the environment (both social and physical) as in opposition to the self (connected through 'occupation') rather than as just one part of the same unified whole, holds profound consequences for whether people of other cultures can share and abide by Western occupational therapists' interpretation of occupation and its supposed essentiality to wellbeing. Thus, Westerners and their ideas about human agency are accused of being overly rational. In this epistemological bent, all phenomena, including human agency and praxis, can be reflexively and systematically investigated and explained by some rational logic. Human performance qualifies as occupation when we interpret it as meaningful, when the means of a task can be tied to some reasonable end.

The importance of tying one's action or 'doing', rationally, to some future objective, orients one temporally toward the future.

The congruence between Western worldviews and occupational therapy theory should be readily evident in that theory, particularly in those conceptual models that purport to explain human agency and its qualities. The Model of Human Occupation[20] (MOHO) (see Ch. 14) and the Canadian Model of Occupational Performance[4] (CMOP) (see Ch. 15), are briefly examined here to illuminate how culture is implicit in the structure of these theoretical models, in contrast to its usual location as a secondary consideration or afterthought. It should be noted that the earliest substantive descriptions of these conceptual models are being purposely referred to in order to situate the genesis of these ideas in a historical and cultural context. That these models undergo adaptations to meet the changing requirements of their respective dynamically changing social contexts is testament to the thesis of this chapter: that meaning and its explanations are culturally situated.

A review of the MOHO[21] reveals that general systems theory[22,23] (GST) was chosen as the framework on which the concepts of this model were to be structured. The model depicts humans as open systems involved in an intercourse with the surrounding physical and social environment. The basic tenet of this interpretation of human action was that humans had an innate drive to master and control their environments. Their subsequent actions in the world were modified by an internal executive order of cognition, which ultimately assembled, modified, and enacted performance. Volition, habituation, and performance comprised the three main occupational performance components residing in the open system.[20] Subsumed in the concept of volition are subconcepts perceived to be resident in the individual, such as 'personal causation', 'values' and 'interests'. In the subconcept of 'personal causation' are contained the concepts of 'self efficacy' and one's 'knowledge of capacity' (to perform). Acting upon the environment would result in feedback and other cues from the environment, which would input into the system, pass through the executive functions, and output again into the environment, forming a loop. Functional states of the individual would be characterized by smooth cycling and equilibrium in the human–environment continuum, while uneven, blocked cycling and imbalance would characterize occupational dysfunctional states. The occupational therapist, in using this model, would endeavor to assist clients to gain better equilibrium with their environments by maximizing performance in any part of the human–environment continuum.

The MOHO's structure and concepts, and the metaphoric representation of human agency depicted in a systems arrangement, reflect virtually all of the descriptors of the modal Western tendencies and cosmologies presented above. The 'self' is depicted as solitary and placed in the center of the 'system'. The transcendence of self over an environment that is distinctly set in opposition is also evident. Successful human agency is conceptualized as a state of efficacy in which one can exercise one's determination to act on the environment and control one's circumstances. 'Control' in this interpretation is set synonymously with 'balance' or order. The compartmentalization of the various concepts and subconcepts systematically working together in logical order is reminiscent of depictions of Western individuals as analytic, materialistic, and rationalistic.

The CMOP[4] is yet another prominent model that has emerged in the latter half of the twentieth century. Three concentric circles representing components of the human–occupation–environment system graphically depict the model (see Ch. 15, Fig. 15.1). The individual is represented by the innermost circle and is conceptualized to consist of four parts: the spiritual, physical, mental, and sociocultural. The outermost circle represents the environment and is conceptualized into four parts: the physical, social, cultural, and institutional. Between the innermost circle (the individual) and the outermost circle (the environment) lies the middle concentric circle, which has been conceptualized as 'purposes of occupation'. These purposes of occupation are divided into three parts: self-care, productivity, and leisure. Occupational performance is depicted in this model as a balance between individual and environment: 'The result of a dynamic, interwoven relationship between persons, environment, and occupation over a person's life-span: the ability to choose, organise, and satisfactorily perform meaningful occupations that are culturally defined and age appropriate for looking after oneself, enjoying life, and contributing to the social and economic fabric of a community.'[4] The interaction between self and environment is through action (occupation). A deficit in one's ability to act according to will results in dysfunction and an upset of systematic balance.

Occupational therapists work to identify the points contributing to imbalance in the system and use activity therapeutically to strengthen and rebalance the system. Thus intervention strategies are geared toward restoring one's mastery over the environment by adjusting individual or environmental attributes. Once again, the primacy of the individual as agent of change in relation to the environment is strongly represented. The conceptualization of both the individual and the environment into limited, discrete components is evident and affords us a view into how the authors constructed the concept of occupational performance along the notions of individual agency, environment, and the utility and meaning of action. What is evident in these constructions of wellbeing is the notion that personal achievement and self-actualization represent the acme of human strivings and that these ideals are derived through a process of exploration and competence. Mastery of self and the environment (nature) becomes equated with healthy states of being. These occupational therapy conceptual models represent and reify Western ideals of health defined along independent, individualistic, and rationalistic proclivities. How appropriate, then, are these depictions of health for societies that abide by very different social and cultural constructions of reality?

THE CHALLENGE OF OCCUPATIONAL THERAPY IN OTHER CULTURAL CONTEXTS

For this discussion, East Asia, and more specifically Japan, is briefly considered. Japan's 120 million people form a part of Asia's collective population, estimated to be over 3.3 billion people,[24] almost half of the world's population. Asia's varied cultures represent a pertinent testing ground for occupational therapy's universality because they have evolved their own distinct philosophies, value patterns, moral and ethical systems, and epistemologies, separate from the Western world.[26] Just as Asian nations have had to be reconciled with the sharp intrusions of modernization and Western cultural forms over the past century, so Japan has had to deal with the systematic transplantation of occupational therapy with all of its subsumed philosophies, values, moral and ethical systems, and epistemology from the West over the past 35 years. Japan has arguably one of the fastest proliferating occupational therapy concerns in the world, with occupational therapy education programs expanding at a near exponential rate in the past decade.

Philosophical underpinnings

An examination of the East Asian version of the cosmological myth[10] discussed earlier (see Fig. 10.1) suggests that Asian peoples may perceive the world quite differently from their Western counterparts. Instead of perceiving the world as rationally separated, the East Asian cosmological perspective places nature, self, and society in a closed, tightly integrated whole. There are no social–structural after-effects of the radical transcendence of a single God, single truth, or single moral code. Rather than ties of loyalty and trust extending linearly and vertically toward a single deity or universal ideal, they settle into a complex, flexible constellation of horizontal relations.

With regard to human behavior, in the absence of an omnipotent deity the social becomes the entity by which all things are valued and judged. Persistence of the Eastern cosmological myth in conceptualizations of nature, self, and society, rather than the predominant Western, transcendent, separated version of it, can be correlated to certain observable social–structural patterns.

This Eastern worldview, for example, may limit the conceptualization of the centrality of 'self' in the universe as well as deflecting reliance on and attribution of accomplishment away from a solitary, centrally situated 'me'. And instead of offering a monotheistic view of an ultimate singular truth, the Eastern cosmological view places deities together with humans and nature in a tightly bound singular entity, creating a polytheism in which multiple truths can exist at the same time. In the Western understanding of the cosmos, the transcendent individual is afforded a perch from which to view and judge all matter according to a single, internally reflected, universally applicable moral code. For the polytheistic Easterner, no such perch exists from which to offer an ultimate judgement. Judgement and interpretation of truth and right are situational, reflected to referent elements in the vicinity of the phenomena rather than to a universal interpretation of truth and moral right, transcending situation and circumstance. In such relational contexts, the notion of grand theories or all-encompassing explanations of phenomena are unimaginable and practically untenable. Such a naturalistic worldview forms the basis of a collectivist social structure and a particular view of meaning that then stands as an awkward substrate in which to set individualistic, independence-oriented constructions of occupation.

In Japanese social contexts, the 'decentralized' conceptualization of self is seen to permit a 'situation ethic'[17,25] to determine behavior, whereby the social situation (referred to as 'frame' or 'ba' by Nakane),[27] and not the centrally constructed self, strongly influences the interpretation, initiation, and shape of human agency. With emphasis placed on horizontal social relations tied to 'frame', a social or group-focused norm gains prominence over an individual-focused norm, where matters pertaining to existentialism and identity are contingent on 'doing'. This is the rationale for Lebra's[17] suggestion that for the modal Japanese person the 'prime mover', which is located internally in most Westerners, is seen to be located external to the self, in the social 'frame'.

So much of the discourse on human occupation is individualistic and therefore reflexive. The notion of deriving meaning from what we do is tacit for most people who abide in a monistic, egocentric view of the world. Most Japanese occupational therapists and their clients have trouble participating in such a perspective of self and of the meaning of action, owing to the lack of such experiences and such interpretation of phenomena in their own realities. For most Japanese people, the meanings attributed to personal agency and phenomena are situational, social group influenced, and vary from circumstance to circumstance. For them, truth and the meaning of doing may be greatly influenced by the social surroundings and the situation of the agent in relation to environment.

In the Japanese collective experience, more than the self, the collective in which one holds membership is agent. When the social frame takes precedence over individual attributes, the realization of personal goals and social roles is constructed to come about by a different dynamic. Achievement is rarely a solitary attribute, rather it is a result of self, the collective, and nature. In the West, there is the notion that we can affect the state of nature (and health) through our actions as energized by mind and will.[3] Hence, the belief persists that we can achieve societal roles and attain success by striving intelligently and unilaterally. The progression of doing, being, and becoming,[2] as Wilcock iterated, need not be questioned. In Japanese social experience, being and becoming are not necessarily contingent on one's effort or skill. Nature, which includes the collective, encompasses the self as a unified whole, and ultimately explains success and failure. In the East, the concepts of fate and karma often provide a powerful explanation for all phenomenal outcomes.

These differences between individualist and collectivist views of occupational performance outcomes can be seen practically in cross-cultural interactions, such as international sporting events. Westerners may find it intriguing to compare the content of interviews given by high performance athletes to television reporters following a successful outcome. Japanese athletes will, almost certainly, begin their interview with expressions of sincere gratitude to the fans, team-mates, support staff, coaches, and practically everyone else, for the success achieved. Although this behavior pattern is seen from time to time in the West, its propensity in almost all public expressions of individual achievement in Japanese settings is noteworthy.

Basking in personal achievement evokes disdain in the Japanese public. This is not only because of social convention in a collectivist society but also because the athlete believes that the success achieved was the result of many factors that coincided at the right time. Victory was not necessarily achieved because the self was able to produce a supreme personal effort or because God had willed it to be. The Western victor's candid, enthusiastic rationalizations, attributing victory to a supreme personal effort or to God, appear brazen and particularly egocentric from a collectivist's vantage-point.

In a collective society where one is accountable to one's social relationships over some single truth, belonging rather than doing becomes the social ethos. Identity and meaning lie within the social collective rather than in personal agency. To be cast out of one's group can result in the invalidation of one's identity and reason for existing. Hence the drive to be independent and autonomous, that is so dominant in modern rehabilitation and occupational therapy, might appear strange or novel, judged from a social backdrop that values social dependence and interdependence. In this context of collective belonging, the progression of becoming, being, and doing is a more convincing model to explain Japanese occupational behavior. Roles are bestowed by the group, and once the role is made explicit, the self emerges to carry out the mandate of the collective. This is fulfillment and the acme of Japanese agency.

CONCLUSION

Often the culture imbedded in our lived realities goes unnoticed. The features of our shared experiences remain unremarked, perhaps because the perch from which we universally judge other elements of the reality around us is itself exempted from scrutiny. If we can, for a moment, lower that perch and descend from our own point of reference in order to view and appreciate other worldviews and perspectives of reality, we gain insight into our own culture and our own particular ways of seeing and knowing.

Currently, critical examination of the culture subsumed in our profession's fundamental thoughts and language remains underdeveloped and there is a particular bias toward shared meanings and interpretations of phenomena germane to Western spheres of experience. This chapter has highlighted some of the more prominent descriptions of Western social proclivities, such as our individualistic, autonomous, analytic, monotheistic, materialistic, and rationalistic tendencies. These limited concepts were also explained in relation to possible differences in worldviews that have a bearing on how one constructs the individual in relation to the social and to elements of the environment. How this fundamental view of reality is configured can have a profound effect on whether and how people ascribe meaning to their actions and place in the world. An open system cosmology that constructs self as equal in status to, and inseparably 'one' with, the environment jeopardizes claims that we occupy our environs through occupation. Self-deterministic notions of unilaterally controlling life circumstances through occupation are meaningless to people who subscribe to more naturalistic viewpoints of reality and who are oriented toward a harmonious existence with nature and its circumstances. What implications, then, might the problem of differing cultures and social constructions of reality hold for the construction of occupational therapy when occupation and occupational therapy are taken out of their original social contexts of meaning and systematically implemented in other differing social contexts? First, we should understand that occupation, the core concept of occupational therapy, may not exist in the lexicons of non-Western societies. Second, the concept could be even more problematic given that the situated meanings ascribed to occupation can differ profoundly, according to the social contexts of particular societies and their constellations of shared experiences. Thus, people in other societies might not attribute the same meanings to their doings as people in the West.

In collective, Confucian, hierarchically-oriented societies like Japan's, a well-meaning therapist working with an elderly woman in a nursing home might unwittingly be negating a lifetime of meaningful experiences and skills for being. Armed with the COPM[28] and a theoretical framework like MOHO,[21] the therapist may be coercing the client into social requirements that are poorly understood by her and run counter to her context for being. The yearning to belong, to depend, to be in harmony with her circumstances, and carry out the role that she has been given in her situation in time (and which others like her may have carried out for centuries) is being intruded upon, frustrated, and dismantled, by an ideology based on the predication of individualism and autonomy, made explicit in concepts like personal causation, occupational performance, and the battery of assessments that follow.

Not all intrusions come in through a side window or back door. Often they come through the front door in the guise of beneficence, emancipation, empowerment, and restoration. Those who are fearful of being left behind in the global economy and the race for technology may actually put out the welcome mat and not necessarily see it as an intrusion. Some may indeed benefit, but the parallels with colonialism from past times are apparent. There is always the danger of importing our own culture and thereby standards of behavior and meanings that can disrupt people's way of life. In the local cultural context, we may actually be modeling and nurturing behaviors that will disadvantage people in their own societies. In this way, occupational therapy can oppress rather than empower, encumber rather than emancipate, and disable rather than restore.

As we contemplate taking occupational therapy into the lives of people living in other geographic locations, and in the margins of our societies, we should rededicate ourselves to allowing the 'insiders' of client groups to understand and dictate the terms by which occupational therapy should be introduced. Occupational therapists are implored to go beyond the requirements of conventional cultural competence and recognize the cultural construction of occupational therapy itself, and all of its situated, subsumed philosophies, theories, and epistemologies. Failure to do so will insure that occupational therapy falls far short of its mandate to enable people through meaningful action. If meaning in occupation is deemed important to members of this profession, then the issue of culture should be of primary concern.

References

1. Dyck I. Multicultural society. In: Jones D, Blair SE, Hartery T, Jones TRK eds. Sociology and occupational therapy. London: Harcourt Brace; 1998:67–80.
2. Wilcock A. Reflections on doing, being, and becoming. Can J Occup Ther 1998; 65(5):248–256.
3. Reilly M. Occupational therapy can be one of the great ideas of 20th century medicine. Am J Occup Ther 1962; 16:1–9.
4. Canadian Association of Occupational Therapists. Enabling occupation: an occupational therapy perspective. Toronto: CAOT Publications; 1997.
5. Marshall R. Review of the myth of Japanese uniqueness. Journal of Japan Studies 1989; 15:266–272.
6. Murphy E. Constructivist epistemology. In: Constructivism: philosophical and epistemological foundations. 1997: Summer. Online. Available: http:www.stemnet.nf.ca/~elmurphy/emurphy/cle2.html 31 May 2002.
7. Christiansen C. Defining lives; occupation as identity: an essay on competence, coherence, and the creation of meaning. 1999 Eleanor Clarke Slagle Lectureship. Am J Occup Ther 1999; 53(6): 547–558.
8. Mead G. Mind, self, and society. Chicago: University of Chicago Press; 1967.
9. Piaget J. The construction of reality in the child. New York: Ballantine; 1954.
10. Bellah R. Beyond belief: essays on religion in a post traditional world. New York: Harper & Row; 1991.
11. Berque A. Identification of the self in relation to the environment. In: Rosenberger N, ed. Japanese sense of self. Cambridge: Cambridge University Press; 1992:93–104.
12. Johnson F. Dependency and Japanese socialization: psychoanalytic and anthropological investigations into Amae. New York: New York University Press; 1993.
13. Porkert M. The Theoretical Foundation of Chinese Medicine. Boston, Massachusetts: Institute of Technology Press; 1974.
14. Gregory-Smith D. Science and technology in East Asia. Philosophy East and West 1979; 29:221–236.
15. DeVos G. Dimensions of self in Japanese culture. In: Marsella A, DeVos G, Hsu F, eds. Culture and self: Asian and Western perspectives. New York: Tavistock; 1985:32–88.
16. Gans H. Middle American individualism. New York: The Free Press; 1988.
17. Lebra S. Japanese patterns of behavior. Honolulu: University of Hawaii Press; 1976.
18. Bandura A. Self-efficacy: toward a unifying theory of behavioral change. Psychol Rev 1977; 84:191–215.
19. DeCharms R. Personal causation: the internal affective determinants of behavior. New York: Academic Press; 1968.
20. Kielhofner G. A model of human occupation. Part three: benign and vicious cycles. Am J Occup Ther 1980; 34:731–737.
21. Kielhofner G. A model of human occupation: theory and application. Baltimore: Williams and Wilkins; 1985.
22. Von Bertalanffy L. An outline of general systems theory. British Journal for the Philosophy of Science 1950; 1:139–164.
23. Parsons T. The structure of social action, New York: McGraw-Hill; 1937.
24. US Census Bureau. Report WP/98; world population profile, Washington, DC: US Government Printing Office; 1998.
25. DeVos G. The relation of guilt toward parents to achievement and arranged marriage among the Japanese. Psychiatry 1960; 23:287–301.
26. Iwama M. The issue is ... toward culturally relevant epistemologies in occupational therapy. Am J Occup Ther 2003; 57(5):582–588.
27. Nakane C. *Tate shakai no ningen kankei.* (Human relations in a vertical society.) Tokyo: Kodansha; 1970.
28. Law M, Baptiste S, Carswell A, et al. Canadian occupational performance measure. 2nd edn. Toronto: CAOT Publications; 1994.

Chapter 11

Social occupational therapy
A socio-historical perspective

Denise Dias Barros, Maria Isabel Garcez Ghirardi, Roseli Esquerdo Lopes (translated by Sandra Maria Galheigo)

OVERVIEW

The aim of this chapter is to discuss the unfolding of a new research area –
seen both as a field for theoretical reflection and as a praxis of intervention:
the so-called 'social occupational therapy', which has been defined as the
body of knowledge related to processes of caring for and dealing with
people lacking an adequate social support network. To that purpose, we
address ourselves to the following tasks: the first is to understand that
occupational therapy has emerged from the main organizing health–disease
framework; the second is to disclose the intertwining relations between
occupational therapy and the society and culture within which it has been
effectively developed. We consider that it is important to outline
methodological principles that allow us to think out our practices beyond
the empirical moment; but we also believe that this has to be done without
narrowing our reflections to the limits of reductionist theories or pre-
established models, a restriction that would make it impossible to
understand fully the movements of the real world, life, and history within
their own contexts. In order to do this, we review the recent history of
occupational therapy and investigate: the emergence of the 'social question'
as a context of intervention for the occupational therapist; the processes of
deinstitutionalization; the importance of territorial actions in occupational
therapy; and, finally, the concepts that allow us to define as a practice of
occupational therapy our attention to social groups undergoing the
breakdown of their supporting social networks.

THE EMERGENCE OF THE SOCIAL FIELD IN OCCUPATIONAL THERAPY

Addressing social issues became a constitutive part of occupational therapy action in Brazil from the time when occupational therapists started to
assume a critical standpoint concerning the foundation of their professional activities.[1–4] This took place as a result of the debate on the role of

professional practice in 'total institutions', as Goffman describes them,[5] or, in Basaglia's[6] description, 'institutions of violence'. These institutions, whether schools, hospitals, asylums, or prisons, are described thus because of their segregative character, based as they are on oppressive relationships that rest upon the divide between powerful and powerless people. This separation has been defended as necessary for education, treatment, or correction. According to Basaglia's perspective, institutional violence may be implicit or explicit and has been justified historically by professional knowledge. At the time when this was happening, several occupational therapists realized that the significance of using activities and developing therapeutic programs in asylums for psychiatric patients went beyond the boundaries of their understanding, at that time, of their daily practice. They realized that explanations focusing on the individual, and based on psychological frames of reference, were neither sufficient nor adequate to respond to that context.[7-10]

Occupational therapists started to question their practice by recognizing first, that their actions took place within a historical process and second, that technical and political dimensions are present in all professional actions. They held to the idea that the problems they were addressing could not be reduced to a discussion on the choice of proper therapeutic resources or on the adequacy of individual programs, since it was evident that some social conditions could not be dealt with on a cure or treatment basis.[11-13]

From this questioning some important positions emerged. The first was the indignation manifested by occupational therapists towards the institutionalization of users of psychiatric services, in which madness was still associated with misery, insistently ignoring the historical separation announced by Pinel.[14] The second was unease with the role occupational therapists were supposed to play, namely keeping the environment calm, preventing manifestations of unusual behaviors, and using activities as a resource for the maintenance of discipline[15,16] and conformity.[17]

As a matter of fact, many Brazilian occupational therapists continued to believe in the prevailing institutional, segregative approach; but even among those who sought for alternatives, dissatisfaction and unease still remained. Others chose to provide psychotherapeutic assistance, in which activity would act, on the one hand, as a mediator in a relationship and, on the other hand, as a resource for self-expression,[7] but this failed to take into account the intolerable living conditions inside the institutions and the larger society.

There was also an expectation for occupational therapists to make use of individual or group activities to conceal the emptiness of life in institutions, places where life is without meaning. Therapeutic objectives were abstract and there was a huge gap between the aim of promoting social inclusion and the feasibility of that intent. The same may be said of the distance between the stated purposes of the institutions and the results of their regimes.[18-20]

Despite the variations in Brazilian occupational therapy reality, many professionals became agents of change along with other social actors and have worked hard for a radical transformation of institutions in Brazil since the end of the 1970s. Their standpoint was sustained by a deeper questioning, which was motivated by the contradictions brought about by institutionalization and the power of the medical view. Their critique was also driven by their awareness of the inadequacies of the reductionist view regarding the processes of falling ill, and by the ill treatment evident in psychiatric wards.[21,12]

Through the influence of Gramsci's ideas concerning the role of the intellectual in class relations,[22] the institutions came to be seen as places for the promotion of hegemonic values. This argument was founded on the notion of society as a place where the values of the ruling classes were reproduced with the help of intellectuals, who might act as agents for the promotion of consensus in the search for social hegemony. Thus intellectuals were supposed to enforce the so-called 'spontaneous' consensus, driving most of the population in the direction imposed by the ruling classes. According to this view, intellectuals are employees of the State apparatus and their function is to promote coercion and maintain discipline, making non-conforming groups submit to hegemonic domination.

Franco and Franca Basaglia,[18] whose ideas were largely influenced by Gramsci,[22] Sartre,[23] and Foucault,[15,16] questioned this view of the role of health workers. These Italian authors argue the need for health workers to understand the relationship between professional and political action. Based on this argument, practitioners, who tend to regard their actions dialectically, should search for a new way of conceiving knowledge that takes into account the needs of the people for whom their actions are designed. In order to get to know what these needs are, professionals should acknowledge that people are able to produce their own interpretations and meanings for the issues that are important to them. The focus was to produce a transformation of the health–disease paradigm through the understanding that therapists' interventions should take into account people's views on their own needs, their culture, and their lives within the community.

These ideas, which were current at the end of the 1970s and beginning of the 1980s in Brazil, underlay the questioning of practice taking place inside the psychiatric hospitals and in many other 'total institutions'. Beatriz Nascimento[24] synthesized the questioning of this period into the assertion that the problem, broadly speaking, was the economic, political, and ideological role that occupational therapists are asked to play in Brazilian society through their professional practice in these institutions. According to Nascimento, it would be important to analyze how, despite the complexity of the social relations involved, occupational therapists are contributing to the maintenance and consolidation of the status quo through their uncritical use of human activity, the status quo being the consolidation of a social order which on the one hand produces, and on the other segregates and punishes people who do not conform to the rational order.

THE SOCIAL FIELD AS A CONTEXT OF OCCUPATIONAL THERAPISTS' INTERVENTION

From the early twentieth century onwards in Brazil, medicine has had an important role in defining the parameters for order in daily life. The notion of social pathology, as described by Carvalho,[25] was applied to two groups: the marginalized (those involved in prostitution, vices, social instability, maladjustment, and social difficulties) and the antisocial (those involved in crime, rule-breaking, and petty antisocial behaviors). The intervention of occupational therapists in the social field in Brazil started by focusing on those groups whose internment[7,26,27] was justified under the category of social pathology.

A debate started to take place toward the end of the 1970s, when occupational therapists, aware of the movements[28] favoring the universalization of social rights, grasped the sociopolitical dimension of their practice. They began to work in social projects and institutions that had previously been outside their usual scope. Some of these professionals offered to participate in projects in educational and correctional establishments – mainly those working with children, adolescents, elders, and prisoners. However, criticism of the use of the medical perspective in social affairs raised new problems, since medicine had played such an important role in creating segregated establishments as a means of sanitizing society.

In response to this, occupational therapists who were concerned about the social dynamics that had produced this reality sought to discuss such issues, asking themselves if they should work with these groups in social institutions.[27,29] This questioning encouraged the emergence of a critical view of occupational therapy, focused on the process of social exclusion. However, it offered little contribution in the sense of proposing an alternative approach that could address the complexity of the situation in which occupational therapists worked. Therefore, some of them continued to reproduce the therapeutic models they were used to, such as moral, behavioral, and neurodevelopmental models.[29,30]

In the case of support provided for children and adolescents, the functionalist view on social marginality and the policies developed in the 1970s still guided professional practice, centered on a reductionist and individualizing approach and developed in the exclusive arena of clinical practice. Taking studies on human development as their reference point, occupational therapists developed their practice from the perspective of concepts such as function/dysfunction, normal/handicapped, and well-behaved/troublesome, revealing an adult-centered, disciplinary, top-down approach. Consequently, in the late 1970s in Brazil occupational therapy did not solve its own contradictions in the social field, restricting its actions to other fields of occupational therapy.[8,27,29]

Concern with the social dimension of service users was slowly incorporated as one aspect among others, dissociated from social and cultural dynamics. However, this concern with the social aspect strengthened the critique of the division between knowledge and practice in occupational therapy fields.

New practices and ideas began to transform the knowledge developed in the area, exposing the fragmented perspective that was used by practitioners to approach the person under treatment, a classification and approach that divided the patient into separate parts of an abstract whole, i.e. into physical, mental, and social aspects.

Criticism of these Cartesian assumptions made room for new professional movements, community action and deinstitutionalization being the most meaningful contributions made by the debate on the social field in occupational therapy. It also encouraged the search for new theoretical sources,[5,15,16,18,31,32] following more historical, dynamic, and complex frames of reference. This favored viewing the patient as a sociopolitical being imbedded in a cultural and historical process, rather than as a sum of fragmented parts.

Occupational therapists need to review the concepts behind and the objectives of their actions if they want to contribute to social change and improve social equality. The essential challenge remains that inequality continues to produce vulnerability, and without a different approach this will lead to the segregation, devaluation, incapacitation, and institutionalization of a significant part of the population. To achieve this social change, it is necessary to transcend the conception of occupational therapy as exclusively a health profession whose founding paradigm restricts its role to the health–disease mediation.

THE PARTICIPATION OF OCCUPATIONAL THERAPISTS IN THE PROCESSES OF DEINSTITUTIONALIZATION

The notion of deinstitutionalization originated in the processes of social and institutional restructuring of European and North American societies after the First and Second World Wars,[31–34] in which modern states started to take official responsibility for their so-called social problems. In other words, the deinstitutionalization movement had its roots in the post-war Welfare State. In this setting, intellectuals developed a growing role in the organization and administration of social life. This was increasingly underpinned by scientific rationalism, the main characteristic of which was to make the link between knowledge and technique in order to solve identified problems.[18,33]

The political and theoretical choice for deinstitutionalization revealed different options and produced different ideas for addressing the problem of 'total institutions', whether they were asylums, prisons, or rehabilitation institutions. Two possibilities were presented: the first, developed in the United States, France, and England, emphasized the creation of community services; the second, restricted to the field of mental health and developed by the Italians, focused on the need to create conditions that would deconstruct the mental asylum from within, overcoming its logic and operation.

According to Basaglia,[6] mental illness should be strategically separated from the notion of madness, and is understood by him as mental suffering or human contradiction. It became important to emphasize this separation in order to question not only psychiatry but also Western rationalism and its operation in the field of Humanities. The concept of deinstitutionalization, according to the view of the Italian democratic psychiatrists,[33,34,35] implies the deconstruction of the culture of the asylum and the creation of strong, non-hierarchical, complex, territorial services responsible for attending people's needs. Thus, in order to address the needs of each person, services such as local health centers, outpatient units, social centers, day hospitals, and night hospitals should be provided. Also, it is important to promote joint initiatives with other institutions in order to create cooperatives, accommodation, and therapeutic companionship programs for those undergoing mental suffering who are in need of these services.

The development of the concept of citizenship became a central concern in the late 1970s and early 1980s in Brazil. At the same time, at the international level, human rights movements were widening their scope of action and providing a frame of reference for social action. A yearning for social and political change gradually developed into various social movements, making demands that ranged from access to public services to the democratization of the country's political life. This included demands for political amnesty, the struggle against the increasing cost of living, and the call for better health and education provision and for improved quality of life. At that time, the social struggle was centered on issues such as access to social rights and the mechanisms of social exclusion. Exclusion became a predominant topic for analysis in popular movements during the 1990s. It comprises the condition of people excluded either from structural processes (such as labor) or from social exchange; it is also used to refer to both the processes that lead to exclusion and the resistance of excluded people to their life predicament.[30] These social struggles, which included the critical movement against institutions such as the asylum and the prison, required deep changes in the understanding and intervention of occupational therapy.

Criticism of the very existence of 'total institutions' produced a growing tendency to understand the user as a valuable interlocutor, i.e. as someone who has a say. The main consequence of this is the idea that health and social workers have to assume full responsibility (*presa-in-carico*)[36] for the care of people within a particular area, called a *territory* by the Italian Democratic Psychiatric Movement,[33,35,37] a concept which will be explained below. It is clear that the processes of deinstitutionalization launched and supported the development of a new practice in occupational therapy, with the following principles:

- Service users have citizen's rights and all their needs should be taken into account.

- Emphasis should be put on transdisciplinary actions and on sociological and anthropological knowledge.

- There is a need for professional training designed to support people in need according to the severity of their condition.

- Occupational therapists should be seen as social and political agents.

- Activity, as a human praxis, should be valued as a means of socialization and interrelationship, and of inclusion within work, life, and economic emancipation.

- Activity should be understood as part of the real life process and should be individually designed for each person, context, and history.

- The approach to the use of activities should disregard the assumption that they are abstract and may be studied and prescribed for particular pathologies, symptoms, and hypothetical situations.

- In places where segregation is still evident, the emphasis of the occupational therapist's work should be on activities which provide socialization and self-expression; and there should also be a focus on situations that promote the deconstruction of the institutional life, followed by the construction of alternative modes of life.

TERRITORIAL ACTION IN MENTAL HEALTH AND THE REBIRTH OF THE SOCIAL QUESTION IN OCCUPATIONAL THERAPY

The notion of territory adopted here, as a methodological proposal, presupposes a geographical space defined historically with social, economic, cultural, and symbolic relations still to be revealed.[3] In this space, different ways of being, dreaming and aspiring, living, working, and accomplishing social interchange may be observed. This notion requires an understanding of health intervention that goes beyond the notion of risk used by the World Health Organization (WHO), which focuses on the isolation and choice of certain variables, mainly biological, for the development of health interventions. Rather, health interventions should address the notion of life possibility, which takes into account the ecological and social environment where people live. Hence life chances are believed to determine people's health chances.[18,37]

The notion of territory thus implies the fundamental idea of recognizing the other, of accepting otherness. For that to happen certain conditions need to be established. First, specialized knowledge should give way to the idea of making use of a plurality of knowledge on social issues. Second, people's actions should be disassociated from the idea that they may be the result of an ill or deviant body or mind, and should rather be viewed as the result of the mediation of culture, from which nobody can be separated. Third, occupational therapy action should be moved from the therapeutic setting to the common settings of everyday life. Finally, the concept of activity as an individual process should be replaced by the view of activity as historical and cultural processes lived by people or groups.

If these steps are not followed, it is impossible to talk about a *social* occupational therapy. It is necessary to break with the discourse that limits health to the medical and psychological model and, instead, engage with the complexity of community life. The task of transforming occupational therapy support has required an interdisciplinary competence that has brought about innovative responses in the newly created services (see the story of João da Viola in Ch. 30). It has also required going beyond the clinical, the dual relationship, transcending the need for a prescribed setting, and facing a new frame reference: the territory.[3,27,38]

A challenge that has emerged from this is the search for new guidelines. In order to construct these, concepts such as occupation, work, and activity have to be deconstructed and newly reconstructed, in order to expand the possibilities of those who are confined within walls and isolated from cultural and social exchanges.

According to Galheigo,[26,29] Brazilian occupational therapists have been invited to re-examine their role as the keepers of social adaptation in the light of the role of social articulators (see Ch. 7). Thus they have been called to think over the specificity of this field of action. Galheigo argues that there is a need to constitute a field of knowledge, both in theoretical and practical terms, which will result in the possibility of thinking about, articulating, and producing the required knowledge according to three domains, namely: the macro-structural and conceptual level; the political and operational level; and the personal and collective assistance level. Such levels are themselves intertwined within daily life, making up the dynamics of professional reality to which social occupational therapy belongs. Such a practice is based upon a dialogue between different social sectors (such as health, education, and social services) and also between different disciplines, through a transdisciplinary frame of reference.[26,29]

SOCIAL OCCUPATIONAL THERAPY AND ITS PRACTICE WITH SOCIAL GROUPS UNDERGOING THE BREAKDOWN OF THEIR SOCIAL SUPPORT NETWORKS

From the sociological point of view, we can identify two target groups of the disciplinary discourse that constitute the population of social occupational therapy. The first target group is composed of those who live in a state of exclusion. Their institutionalization is justified by the fact that they are considered dangerous to society; in other words, they are undergoing a process of social exclusion to facilitate their recovery, education, and/or repression. Among others, these include people who still occupy 'total institutions' that are isolated from the community, such as asylums, psychiatric hospitals, institutions for the handicapped, and prisons; institutionalized children and adolescents in youth custody centers; and elders who are inmates of asylums and who are deprived of social rights. The second target group is composed of those who are exposed to insecurity in work, due to social changes in labor relations, to relational vulnerability and, consequently, to marginalization and the breakdown of their social support networks. For this group, the failure of integration is associated with the deterioration of the world of work and its consequences for quality of life, such as poor access to housing, education, sociability, and culture, leading to processes of disaffiliation.[39,40] They live under constant threat of exclusion.

Thus, occupational therapy is able to make a contribution in fields that have until recently remained outside its remit. In doing so, it is important for occupational therapists to keep in mind that the struggle against exclusion implies the struggle that is under way against the deregulation of work and in favor of the redistribution of wealth. It is also necessary to consider that actions should be imbedded in an aware, political process. This new role for occupational therapy in Brazil has been made possible by its history, by the magnitude of the critical debate on the total institutions and, above all, by a new understanding of the use of activity as a resource for mediation in social processes.[29,38] The adoption of this role requires a review and reformulation of the concepts developed above and a redirection the professional praxis.[41–43]

Analyzing the strategies and resources used for the promotion of inclusion and participation in different social groups, we notice that activities (related to either craftsmanship, art, culture, or income generation) have become an organizing axis for intervention (see Ch. 30). Society acknowledges activities as valuable resources; however, few occupational therapists have been attentive to this new sort of demand. In Brazil, new social agents, such as the street educator, the craftsman, and the cultural agent[44] have appeared, showing that activities are considered as essential resources. Social occupational therapy may reinvent itself by accepting the challenge of making a link between this social demand and the accumulation of knowledge on the use of activity as a mediator of support.

The proposal of a social field in occupational therapy, which has emerged from the abandonment of reductionist models and simplistic perspectives, has taken on new meanings and commitments since the late 1990s. Its rise has been an outcome of seeking an approach to problems by learning to recognize social needs and to develop creative solutions. This has made the methods used dependent upon the comprehension and interpretation of social reality, and not the other way around. In addition, it has resulted in a redefinition of aims and means of intervention, establishing occupational therapy over broader frames of reference.

A new outline for addressing social issues, highlighted by Castel,[40] has defined another type of demand. During the 1980s and 1990s changes in work led to the degradation of work relations and of associated systems of social protection. Changes in social rules have led to the emergence of individuals who undergo disqualification, social disability, and breakdown of personal or social bonds, who are under threat of being socially excluded or discriminated against. However, at the same time, organized civil society has gradually turned against these excluding processes. Civil society is broadly understood here as all of those who do not work for the Government or the State and who work on behalf of the community: the popular movements, churches, unions, and associations. Even so, there are contradictions in the role these organizations play; many of them have strongly criticized the lack of public policies and have struggled in favor of social rights.

SOCIAL OCCUPATIONAL THERAPY: REVIEWING CONCEPTS

Occupational therapy is mainly based upon communication processes and actions, simultaneously operated by different language and thought forms. In other words, talking about activity is the same as talking about the processes of communication and interpretative mediation that take place between the phenomenon and the person involved.[45–48] After all, to act, to react, to interact and to do are significant means of saying something about the world in a concrete and material way, i.e. these activities represent the interaction of mankind with his historicity. This interpretative mediation is, therefore, tied up with the representations of the world determined by history. It is the comprehension of the inseparability between mankind and world and between personal history and social history that gives identity to social occupational therapy. Our reactions to reality, and our physical and living interactions with the material world, are signs of multiple and complex communications. In this context it is important to consider experience alongside historicity. Attributed senses and meanings are apprehended by persons within the social and historical context to which they belong.

This view is contrary to the dominant assumption that establishes a dichotomy between individual and society, mankind and nature, mankind and culture, body and mind, and because of which occupational therapists are tricked into the illusion that their subjects are separated from the environment and from society. For that reason, social occupational therapy is only defined within the social and historical context and interrelation. Social occupational therapy understands people in the space between the objectivity of their problems and the subjectivity of the interpretation of their needs; in the space between their perception of their own lives and the point of view of the occupational therapist; in the space between the use of technique and the difficulties of everyday life.

The role of occupational therapists is defined by the characteristics, problems, and concrete needs of the population with whom and for whom they work; moreover, this role is delineated by their social responsibility as health professionals within a changing system.

We believe that giving priority to the point of view of the user in defining professional interventions is not a usual procedure and this causes difficulties in understanding, carrying out, and accepting this approach. The same can also be said of the way that this approach does not accept the activity as an abstraction, empty of a concrete sense for the persons involved. Activity should be defined according to existential meaning and to people's motivation, rather than being technically prescribed. This concept of activity assimilates the unconscious dimension from psychology, but it also becomes a concept full of historicity, since as it is an instrument for emancipation, it has to be sustained by a social, cultural, and political dimension. It is actually an unfinished concept, based on evidence; it is universal because it moves through different situations; it also has different meanings for each particular situation, and it only makes sense within the context of the exchanges and practices wherein it takes place.

The activity becomes meaningful at the crossroads of kaleidoscopic interpretations: it is apprehended, lived, and acted by each of its actors and it is modified by the intention of transformation existent in the aims of the program in which the activity is imbedded. That is the reason why the concept of activity in social occupational therapy is a construct, a mediation of multiple relationships placed in time and within cultural references. As has been said above, it is unfinished and embodies its own incompleteness; it is dynamic and constitutes itself by the process of communication in the form of verbal or non-verbal language that is symbolic, iconic. The notion of activity is materialized through experience and is linked to the way people feel it, and the meanings they attribute to it. The activity is built by communication, experience, and lived situations, according to the history, social practices, and cultural values of particular persons or social groups. For that reason, it is both singular and plural, and it may become an instrument of emancipation or alienation. As a matter of fact, the chosen purposes and processes characterize the activity as a promoter of emancipation and citizenship.

Occupational therapy includes fields of knowledge and intervention from health, education, and the social domain, and should develop adequate methodologies for community and territorial actions. Therefore the occupational therapist is required to accept challenges and try to contribute to the formulation and development of actions that may help to solve problems associated with the process of the breakdown of the social support networks. There is a case for encouraging an epistemological attitude in occupational therapy, wherein the choice of interventions should be considered by comprehension of the demand and by the use of activities as a centralizing and guiding element for the construction of a complex and contextual process.[49]

It seems essential to seek connections in order to explain an occupational therapy that has been developed out of the health–disease structural axis. In order to envision the practice of social occupational therapy, the relationship between occupational therapy, society, and culture has to be argued and methodological principles have to be delineated. However, we should insure that this debate does not inhibit reflection or establish pre-defined models that lack the ability to take into account the flux of reality, history, and life in context.

References

1. Nascimento BA. *O mito da atividade terapêutica.* Revista de Terapia Ocupacional da USP 1991; 1(1):17–21.
2. Oliver FC, Barros DD, Medeiros H, Paganizzi L. *La función social-diálogo entre colegas (Brasil y Argetina) acerca de la función social de la terapia ocupacional. Materia Prima.* Primera Revista Independiente de Terapia Ocupacional en Argentina 2000; 4:5–8.
3. Oliver FC, Barros DD. *Reflexionando sobre desinstitucionalización y terapia ocupacional. Materia Prima.* Primera Revista Independiente de Terapia Ocupacional en Argentina 1999; 4(13):17–20.
4. Mângia EF. *Psiquiatria e tratamento moral: o trabalho como ilusão da liberdade.* Revista de Terapia Ocupacional da USP 1997; 8(2/3):91–97.
5. Goffman E. *Prisões, manicômios e conventos.* São Paulo: Perspectiva; 1974.
6. Basaglia F. *Le istituzioni della violenza e le istituzione della toleranza.* In: Basaglia F. *Scritti II: 1968–1980.* Torino: Einaudi; 1982:80–86.
7. Benetton MJ. *Uma abordagem psicodinâmica em terapia ocupacional.* Revista de Terapia Ocupacional da USP 1991; 1(2/3):55–59.
8. Nascimento BA. *Loucura, trabalho e ordem: o uso do trabalho e da ocupação em instituições psiquiátricas.* São Paulo; 1991. *(Dissertação de mestrado – Ciências Sociais, PUC).*
9. Medeiros MHR. *A terapia ocupacional como um saber: um enfoque epistemológico e social.* São Paulo: Hucitec/EduFSCar; 2003.
10. Mângia EF. *Apontamentos sobre o campo da terapia ocupacional.* Revista de Terapia Ocupacional da USP 1998; 9(1):5–13.
11. Lopes RE. *Cidadania, políticas públicas e terapia ocupacional, no contexto das ações de saúde mental e saúde da*

pessoa portadora de deficiência, no Município de São Paulo. Campinas; 1999. *(Tese de doutorado – UNICAMP).*

12. Nicácio MFS. *O processo de transformação da saúde mental em Santos: desconstrução de saberes, instituições e cultura.* São Paulo; 1994. *(Dissertação de mestrado – Ciências Sociais, PUC).*

13. Barros DD. *Cidadania versus periculosidade social: a desinstitucionalização como desconstrução de um saber.* In: Amarante P. *Psiquiatria social e reforma psiquiátrica.* 2nd edn. Rio de Janeiro: Fiocruz; 1998:171–195.

14. Pinel P. *Traité médico-philosophique sur l'aliénation mentale.* 2nd edn. Paris: JA Brosson; 1809.

15. Foucault M. *História da loucura na idade clássica.* São Paulo: Perspectiva; 1987.

16. Foucault M. *Vigiar e punir. Nascimento da prisão.* Petrópolis: Vozes; 1983.

17. Cohen S. Visions of social control: crime, punishment and classification. Cambridge: Polity Press; 1985.

18. Basaglia F, Basaglia FO. *Los crímenes de la paz: investigación sobre los intelectuales y los técnicos como servidores de la opresión.* México: Siglo XXI; 1977.

19. De Leonardis O. *Il terzo escluso. Le istituzione come vinculo e come risorce.* Milano: Feltrinelli; 1990.

20. Barros DD. *Os Jardins de Abel: desconstrução do manicômio de Trieste.* São Paulo: EDUSP/Lemos Editorial; 1994.

21. Barros DD. *Habilitar–reabilitar … o rei está nu? Revista de Terapia Ocupacional da USP* 1991; 2(2):100–104.

22. Gramsci A. *Quaderni del cacere: gli intellectuali e l'organizzazione della cultura.* Torino: Eunaudi; 1955.

23. Sartre JP. *Em defesa dos intelectuais.* São Paulo: Ática; 1994.

24. Nascimento BA. *A saúde e a saúde.* São Paulo: Pontifícia Universidade Católica de São Paulo; 1986. [unpublished work]

25. Carvalho B. *Medicina social.* São Paulo: EDUSP; 1964.

26. Galheigo SM. *Repensando o lugar do social: a constituição de um campo de conhecimento em terapia ocupacional.* Águas de Lindóia: Programas e Resumos do VI Congresso Brasileiro de Terapia Ocupacional 1999; 1:24.

27. Barros DD. *Operadores de saúde na área social. Revista de Terapia Ocupacional da USP* 1990; 1:11–16.

28. Gohn MG. *Teorias dos movimentos sociais. Paradigmas clássicos e contemporâneos.* São Paulo: Loyola; 1997.

29. Galheigo SM. *O social: idas e vindas de um campo de ação em terapia ocupacional.* In: Pádua EMM de, Magalhães LV. *Terapia ocupacional, teoria e prática.* Campinas: Papirus; 2003:29–48.

30. Teixeira LB. *Terapia ocupacional: lógica do capital ou do trabalho?* São Paulo: Hucitec; 1991.

31. Castel R. Decentralization of social interventions. *Per la Salute Mentale/For Mental Health* 1988; 1:205–210.

32. Gallio G. *A transformação da psiquiatria italiana: história, teoria e prática. Cidade Universitária – Universidade de São Paulo.* São Paulo, 20 de março de 1990. [unpublished work]

33. Rotelli F, De Leonardis O, Mauri D. *Desinstitucionalização, uma outra via.* In: Nicácio F. *Desinstitucionalização.* São Paulo: Hucitec; 1990:17–59.

34. Bachrach L. Deinstitutionalization: an analytical review and sociological perspective. Rockville: National Institute of Mental Heath; 1976.

35. Rotelli F, De Leonardis O, Mauri D. *Itinéraire d'un mouvement.* Perspectives *Psychiatriques* 1982; 5(89): 387–394.

36. Dell'Acqua G, Mezzina R. *Risposta alla crisi: strategie ed intenzionalità dell'intervento nel servizio psichiatrico territoriale.* Per la Salute Mentale/For Mental Health 1988; 1:3–23.

37. Rotelli F. The invented institution. *Per la Salute Mentale/For Mental Health* 1988; 1:189–196.

38. Barros DD, Lopes RE, Ghirardi MIG. *Terapia ocupacional e sociedade.* Revista de Terapia Ocupacional da USP 1999; 10(2/3):71–76.

39. Castel R. *Da indigência à exclusão, a desfiliação. Precariedade do trabalho e vulnerabilidade relacional.* In: Lancetti A. *Saudeloucura 4.* São Paulo: Hucitec; 1994:21–48.

40. Castel R. *As metamorfoses da questão social: uma crônica do salário.* 2nd edn. Petrópolis: Vozes; 1999.

41. Freire P. *Ação cultural para a liberdade e outros escritos.* Rio de Janeiro: Paz e Terra; 1978.

42. Freire P. *Pedagogia do oprimido.* Rio de Janeiro: Paz e Terra; 1979.

43. Vásquez AS. *Filosofia da práxis.* Rio de Janeiro: Paz e Terra; 1990.

44. Graciani MSS. *Pedagogia social de rua.* São Paulo: Cortez/Instituto Paulo Freire; 1997.

45. Lima EA. *Terapia ocupacional: um território de fronteira?* Revista de Terapia Ocupacional da USP 1991; 2(2):100–104.

46. Ghirardi MI. *Educação inclusiva, processos psicológicos e a terapia ocupacional.* Revista de Terapia Ocupacional da USP 2000; 11(1):13–16.

47. Brunello MIB. *História de vida: uma técnica de aproximação da realidade.* Revista de Terapia Ocupacional da USP 1997; 8(2/3):87–90.

48. Brunello MIB. *Loucura: um processo de desconstrução da existência.* Revista de Terapia Ocupacional da USP 1998; 9(1):14–19.

49. *Centro de Docência e Pesquisa em Terapia Ocupacional. O Curso de Terapia Ocupacional da Faculdade de Medicina da Universidade de São Paulo.* São Paulo; 1997.

Chapter 12

The presence of child spirituality
Surviving in a marginalizing world

Imelda Burgman, Abigail King

OVERVIEW

The contribution of spirituality to children's sense of self and sense of agency is a neglected area of knowledge in our understanding, and children surviving marginalization have had limited opportunities to voice their knowing of themselves and their lives. In this chapter the presence of spirituality in contributing to the resilience of these children through qualities such as hope, trust, and faith is explored from philosophical, theoretical, and research perspectives. Children's connections to their own dreams and desires, to others, to nature, and to meaningful cultural experiences all contribute to giving them a sense of purpose and meaning in an often difficult world. As occupational therapists we need to be mindful of the presence and the expression of spirituality in the lives of children surviving marginalization so that we can connect with and assist them in ways that have meaning and power for each of them in the community, society, and world in which they live.

INTRODUCTION

The aim of soul work is not adjustment to accepted norms or to an image of the statistically healthy individual. Rather, the goal is a richly elaborated life, connection to society and nature, woven into the culture of family, nation and globe.[1] (p. xvii)

Children need access to meaningful occupations in order to connect with their spirituality, finding purpose and therefore meaning in their lives. Spirituality is expressed in the daily activities of children; communicated in their self-care, play, connections with nature, conversations, and participation in educational, religious, and work contexts. When children experience occupational apartheid (see Ch. 6) through isolation from meaningful cultural practices, they are facing disconnection not only from their community but also from their own spirit. The contribution of recent occupational therapy theory[2,3] has highlighted the need for occupational therapy practice to undertake a paradigm change[4] that includes spirituality within daily practice. The core component of spirituality[2] in the lives of children is ultimately a primary enabler for successful adaptation to the challenges in their lives. Their ability to utilize spiritual qualities such as hope, courage, and trust underlies their potential across all aspects of their lives.

Traditional theories of childhood position children as unknowing and powerless. They place the understanding of childhood and the needs of children within adult narratives that do not enable children to live out their own truths. Dominant cultural narratives also fail to support the spirituality and meaningful lived experiences of children surviving marginalization. When children are valued and supported through alternative narratives, they are enabled to express their self-agency and are empowered to realize their potential as contributing members of their communities. The spirituality of children surviving marginalization is seen in their emotional resilience to the adversities in their lives and their continuing engagement in life. To assist children who are at risk and who are vulnerable because of the overwhelming nature of their circumstances, we need to develop our understanding and ability to assist them to identify and connect with their spiritual qualities, to engage the power of their spirits in the meaning-making of their lives. We also need to assist them in building a sense of connection within their own communities and within the world in which they live, enabling them to draw on the collective power and resilience of those connections. Within the cultural and daily rituals and activities of life, children surviving marginalization can find peace and connection to be able to sustain, nurture, and heal their spirits.

THE MAKING OF MEANING

Meaninglessness inhibits fullness of life and is therefore equivalent to illness. Meaning makes a great many things endurable – perhaps everything.[5] (p. 373)

Spirituality refers not only to the way children construct meaning,[6] it is also their source of motivation for daily activity.[7] The way in which children enact their lives and thereby make meaning is a basic tenet of the work of occupational therapy. Children's inner worlds, truths, and experiences are projected into their daily activities and interactions with others and with nature. The use of language, play, art, music, humor,[8–10] and daily activity reflects and connects children with what is meaningful in their lives. Two theoretical models that present the concept of spirit or spirituality as being central to each person are the Canadian Model of Occupational Performance (CMOP)[2] and the Occupational Performance Model (Australia) (OPM (Aust)).[3] Each of the models presents its own broad conceptualization of spirituality and the understanding of its centrality and importance in people's lives. The CMOP places spirituality as the central essence of each human being. Spirituality is conceptualized as providing personal meaning to everyday life and life choices.[2] The OPM (Aust) views spirit as one of three fundamental elements of the person (the others being mind and body), which 'is imbedded in all aspects of occupational existence'.[3] (p. 12) Children's access to spirituality and hence participation in meaningful activity is restricted or denied in all societies where the injustice of occupational apartheid exists.

As occupational therapists and as a profession, what do we then bring to our relationships with these children? We bring our values and principles, our professional knowledge and skills, our valuing of our professional knowing, our beliefs about childhood and wellbeing, our experience with other children, our successes and failures and what we have understood of them, and our experiences of life and of having been a child. But we are also capable of bringing our joy in working with children, our belief in their power and agency, our belief in their potential (and ours), our interest in who they are and what they feel and want. How these are woven together within each of us contributes to the creation of who we are as occupational therapists. The ways of thinking promoted by our universities and schools contribute to a collective enactment of a therapeutic culture.[11–16] We need to be mindful of how our ways of thinking about childhood affect the ways we make our own meanings and communicate these to the children we are serving. Providing meaningful interventions demands cultural and spiritual sensitivity that will not marginalize children within an adult-centered medical or problem-focused system. It also demands that we consider and come to know our own spirituality and personal values and the impact that these have on our relationships with children. If we do not understand our professional and personal selves, then how can we understand the influence that these identities have upon the children that we seek to help?

Occupational therapists' understanding and application of therapy is traditionally based upon prescribed Western understandings of children's social and emotional needs and resources.[15,17–19] If we do not critically reflect on these understandings we are at risk of positioning children as lesser; lesser than our adult selves, and certainly lesser than they are capable of being. If we consider children to be always in need of adult guidance, in aspects of their lives from the physical to the spiritual, then we will also develop a relationship with them that positions them as powerless and will perceive them primarily in that role. We can choose to sustain the therapeutic relationship at the professional level, defined by the medical and psychological models of childhood, but we would be doing so at a cost to a child's self that we may never understand. If, however, we choose to see children as knowing themselves far better than we ever will, then we can approach our relationships with them with a greater openness to what may happen and what we will learn.[20–24] Children bring much to the therapeutic relationship: knowing of their identity, knowing of their self, knowing of their spirit, knowing of the difficulties and pleasures of *their* world, and *their* wishes for what is important to face, to leave, or to consider.

Enacting therapy

In order for occupational therapists to gain insight into and address the spiritual beliefs and values held by children and the way these impact on their lives and wellbeing,[25] it is important to understand the stories of their lives.[24,26] In order to facilitate change in the lives of children, occupational therapists need to remain cognizant of the power of children's perceptions and their understandings of themselves in relation to their ability to achieve. Theorists have explored and offered explanations for motivation and suffering.[27,28] However, the meanings that motivate children and adults are often indescribable and intangible. We do know that spirituality finds expression through connection – be it through action, through another person or group of people, through art, nature, or religious practice. We all evoke each other's presence and it is this that is fundamental to our therapeutic relationships.[29] As therapists we must try to understand the way that children construct and express meaning. The importance of spiritual expression then becomes paramount to the success of our interventions.

The purpose of facilitating therapeutic change is to bring positive influences to bear on children's abilities and desires to attempt and pursue new roles and tasks – awakening confidence and spiritual power.[30–34] By listening with interest[35] and respect,[6,10] and demonstrating spiritual qualities ourselves, we demonstrate qualities for children to identify with within themselves. It is important to become familiar with the language of emotional distress across cultures and to understand cultural beliefs imbedded in expressions of spirit.[36–42] It is our responsibility to acknowledge and facilitate access to and expression of this inner essence in helping children in their journey towards wellbeing. Thus we need to understand what spirituality may mean and how it may be expressed in the lives of children surviving marginalization.

THE PRACTICE OF SPIRIT

Spirituality is the practice of spirit – the conscious, goal-directed activity which brings spirit and soul into being.[43] (p. 198)

Embodiment of spirituality

The expression of spirituality for children is wrapped within their reality and the meanings of their lives. The connection of children to their own spirituality and to the world's spirituality highlights the meaning of spiritual inclusiveness, within which they embrace, and are embraced by, the world. This spirit of inclusiveness reflects Townsend's[44] community spirituality within which each person's uniqueness is honored and in turn contributes to the psychological health and strength of the community. In the philosophical and theological works of those who have attempted to define its meaning, spirituality has come to encompass many qualities, including faith, courage, trust, hope, belonging, compassion, purpose, joy, awe, wonder, creativity, awareness, and transcendence.[45–51] What is central to all these works is the acknowledgement that each of us is a spiritual being who is trying to construct meaning in our life. When spiritual qualities are expressed through the self they become qualities such as resilience, self-esteem, playfulness, humor, enthusiasm, curiosity, adaptive behavior, engagement, connection with others, forgiveness, and meaning.[1,51-55] For example, the spiritual qualities of belonging, trust, and faith (in oneself and others) are evidenced in the connections children make with others. Thus spiritual qualities affect personal reality, and consequently the wider realities of family, community, and society.[55] Being able to find meaning in daily life assists in the strengthening of positive coping behaviors and resilience to the experience of occupational apartheid.[54,57-60]

Resilience and survival of the self encompass coping and optimism,[14,61,62] which are built on a foundation of hope[63] and faith in life's meaning and purpose.[64,65] The more tenuous children's beliefs and understandings are, or the more dependent they are on others for validation, the more vulnerable they are to outside stresses.[1,54,59,66] Children's ability to draw on the courage and power of the spirit facilitates healing through the positive expression of emotions, which in turn influences positive actions.[53,66] The embodiment of the spiritual qualities of love, joy, and connection assists in building resilience and self-esteem[59] while alleviating the impact of emotions such as despair, anger, and hopelessness. The expression of humor is also an embodiment of joy, and supports connection with others and coping in times of stress.[8,9,38,67,68] Psychological and physical health have been shown to be intricately linked with the 'health' of the spirit's expression through the self.[1,53,63,65,69,70] In the pursuit of meaningful outcomes with children, it is important that we help them to access and utilize spiritual qualities in their everyday lives.

Engagement and wholeness

Each child's ability and opportunity to respond to life experiences creates the possibility of engagement or disengagement in life. Persistence in the face of daily struggle, through hopefulness, promotes engagement and wholeness of the self through integration with the spirit. Subjugation of the self, through feelings of hopelessness, creates disengagement and splintering of the self from the spirit.[48,55,65,69,71] Continuing to engage in life's experiences despite difficulties encourages the development of cognitive, physical, and emotional skills through openness to experiences, thereby supporting the development of the self[14,59] and consequently the spirit. Levels of engagement and disengagement in daily life are often observed in the level of curiosity and motivation invested by children in their play and learning. In many religions and cultures response to severe trauma can be influenced by a profound spiritual belief in the purpose of suffering, supporting a continuing engagement and hopefulness in life.[51,72-77] A strong connection of the self to the spirit, and the ability of the self to draw on the nurturance of the spirit, is shown in children's and adults' ability to survive extreme suffering and to continue to hope in spite of overwhelming tragedy.

Connection

Children's connection to their own dreams and desires, continuing to have hope and faith despite living in an unforgiving world, gives them purpose and therefore meaning in their lives. This foundation enables them to remain resilient to the stresses and sorrows of their lives. The need to belong through connection with others is strongly evident in children's participation in community experiences,[36,67,78,79] and for children surviving marginalization, such as homeless children, in their membership in the gangs which form their families.[60,80] In the myriad of relationships that children have with others in their lives, at an individual and collective level, connection to others through love and trust[69] creates respectful and nurturing relationships. Connection with others provides additional support in times of emotional and thus spiritual need, aiding children's resilience to life's challenges and enabling them to respond knowing that their efforts are valued and supported.[63,81–85] Children who feel disconnected experience loneliness, a sense of rejection, feelings of alienation from others, and they are more at risk of depression and suicidal behaviors.[57,63,81,82,86] If we consider children's need for connection with others, then we are considering the importance of the love of family and friends. The meeting of community, society, and culture then supports these connections in a spirituality of inclusiveness[44] within which children are valued. Collective resilience is experienced through supportive relationships with others.[63,87] The collective power[88] of this resilience aids children in sustaining themselves within their daily reality, offering courage and hope to their spirits.

The lived spiritual experience of children seeks expression that is accepted and fostered by others, and in turn seeks to connect with others in ways that are meaningful. Children's perceptions of the world influence their responses and are unique to each child.[89–91] Whether children find their environment and interaction with others to be enriching or limiting will also call upon intrinsic resources, and will assist or hinder the ongoing development of the self.[92,93] The limitations and exclusions of occupational apartheid may occur through dominant societal, religious, or cultural narratives, and will impact on children's ability to sustain their spirit without the nurturance of their world. For these children, including the poor,[91] the homeless,[32,80,94] the displaced,[79] the victims of war,[31,95] and many culturally distinct minorities,[41,96,97] the reliance on the strength of the spirit is an important enabler to an ongoing belief in the value and power of the self.

Spiritual distress

Spiritual distress is experienced when children are not allowed to express their knowing, or their expression is not accepted by others.[98,99] The occupational apartheid experienced by children surviving marginalization leads to an exclusion where their spiritual expression is often not seen, heard, understood, or respected in their dominant society. Subjugation of the spirit, in an effort to survive in a hostile world, may be seen in vulnerable children who live with occupational apartheid because of political or religious oppression, or ethnic hatred.[63] For children who are victims of ongoing conflict, such as the children of Palestine and Northern Ireland, spiritual distress may lead to acts of aggression in an effort to be heard. If distress is not given a voice then children may never heal from the trauma they have experienced.[100] As the 'language' of children surviving marginalization may be different not only from that of adults but also from the dominant understandings of children,[63] we need to broaden our perception of how spirituality is expressed. This means asking, listening carefully, watching closely, and respecting ways of life and meanings much different from our own.[6,36,37,40,42,81,87] When this is done successfully, as in Tenberken's[94] work in Tibet (see Ch. 3) children are released from distress through understanding. Children creating change together speaks of collective power and resilience, supported through hope and trust, which is transformed into creative power that changes their lives.

Children who are perceived by society as marginalized are not generally perceived as resilient, nor are they perceived as beings of self-agency. In contradiction to the *United Nations Convention on the Rights of the Child*,[101] they are not listened to, protected, or valued on a global scale. Therefore, they must deal with the injustices of displacement (from families, from culture), armed conflict, imprisonment, economic hardship, political and cultural oppression, and social and physical exploitation. Dominant cultural narratives do not allow children sociopolitical power, and curtail their freedom to express themselves and to experience a sense of empowerment within their own lives.[12] These children are vulnerable to societal discrimination, environmental dangers, physical illness, and psychological trauma.[42,63,95,102,103]

Children's expressions of their spiritual strength are as varied as their lives, and because of this, in our relationships with children, we need to pay attention to their unique narratives and worldviews. Their spiritual knowing is not tied to religious education, or to cognitive or emotional development.[84,104,105] The unique worldviews of children, meanings that encompass the influences of community, society, and culture (their own and the one in which they live), must be respected in helping them to maintain and regain their sense of spiritual strength. We, as fellow human beings and as a professional body, are in a strong position to advocate for and facilitate the power of children's spirituality as a basis for health and wellbeing.[16]

THE MOVEMENT OF EXISTENCE

The union of soul and body is not an amalgamation between two mutually external terms, subject and object, brought about by arbitrary decree. It is enacted at every instant in the movement of existence.[106] (pp. 88–89)

In Western and non-Western cultures, interactions with people, art, music, stories, and nature, and the motivation for achieving goals and dreams, all manifest children's spirituality in daily life. Coles[84,96,107] has spent many years interviewing children on their experiences and the meanings of their lives. These children have lived in segregated societies, rich and poor neighborhoods, rural and urban landscapes, in war and peace times, and demonstrate the influence of their cultural and religious backgrounds. The lives of these children have been challenged by the changing cultures in which they lived, and were nourished by their sense of purpose and opportunities to express themselves. Opportunities for expression gave children emotional and spiritual strength to pursue the meaning of their lives. Expression through art and nature, and participation in music and stories, are time honored ways of exploring and deepening the connection to one's own spirit (and the spirit of the world) in many cultures.[32,74,96,107–112] The joy and creativity of play is spiritual by nature, manifested through the dimensions of intrinsic motivation, the suspension of reality and an internal locus of control.[113] Play helps children to uncover meaning in daily life and thus is meaning-making.

The extensive work of Kubler-Ross[114–116] and her colleagues was instrumental in challenging Western society's beliefs regarding the understanding and needs of children. Her work presented the ability of children to express their philosophical understanding and spiritual connections in the midst of deep suffering through the use of 'non-verbal symbolic language',[116] (p. 19) such as drawing/painting and play with representational objects. Her work reflects the need for adults to remember once again the language of childhood if we are to understand the depth of children's knowing, in order to be able to respect and converse with that knowing. Children's use of symbols and non-language-based expression of thoughts and experiences is often forgotten by the world of adults and begs the respect of closer attention and understanding if we are to assist children in expressing their spirituality within the meaning of the daily occupations of childhood.

The search for meaning and the exploration of understanding of the self, and of others and the world, are integral to spiritual development.[117–119] That there is more to understand and become known is made explicit through the child's need for time outside the world in order to consider it and reframe it and then to re-enter it. Children need access to a 'space' where they can explore the personal meaning of both positive and negative experiences. For children exposed to war, poverty, sexual abuse, or simply a lack of caring from the world in which they live, this 'space' can enable a much greater healing of a damaged spirit. Simó Algado and colleagues,'[31] work with children in a Kosovo refugee camp (see Ch. 18), Kronenberg's[108] engagement with clowns and street children ('survivors of the street') in Guatemala (see Ch. 19) and the Georgian occupational therapy students'[120] pilot experiences with orphans and internally displaced people in Tbilisi (see Ch. 31) highlight the power of this 'space' to help children reclaim themselves and to find the strength of spirit to continue their lives with hope. Be it via the mediums of daydreaming, play, or the practice of faith and its rituals, children can find a sense of connection and meaning through opportunities to reflect on their daily lives.

Healing spaces

Play

Play as a vehicle for expression and connection to the spirit and to the world also provides a space away from the world, for the consideration and reframing of the world. Children engaging in pretend war play in

Bosnia are dealing with the meaning of ethnic cleansing in their lives and their emotional reactions to its impact, helping themselves to heal. Children making toy boats from scraps and floating them in a drain are removing themselves for a time from the harsh realities of their Manila shanty town and reconnecting with their imaginative and joyful spirits. Play without rules, for expression of the spirit outside of the confines of society, is necessary for the sustaining of the spirit and for its growth.[109,121] Csikszentmihalyi[122] considered the concept of flow as most evident in children when they are at play, where the self is absorbed within the activity and also forgotten. In play, as in leisure, the spirit can be fully expressed through the self, entering into a state of serenity where the world can unfold.[123,124] That this unfolding world can be very different from the lived world gives children respite from their cares and sorrows. Children can be anything or anyone they want to be, can express their dreams and desires, and can create meaning for their lives that they can carry with them into their day-to-day world.

Cultural rituals

The connection of flow experiences with other activities that are not play moves towards spiritual or transcendental experiences that engage the self in a way whereby the self is no longer significant. The immersion of the self and the expression of the spirit are the intrinsic rewards of the experience. This can be seen in the cultural rituals of Aboriginal Australians and the First Nations People of North America where communal spirituality supports the transcendence of the individual.[87,109,125,126] Children and young people may create gang rituals to replace the loss of meaningful cultural rituals of transition to a stronger self and immersion in a self that is greater than the power of one. In response to spiritual distress or feelings of spiritual alienation, children may also engage in substance abuse or sexual promiscuity to remove themselves from their reality, in an attempt to find a better one where their sense of aloneness and despair is eased for a time.[32,86,127–129] These ways do not ultimately support the spirit but can be seen as an attempt to find relief from spiritual distress.

The practice of rituals that reflect inclusiveness of children within their communities, such as the corroborees of Aboriginal Australians,[111] supports children in learning ways to connect: to themselves, their community, and the supportive beliefs of their culture. This inclusiveness has been strong in many cultures,[87,126] helping children to sustain their spirits and to contribute to an ongoing communal spirituality, which they can draw upon in times of need. Children who experience ethnocultural marginalization within the dominant culture, such as the First Nations People, African Americans, or the Sami of Norway, may become emotionally torn between theirs and the dominant culture. Their connections to the nurturance of their own culture may be set aside in an attempt to be accepted and valued by the dominant culture.[97,103,130] For children who are displaced, such as refugees, or otherwise marginalized, such as homeless children, cultural alienation, including the absence of cultural rituals, places them at risk of emotional vulnerability.[100,128,131] Inclusive spirituality needs to be (re)created to offer children the opportunity to experience a sense of wider community, and (re)built in a way that is culturally and personally meaningful. The work of Simó Algado and colleagues[79] with Mayan refugees (see Ch. 25) and children survivors of war in Kosovo[31] (see Ch. 18) reflects the concept of rebuilding in a way that was meaning-making for the community's youth.

Daily rituals   The rituals that lend meaning to daily life, such as tending to a garden, caring for animals, or sharing a meal with the family, are meaningful for children in many cultures,[41,67,96] speaking as they do to a sustained connection to others and nature. The flow of daily rituals offers its own peace to sometimes fractured and terrifying lives. The learning of traditional ways of living and being, in cultures such as those of the Mayan and First Nations People, provides children with connection not only with the time-honored daily rituals of the community as a whole, but also with nurturing connections to the land, nature, and the cosmos.[40,73,87,125,126] The importance of these activities lies not only in their immediate value, but also in their contribution to the laying down over time of experiences and perceptions.[90] This empowers children to find effective and meaningful ways of developing their own sense of self and spirituality. For many refugee children there is a need to reconstruct meaningful daily activities which foster and heal the spirit.[31,79,95] Being traumatized, displaced, and with an uncertain future, these children are at risk of developing perceptions of the world as only a dangerous and uncaring place. Re-establishing daily rituals that provide a peaceful rhythm and a sense of identity, in the home, at school, and in leisure, are vital to replenishing the spirit. For all children surviving marginalization to experience these feelings, we need to enable them through occupational justice, which gives them access to experiences that have personal meaning for them. These meanings will be influenced by cultural preference. For example, what has personal meaning and spiritual power for a child in Tibet[94] may have a different means of expression within the life of a child on the streets of Guatemala,[32] in the favelas of Brazil,[96] or in an urban neighborhood in America.[78] What is important is that we listen to children and that we respect their stories and the meanings that they find in their lives. If we also honor those meanings through our actions, then we will truly be enabling them to access their spirits.

CONCLUSION

Within our relationships with children surviving marginalization we must allow their spirituality to reveal itself and not be defined by us. We have an ethical responsibility to meet children at the places of their being, doing, and knowing, thus meeting the challenge of the paradigm change that acknowledges and incorporates spirituality in the heart and practice of occupational therapy. The influence of spirituality on wellbeing directs our attention to the price we ask of children's physical and emotional selves when we do not heed their spiritual needs. It is manifested in their difficulty in remaining engaged in life, in the seeking of opportunities, and in their determination to pursue their dreams. The finding of meaning can create hope for things to come, that each ending or loss is also a beginning of the new. If we wish to serve children surviving marginalization, and the families, communities, and societies in which these children live, we must support children's connection to themselves, their communities, nature, and the world, in ways that are meaningful and empowering for them.

References

1. Moore T. Care of the soul. New York: Harper Collins; 1992.
2. CAOT, ed. Enabling occupation: an occupational therapy perspective. Ottawa, ON: CAOT; 1997.
3. Chapparo C, Ranka J. Occupational performance model (Australia). Monograph 1. Sydney: Occupational Performance Network; 1996.
4. Dunn W. Independence through activity: the practice of occupational therapy (pediatrics). Am J Occup Ther 1982; 36(11):745–747.
5. Jung CJ. Memories, dreams, reflections. London: Random House; 1961.
6. Unruh AM, Versnel J, Kerr N. Spirituality unplugged: a review of commonalities and contentions, and a resolution. Can J Occup Ther 2002; 69(1):5–19.
7. Egan M, DeLaat MD. Considering spirituality in occupational therapy practice. Can J Occup Ther 1994; 61(2):95–101.
8. Sheldon LM. An analysis of the concept of humor and its application to one aspect of children's nursing. J Adv Nurs 1996; 24(6):1175–1183.
9. Astedt-Kurki P, Isola A, Tammentie T, Kervinen U. Importance of humor to client–nurse relationships and clients' well-being. Int J Nurs Pract 2001; 7(2):119–125.
10. Ward SL. Caring and healing in the 21st century. Am J Matern Child Nurs 1998; 23(4):210–215.
11. Foucault M. The birth of the clinic. London: Routledge; 1973.
12. Merleau-Ponty M. Primacy of perception. USA: Northwestern University Press; 1964.
13. Lupton D. Foucault and the medicalisation critique. In: Petersen A, Bunton R, eds. Foucault, health and medicine. London: Routledge; 1997:94–110.
14. Masten AS. Ordinary magic: resilience processes in development. Am Psychol 2001; 56(3):227–238.
15. Galheigo S. Challenging the constructions of childhood used by therapeutic models. In: 12th WFOT Conference. Paris: 1998.
16. Townsend E. Reflections on power and justice in enabling occupation. Can J Occup Ther 2003; 70(2):74–87.
17. O'Brien V. Early childhood: the social domain. In: Zemke R, Clark F, eds. Occupational science: the evolving discipline. Philadelphia, PA: FA Davis; 1996.
18. James A, Jenks C, Prout A. Theorizing childhood. Cambridge, UK: Polity Press; 1998.
19. Prout A. Childhood bodies: social construction and translation. In: Williams S, Gabe J, Calnan M, eds. Health, medicine and society: key theories, future agendas. London: Routledge; 2000:109–122.
20. Rogers CR. Client-centered therapy. Its current practice, implications, and theory. Boston, MA: Houghton Mifflin; 1951.
21. Rogers CR. On becoming a person. A therapist's view of psychotherapy. London: Constable; 1961.
22. Howard BS, Howard JR. Occupation as spiritual activity. Am J Occup Ther 1997; 51(3):181–185.
23. Spencer J, Davidson H, White V. Helping clients develop hopes for the future. Am J Occup Ther 1997; 51(3):191–198.
24. Mattingly C. Healing dramas and clinical plots. Melbourne: Cambridge University Press; 1998.
25. Barnes LL, Plotnikoff GA, Fox K, et al. Spirituality, religion and pediatrics: intersecting worlds of healing. Pediatrics 2000; 106(4):243–252.
26. Clark F. Occupation imbedded into real life: interweaving occupational science and occupational therapy. Am J Occup Ther 1993; 47(12):1067–1077.
27. Freud S. On metapsychology: the theory of psychoanalysis. Ringwood, VIC: Penguin; 1984.
28. Kielhofner G. A model of human occupation. Theory and application. Baltimore: William & Wilkins; 1995.

29. Van Amburg R. A Copernican revolution in clinical ethics: engagement versus disengagement. Am J Occup Ther 1997; 51(3):186–190.

30. Dugan TF, Coles R, eds. The child in our times. Studies in the development of resiliency. New York: Brunner/Mazel; 1989.

31. Simó Algado S, Mehta N, Kronenberg F, et al. Occupational therapy intervention with children survivors of war. Can J Occup Ther 2002; 69(4):205–217.

32. Kronenberg F. Street children: being and becoming. Research study. Heerlen, The Netherlands: Hogeschool Limburg; 1999.

33. Maslow A. Toward a psychology of being. 3rd edn. New York: John Wiley; 1999.

34. Moustakas C, ed. The child's discovery of himself. New York: Jason Aronson; 1973.

35. Farrar J. Addressing spirituality and religious life in occupational therapy. Phys Occup Ther Geriatr 2001; 18(4):65–85.

36. Leininger M. Transcultural nursing research to transform nursing education and practice: 40 years. J Nurs Scholarsh 1997; 29(4):341–347.

37. Leininger M. A mini journey into transcultural nursing with its founder. Nebr Nurse 2001; 34(2):16–17.

38. Lang M. Then and now: how being Jewish has influenced my work as a psychotherapist. Psychother Aust 2002; 8(3):22–29.

39. Watson MJ. Watson's theory of transpersonal caring. In: Walker PH, Neuman B, eds. Blueprint for use of nursing models: education, research, practice and administration. New York: National League for Nursing Press; 1996:141–184.

40. Darnell R. Occupation is not a cross-cultural universal: some reflections from an ethnographer. J Occup Sci 2002; 9(1):5–11.

41. Thibeault R. Fostering healing through occupation: the case of the Canadian Inuit. J Occup Sci 2002; 9(3):153–158.

42. Hubbard J, Realmuto GM, Northwood AK, et al. Comorbidity of psychiatric diagnoses with post-traumatic stress disorder in survivors of childhood trauma. J Am Acad Child Adolesc Psychiatry 1995; 34(9):1167–1173.

43. Kovel J. History and spirit. Boston: Beacon Press; 1991.

44. Townsend E. Inclusiveness: a community dimension of spirituality. Can J Occup Ther 1997; 64(3): 146–155.

45. Dalai Lama. The good heart. Sydney: Rider; 1996.

46. Fowler JW. Religious institutions. I. Toward a developmental perspective on faith. Relig Educ 1974; LXIX(2):207–219.

47. Hardy SA. The spiritual nature of man. A study of contemporary religious experience. Oxford: Clarendon Press; 1979.

48. Hillman J. A blue fire. New York: Harper & Row; 1989.

49. McGrath AE. Christian spirituality. Oxford: Blackwell; 1999.

50. Weil S. Gravity and grace. London: Routledge & Kegan Paul; 1952.

51. Dalai Lama. An open heart. Sydney: Hodder Headline Australia; 2001.

52. Burkhardt MA. Spirituality: an analysis of the concept. Holist Nurs Pract 1989; 3(3):69–77.

53. Goleman D. Afflictive and nourishing emotions: impacts on health. In: Goleman D, ed. Healing emotions. Boston, MA: Shambala; 1997:33–46.

54. Yahne CA, Miller WR. Evoking hope. In: Miller WR, ed. Integrating spirituality into treatment. Resources for practitioners. Washington, DC: American Psychological Association; 1999:217–234.

55. Zukav G. The seat of the soul. New York: Simon & Schuster; 1989.

56. Dalai Lama. Medicine and compassion. In: Goleman D, ed. Healing emotions. Boston, MA: Shambala; 1997:243–250.

57. Rew L, Taylor-Seehafer M, Thomas NY, et al. Correlates of resilience in homeless adolescents. J Nurs Scholarsh 2001; 33(1):33–40.

58. Miller WR, Thoresen CE. Spirituality and health. In: Miller WR, ed. Integrating spirituality into treatment. Resources for practitioners. Washington, DC: American Psychological Association; 1999:3–18.

59. Fredrickson BL. Cultivating positive emotions to optimize health and well-being. Prevention & Treatment 2000; 3: Article 1. Online. Available: http://journals.apa.org/prevention/volume3/ pre0030001a.html 14 April 2001.

60. Felsman JK. Risk and resiliency in childhood: the lives of street children. In: Dugan TF, Coles R, eds. The child in our times. Studies in the development of resiliency. New York: Brunner/Mazel; 1989:56–80.

61. Friesen MF. Spiritual care for children living in specialized settings. Breathing underwater. New York: Haworth Press; 2000.

62. Seligman MEP. The optimistic child. Sydney: Random House; 1995.

63. Hall J. Marginalization revisited: critical, postmodern, and liberation perspectives. Adv Nurs Sci 1999; 22(2):88–102.

64. Schulz ML. Awakening intuition. Sydney: Bantam; 1998.

65. Frankl VE. Man's search for meaning. London: Hodder and Stoughton; 1959.

66. Myss C. Anatomy of the spirit. Sydney: Bantam; 1996.

67. Hanson I, Hampton MR. Being Indian: strengths sustaining First Nations Peoples in Saskatchewan residential schools. Can J Commun Ment Health 2000; 19(1):127–142.

68. Spitzer P. The clown doctors. Aust Fam Physician 2001; 30(1):12–16.

69. Borysenko J. Guilt is the teacher, love is the lesson. New York: Warner; 1990.

70. Carlson R, Shield B, eds. Healers on healing. New York: Jeremy P Tarcher/Putnam; 1989.

71. Jung CG. Modern man in search of a soul. London: Routledge & Kegan Paul; 1933.

72. Holtz TH. Refugee trauma versus torture trauma: a retrospective controlled cohort study of Tibetan refugees. J Nerv Ment Dis 1998; 186(1):24–34.

73. Napoli M. Holistic health care for Native women: an integrated model. Am J Public Health 2002; 92(10):1573–1575.

74. Newlin K, Knafl K, Melkus G. African-American spirituality: a concept analysis. Adv Nurs Sci 2002; 25(2):57–70.

75. Frank G, Bernardo CS, Tropper S, et al. Jewish spirituality through actions in time: daily occupations of young orthodox Jewish couples in Los Angeles. Am J Occup Ther 1997; 51(3):199–206.

76. Ali AY, tr. The Holy Qur'an. Hertfordshire, England: Wordsworth Editions; 2000.

77. Mascaro J, tr. The Baghavad Gita. London: Penguin; 1962.

78. Rappaport J. Community narratives: tales of terror and joy. Am J Community Psychol 2000; 28(1):1–24.

79. Simó Algado S, Gregori JMR, Egan M. Spirituality in a refugee camp. Can J Occup Ther 1997; 64(1):138–145.

80. Glauser B. Street children: deconstructing a construct. In: James A, Prout A, eds. Constructing and reconstructing childhood: contemporary issues in the sociological study of childhood. London: The Falmer Press; 1990:138–156.

81. Fazel M, Stein A. The mental health of refugee children. Arch Dis Child 2002; 87(5):366–370.

82. Rew L, Thomas N, Horner SD, et al. Correlates of recent suicide attempts in a triethnic group of adolescents. J Nurs Scholarsh 2001; 33(4):361–367.

83. Humphreys JC. Turning and adaptations in resilient daughters of battered women. J Nurs Scholarsh 2001; 33(3):245–251.

84. Coles R. The spiritual life of children. Boston: Houghton Mifflin; 1990.

85. Coles R. Moral energy in the lives of impoverished children. In: Dugan TF, Coles R, eds. The child in our times. Studies in the development of resiliency. New York: Brunner/Mazel; 1989:45–55.

86. Tsey K, Every A. Evaluating Aboriginal empowerment programs: the case of family well being. Aust N Z J Public Health 2000; 24(5):509–514.

87. Waller MA, Patterson S. Natural helping and resilience in a Dine (Navajo) community. Fam Soc 2002; 83(1):73–84.

88. Kulig J. Community resiliency: the potential for community health nursing theory. Public Health Nurs 2000; 17(5):374–385.

89. Jacelon CS. The trait and process of resilience. J Adv Nurs 1997; 25(1):123–129.

90. Bronfenbrenner U, Morris PA. The ecology of developmental processes. In: Damon W, Lerner RM, eds. Handbook of child psychology. Theoretical models of human development. 5th edn. New York: John Wiley; 1998:993–1028.

91. Garmezy N. Reflections and commentary on risk, resilience, and development. In: Haggerty RJ, Sherrod LR, Garmezy N, Rutter M, eds. Stress, risk, and resilience in children and adolescents. Processes, mechanisms, and interventions. Cambridge, UK: Cambridge University Press; 1996:1–18.

92. Bronfenbrenner U. The ecology of human development. Experiments by nature and design. Cambridge, MA: Harvard University Press; 1979.

93. Fine SB. Resilience and human adaptability: who rises above adversity? Am J Occup Ther 1991; 45(6):493–503.

94. Tenberken S. My path leads to Tibet. New York: Arcade; 2003.

95. Weine S, Becker DF, McGlashan TH, et al. Adolescent survivors of 'ethnic cleansing': observations on the first year in America. J Am Acad Child Adolesc Psychiatry 1995; 34(9):1153–1159.

96. Coles R. The moral life of children. New York: Atlantic Monthly Press; 1986.

97. Kvernmo S, Heyerdahl S. Acculturation strategies and ethnic identity as predictors of behavior problems in Arctic minority adolescents. J Am Acad Child Adolesc Psychiatry 2003; 42(1):57–65.

98. Ryan M, Stower L. A vision of the whole child: The significance of religious experiences in early childhood. Aust J Early Child 1998; 23(1):1–4.

99. Carpenito LJ. Spiritual distress. In: Carpenito LJ, ed. Nursing diagnosis: application to clinical practice. Philadelphia: JB Lippincott; 1995:886–905.

100. Berman H. Children and war: current understandings and future directions. Public Health Nurs 2001; 18(4):243–252.

101. United Nations. United Nations Convention on the Rights of the Child. United Nations General Assembly (Resolution 44/25). New York: United Nations; 1989.

102. Masten AS, Miliotis D, Graham-Bermann SA, et al. Children in homeless families: risks to mental health and development. J Consult Clin Psychol 1993; 61(2):335–343.

103. Phinney JS. When we talk about American ethnic groups, what do we mean? Am Psychol 1996; 51(9):918–927.

104. Robinson E. The original vision. Oxford: The Religious Experience Research Unit; 1977.

105. Farmer LJ. Religious experience in childhood: a study of adult perspectives on early spiritual awareness. Relig Educ 1992; 87(2):259–268.

106. Merleau-Ponty M. Phenomenology of perception. London: Routledge & Kegan Paul; 1962.

107. Coles R. Their eyes meeting the world. The drawings and paintings of children. Boston: Houghton Mifflin; 1992.

108. Kronenberg F. Juggling with survivors of the street – occupational therapy, clowns and street children. Paper presented at the 13th WFOT Conference. Stockholm. 2002.

109. Campbell J. The masks of God: primitive mythology. New York: Penguin; 1959.

110. Campbell J. The masks of God: occidental mythology. New York: Penguin; 1964.

111. Yalmambirra. Black time … white time: my time … your time. J Occup Sci 2000; 7(3):133–137.

112. Bradley J. Mapping the sacred. Cultural Survival Quarterly 2002; Summer: 8–10.

113. Levy J. Play behavior. New York: Wiley; 1978.

114. Kubler-Ross E. On death and dying. London: Tavistock; 1969.

115. Kubler-Ross E. Death. The final stage of growth. Englewood Cliffs, NJ: Prentice-Hall; 1975.

116. Kubler-Ross E. Living with death and dying. How to communicate with the terminally ill. New York: Touchstone; 1981.

117. King U. Spirituality in secular society: recovering a lost dimension. British Journal of Religious Education 1985; 7(3):135–139.

118. Langeveld MJ. The stillness of the secret place. Phenomenology + Pedagogy 1983; 1(1):11–17.

119. Rowe D. The construction of life and death. Chichester, England: John Wiley; 1982.

120. Arganashvili A, et al. Occupational therapy with street children and internally displaced people in Georgia. European Network of Higher Education in Occupational Therapy, Module 7, unpublished final assignment reports. Tbilisi, Georgia: 2003.

121. Moustakas CE. Psychotherapy with children. New York: Harper & Row; 1959.

122. Csikszentmihalyi M. Beyond boredom and anxiety. San Francisco: Jossey-Bass; 1975.

123. Ackerman D. Deep play. New York: Vintage; 1999.

124. Pieper J. Leisure. The basis of culture. Markham, Ontario: Penguin; 1963.

125. Gold P. Navajo and Tibetan sacred wisdom. The circle of the spirit. Rochester, VE: Inner Traditions International; 1994.

126. Tripcony P. Too obvious to see: Aboriginal spirituality and cosmology. Journal of Australian Indigenous Issues 1999; 2(4):7–14.

127. Choi H. Understanding adolescent depression in ethnocultural context. Adv Nurs Sci 2002; 25(2):71–85.

128. Whitworth Wittig MC, Wright JD, Kaminsky DC. Substance use among street children in Honduras. Subst Use Misuse 1997; 32(7&8):805–827.

129. Jutkowitz JM, Spielmann H, Koehler U, et al. Drug use in Nepal: the view from the street. Subst Use Misuse 1997; 32(7&8):987–1004.

130. Phinney JS. Ethnic identity in adolescents and adults: review of research. Psychol Bull 1990; 108(3):499–514.

131. Hodes M. Refugee children: may need a lot of psychiatric help. BMJ 1998; 316(7134):793–794.

Chapter **13**

Challenges for occupational therapy in community-based rehabilitation

Occupation in a community approach to handicap in development

Hetty Fransen

OVERVIEW

An encounter with other cultures can lead to openness only if you can suspend the assumption of superiority, not seeing new worlds to conquer, but new worlds to respect.[1]

The promotion of the participation of people with disabilities in society is a world-wide development. The concept of participation has its own meanings in so-called developing countries where, rather than how to get people with disabilities out of the institutions, the question is how to provide non-institutional services for the many people who have no access to any care at all.[2] Disability and handicap are poverty-related in so-called developing countries and their 'hidden dimensions' are only starting to be recognized.[3,4] Community-based rehabilitation (CBR) was created specially for people with disabilities in these poor and underserviced areas. Pioneering occupational therapists, along with other professionals, have contributed to this strategy within community development for the rehabilitation, equalization of opportunities, and social integration of all people with disabilities. Published information, however, is still limited in mainstream occupational therapy literature. This chapter attempts to look at the present situation with regard to CBR, and the practice of the art of occupational therapy in CBR, in terms of the creative opportunities they present. The aim is to elaborate critically on the possible roles for occupational therapists, paying special attention to problematical issues such as cultural compatibility, community participation, sustainability and evaluation, and power relationships and collaborative partnerships. The chapter ends with suggested actions for the occupational therapy profession that will help to develop this challenging field dealing with survival, human dignity, and inclusive development.

Although in the rest of this chapter the terms developing and developed countries are used, the controversial nature of these descriptions and the assumptions they contain is recognized and acknowledged.

UNDERSTANDING CBR

There is a wide range of opinions and philosophies about what CBR actually is or what it should be. Projects and programs that are referred to as CBR can cover very diverse disability-related practices. Although the CBR concept may be attractive in the developed world too, this chapter focuses on the specific context of the developing world, where the concept emerged and where 80% of the world's people with disabilities live.[5]

Historical development and definition

The concept of CBR emerged in the late 1960s in developing countries in the same period as primary health care (PHC). PHC services are essential healthcare services (such as immunization, maternal and child care, health education, family planning, etc.) delivered in the community, accessible for all people, and bringing health care as close as possible to where people live and work.[6] PHC services were supposed to include rehabilitation services for people with disabilities. The World Health Organization (WHO) introduced the CBR concept officially in 1978 at the Alma Ata conference,[7] declaring the urgency of addressing the overwhelming problem of disability in developing countries. Similar initiatives by non-governmental organizations (NGOs) and governmental organizations (GOs) took place in different countries with diverse socio-economic conditions, cultures, and political systems, each of them using the same basic principles of transfer of knowledge and skills to people with disabilities and their families, and valorizing the role of the community in order to create access to education, vocational training, and employment.[5]

In 1994 the following approach to CBR was agreed on by the International Labor Organization (ILO), the United Nations Educational, Scientific and Cultural Organization (UNESCO), the United Nations Children's Fund (UNICEF) and the WHO:

> *CBR is a strategy within general community development for rehabilitation, equalization of opportunities and social inclusion for all children and adults with disabilities. CBR is implemented through the combined efforts of people with disabilities themselves, their families and communities, and the appropriate health, education, vocational and social services. The major objective of CBR is to insure that people with disabilities are empowered to maximise their physical and mental abilities, have access to regular services and opportunities and become active, contributing members of their communities and their societies.[8]*

Its core ingredients include being community based, providing rehabilitation, being culturally compatible and using local resources.[9,10] CBR shares most of its inherent values with the principles of health promotion, briefly outlined as empowerment, enablement, social justice, importance of an active and meaningful lifestyle, and respect for cultural differences.[11]

In recent years the multisectoral approach has been accentuated, emphasizing cooperation and collaboration by all relevant actors (or stakeholders) in contributing resources, skills, and initiatives to start and sustain a CBR program. Stakeholders are people with disabilities, their families, their communities, governments (local, regional, national), NGOs, and organizations of people with disabilities, professionals (medical and allied health professionals, educators, social scientists, and others), and the private sector. A CBR program, defined as a model for community development and partnership, should include the following components:[12]

1. The creation of a positive attitude toward people with disabilities
2. The provision of rehabilitation services
3. The provision of education and training opportunities
4. The creation of micro and macro income generation opportunities
5. The provision of care facilities
6. The prevention of the causes of disabilities
7. The management, monitoring and evaluation of the program.

A community approach to handicap in development

In some countries CBR projects gradually moved from being pilot projects to being included in national policies such as PHC,[6] but many other CBR projects were established in isolation from other development activities rather than being integrated with them.[3] Despite the progress made in the past 25 years, it is estimated that only 2% of the 480 million people with disabilities living in developing countries currently receive assistance.[4,5] The vast majority of people with disabilities still can not access even basic rehabilitation services and are not enabled to participate in school, training, work, recreation, or other social activities.[5] Only 2% of children with disabilities receive any education or rehabilitation.[4,13] Women and girls with disabilities often have significantly fewer opportunities than men and boys with disabilities. The few relevant statistics illustrate that women and children receive less than 20% of rehabilitation services,[14] and the number of girls with disabilities enrolled in schooling is estimated at less than half the number of boys with disabilities.[15] There are many 'missing disabled people' dying prematurely due to their exclusion from the developmental process and lack of adequate services.[4] Awareness of these 'hidden dimensions' of handicap has resulted in a shift to a focus on the causes of the problems. Increasing emphasis is placed on inclusion in development, equalization of human rights,[16] and full access to community participation.[5] Theoretically and ideally, basic rehabilitation for people with disabilities is a matter of human rights. However, in practice in low-income countries, this human right may not constitute a priority because of the scarcity of available resources, which are not even able to meet the basic needs for survival such as food and shelter. Basic rehabilitation facilities remain non-existent or inaccessible in many places, being viewed rather as a humanitarian target, or sometimes even a luxury.[17]

Literature in the field of development studies has pointed out the very significant role poverty plays in disability. As a measure of the difference between developing and developed countries, the average Gross National Income (GNI) per capita in 2002 was $430 a year for low-income countries compared to $26 310 for high-income countries.[18] For the group of least developed countries the GNI per capita is estimated at $280. Although progress has been made in some countries, many poor nations suffer severe and continuing socio-economic reversals, increasing the gap between rich and poor countries.[19] The link between disability, poverty, and social exclusion is direct and strong all over the world. Poverty results in increased risks, identified as conflicts (domestic, communal, interfamily, inter-religious and even international), malnutrition, poor or absent education services, inadequate communication and transportation infrastructure, increased level of hard physical labor, increased family and stress levels, increased exposure to natural disasters, increased exposure to environmental hazards and disasters, little or no access to disability prevention information and activities, and inadequate health and rehabilitation services.[3] Another significant link between poverty and disability is the impact on families. In families who live in poverty, each member has to contribute to meeting the family's needs or the survival of other family members is put at risk. Poverty is one of the major causes of impairment and disability, and impairment and disability create poverty, in a negative cycle.[3] Considering CBR as a part of general community development places disability in the wider context of inclusive development and social justice, with an emphasis on dignity, equal opportunities, and equal rights.

Recently, various CBR initiatives and programs have been subject to evaluation, the hitherto scarce literature on CBR has expanded, and a critical debate is taking place in interdisciplinary journals.[3,6,17,20-24] One of the critiques is that the development projects have largely failed the poor, because of the emphasis placed upon the roles of professionals, most of whom are expatriates with values and modes of thought based in Western professional culture. Another often reported obstacle for successful implementation is the difficulty of multisectoral collaboration. This results in initiatives remaining restricted to pilot areas, with little or no integration in national policies, and in lack of resources for training community workers and sustaining the programs. In practice, community ownership (the power to have fundamental control of a program), so important in its theoretical concept, is still barely a reality. Furthermore, poor links between community and referral systems, the lack of participation of disabled people's organizations, and the difficulty of including all disability groups have also been identified as barriers to successful outcomes.

The shift in vision of CBR may be summarized as follows:

- No one model can serve for the whole world, given the diversity of communities.
- There is a shifting emphasis from a medical model to a sociopolitical model of disability, resulting in the expansion of the focus from medical rehabilitation toward more comprehensive multisectoral approaches.
- An increased emphasis on human rights and equal opportunities for people with disabilities is apparent.
- CBR is considered as an essential part of community development, with the goal of empowerment of the whole community.
- Effective management has come into focus to improve service delivery.

As a prerequisite for effective development, the adoption of a people-centered and community centered approach is advocated, with the formulation of priorities for development set by those who will benefit from such services.[3,5,6,9,10,16]

OCCUPATIONAL THERAPY AND CBR

Pioneering occupational therapists have been working in CBR programs in developing countries, though no estimate is available of the number or distribution of expatriates and local practitioners. Most of them work as trainers and educators (mid level), with the aim of facilitating and developing programs and passing on knowledge and skills to community members. Some work 'hands-on' in the community, others are accessible on a referral basis or work as program leaders.

The current roles of occupational therapists in CBR can be summarized as follows:[25-31]

- transfer of basic rehabilitation skills to community members (community workers and/or families), creation of positive attitudes, and limitation of burden (through training, education, and supervision)

- provision of therapy when needed in preparation for participation (basic rehabilitation, e.g. assistive technology, wheelchairs, aids and skills for interaction, building self-esteem, teaching basic skills for advocacy)

- provision of first line referral services and guidance to help people find their way into the system and become their own advocates (bridging the gap between community and institution)

- facilitation of program implementation, establishing program development at both government and community level

- insuring and facilitating effective and efficient collaboration among the many sectors that contribute to CBR, for example integrating services in PHC.

The analysis of what occupational therapists effectively do (*transfer, create, limit, provide, facilitate, bridge, teach, integrate, establish, guide, insure, prepare*) demonstrates a large degree of congruence with PHC and health promotion.

Several occupational therapists with CBR practice experience have pointed out that characteristics in the core of occupational therapy are essential to the practice of CBR.[10,25-29,32] The first characteristic is our central concept of 'occupation' with its focus on level of activity and participation in daily life. The view of occupational performance as a dynamic interaction between people and their environments is central in the contemporary occupational therapy models. Although an individual, medically oriented approach (more cure than care) has dominated occupational therapy in the Western world since the Second World War, renewed focus on its social vision has arisen within the profession.[33,34] Currently, new concepts such as occupational justice[35,36] (see Ch. 9), proposed as the foundation and fundamental purpose of occupational therapy, and occupational apartheid (see Ch. 6) are being introduced and explored. Similarly, the international community has broadened the definition of health to encompass more than the absence of illness. The *International Classification of Functioning, Disability and Health* (ICF)[37] refocuses on the *abilities* of people with disabilities, and their social inclusion. In particular, occupational therapists are in a position of skill transfer, as their usual work is focused on the daily occupations of people. The second characteristic essential to CBR is the problem-based approach to daily life occupations in occupational therapy, which values the process of becoming able.[38] Third, is occupational therapy's very practical approach to rehabilitation issues, with its emphasis on creativity in tailoring the solution of problems to the person's needs, an important skill for creating possibilities in a context of limited resources (both economic and human). Finally, occupational therapy's emphasis on sharing information and collaborating with clients, viewing them not as passive recipients but as active citizens and co-creators of the future, is an essential characteristic of CBR.

Various authors have pointed out the urgent need for people with disabilities to take on directive and protagonist roles within CBR.[5,8,9,10,39] In their professional role occupational therapists also have an opportunity to be valuable contributors and to take leading positions in CBR programs, in supportive ways that do not undermine the positions of people with disabilities. Our eclectic education (grounded in a broad vision of health which is in line with the new definitions in the ICF),[37,40] which includes knowledge from medical, psychological, sociological, and technical arenas, along with broad, hands-on experience and graduate level entry, provides a good basis for supervision roles, since we have understanding across many disciplines. The shift in focus from service delivery to management requires continuing development of skills in interpersonal relationships, leadership, monitoring, and management, besides competence in delivering professional services. The personal characteristics and attitudes of the professional may be more important than the professional background. Management skills and sociopolitical skills, generally acknowledged as still underdeveloped in occupational therapy, are challenged.[10,41]

An occupational perspective on community development

Discussions on disability often consist of dialectic opposing the individual medical model and the social model. However, not all problems faced by people with disabilities stem from negative social attitudes, nor can impairment be denied as a factor, especially in countries where people don't have access to basic health and education services. The relationship with poverty must be recognized. To equate CBR with a 'biopsychosocial' model as an integration of the medical and the social models may still be reductionist, since both models perceive people with disabilities as essentially passive subjects,[42] and fail to reflect the human potential to influence the course of life.[38,42,43] In its latest definition, CBR is placed within the perspective of inclusive development, with development defined as 'a process by which the members of a society increase their personal and institutional capacities to mobilise and manage resources to produce sustainable and justly distributed improvements in their quality of life consistent with their own aspirations'.[17] Disability has to be re-thought as a development and social issue in which the rights and needs of the disabled person can be met by inclusive rather than exclusive social attitudes, coupled with an individually focused rehabilitation process when necessary.

There have been many influencing factors, including those of international declarations such as the ILO proclamation which views disability as a condition of occupational disadvantage.[5] Occupational therapists are called upon to implement their knowledge about the broad meanings of the construct of 'occupation' related to occupational disadvantage (see Ch. 6), occupational justice (see Ch. 9),[36] and occupational development, in order to build inclusive communities wherein all citizens (disabled and non-disabled) may benefit. The challenge for occupational therapists in CBR is to use occupation in the local context as a tool for social and community development, bridging the gap between disadvantage, deprivation, and potential.

CRITICAL ISSUES

An international consultation on reviewing CBR was held in 2003 to discuss relevant issues and prepare recommendations for the strengthening of CBR programs.[5,8,10,44–46] How can the occupational therapy profession contribute positively to problematical issues such as cultural compatibility, community participation, sustainability and evaluation, and power relations and collaborative partnerships? Some suggestions are offered below.

Cultural compatibility

CBR originated in the minds of Western educated specialists and is usually proposed and propelled by development workers who are not from the target culture. It should be an example of positive cross-fertilisation in the marketplace of ideas, rather than an imposed system from outside the local culture.[20]

Culture may be defined as learned, shared experience that provides 'an individual and the group with an effective mechanism for interacting both with others and with the surrounding environment'.[47] Culture is a very important element in the meaning construction of reality; it is context related and ever changing. Although culture is mentioned as a major element in contemporary professional models, it is addressed in a general way. Moreover, most of the occupational therapy models are developed in Western countries and incorporate Western middle-class values in theory and practice (see Ch. 10).[48,49] The main concern of the literature on 'culture' is with the definition of the different needs of immigrants in Western societies and the difficulty health care has in responding to these needs.[50] A second concern of the literature is the cross-cultural validity of assessments and analysis of occupational performance differentials that have shown that assessment protocols and evaluations of performance are always cultural constructions (see Ch. 10).[50] Furthermore, most accounts in the literature are written by Western occupational therapists studying the culture of 'others' (as in the early days of cultural anthropology, which was then called 'the sociology of non-Western societies'). These cultural groups may be marginalized by the fact that they are not mainstream and generally belong to socio-economically and politically disadvantaged groups (immigrants, people with lower socio-economic positions, victims and survivors of war, refugees, citizens of previous colonies). Their difficulties need not always be a matter of culture. A critique of the concept of culture is that if misused (deliberately or not), it tends to essentialize and mystify human differences, disguising underlying socio-economic and political issues (see Ch. 6).

Cultural compatibility is obviously an important issue in CBR. Since many CBR programs place 'changing attitudes' among their main objectives, an understanding of how different impairments are viewed is essential. Coleridge[21] explained concisely how all development interventions must be rooted in a thorough understanding of the local culture: first of all because all developmental activities take place within a cultural context; and secondly because in poor communities, where people with disabilities are not seen as a priority for development nor included in most mainstream development programs, an awareness of the cultural issues surrounding disability is a key factor for integrating disability into the general developmental process.

Some development planners see culture as a hindrance to development. Chambers[22] attributes the apparent failure of the development industry to its inappropriate thought processes and values. With Miles,[51] he argues for a fundamental reorientation for professionals toward respect for and belief in the validity and inherent worth of locally generated knowledge. Where CBR has been initiated and guided by local initiators or by the combined efforts of expatriates and local development workers, the cultural issue does not come to the fore.[26–29] The themes treated in these authors' accounts do not primarily concern cultural perspectives, but rather community development questions from socio-economical, educational, or political perspectives. It may be that lack of cultural competence sometimes overshadows the fundamental emancipatory mission of providing basic rehabilitation and social inclusion.

Community participation

It has become evident that community involvement is a necessary condition for success.[3,6,8,9,10,17,22,52] But what is understood by 'the community' and how and to what level should this 'defined' community be involved?

Community has different meanings. Its construct is studied by many scientific disciplines. In the natural world, our community is the unit that orchestrates individual movements in space over time. In the cultural world, community is the setting in which, from one generation to the next, human beings learn how to be fully human.[53] Community relates to connectedness. It is a unit with historical depth in time. Within the occupational therapy literature, Grady[34] elaborated on the concept of community and distinguished between established communities such as towns, neighborhoods, schools, and workplaces, and the personal communities we create ourselves, which include family, friends, and acquaintances. Townsend[33,43,54] pointed out the importance of the spiritual dimension in relation to the inclusiveness of communities. For the international consultation of the WHO on CBR, 'community' refers to the smallest administrative area where people live.[5]

Several difficulties surround the practice of community participation in CBR and community participation is still very limited in many programs. Vanneste[17] exposes examples from Africa: some programs do not involve the community at all, while others that rely almost completely on existing resources are overtaxing communities. It is precisely the 'lack of community' i.e. the breakdown of traditional structures (for example in areas with high AIDS prevalence) that contributes to the multitude of problems facing African countries. Such weakly constructed communities cannot organize appropriate services for their people with disabilities, and in these cases the assumption of CBR that the local community, characterized by benevolence and viewed as a homogeneous entity, will play a pivotal role must be critically questioned.[17,32] CBR and occupational therapy have to insure that individuals' needs as well as those of the community are included. Occupational therapists should assist and facilitate individuals to participate and try to limit occupational deprivation, disability, and exclusion. Sustainability will only be achieved when the entire community is the beneficiary.

To view community as uniform will inevitably lead to misunderstandings. In the field of CBR there are definitely different interests and different needs (people with disabilities, family members, professionals, bureaucrats). Communities do not reflect a consensus, nor are they static. Communities have a past, a present and a future. Like people and cultures, communities also have their story.[55] A meaning centered perspective is proposed, in which the life situation of people with disabilities and their community is understood, and the unique way in which disabilities injure and shape community life is addressed. Miles[51,56] advocates that the most durable solutions are likely to have long roots in the culture and perceptions of the people and their communal histories. Just as it is important for occupational therapists to understand 'the story they enter' of an individual client, so it is important to understand 'the story of the community they come into'. The widely varying needs, such as independence, interdependence, support, management, and resource development, then require unique and diverse methods of mobilization (such as technical equipment, advocacy, self-help, training, awareness raising).[23] The challenge for occupational therapy in CBR is to understand the significant actors in each community story and to address the broadness of these community interests and needs. The mobilization methods should open ways of involving local stakeholders in becoming active in CBR, eventually leading to community participation and ownership.[32] Enabling occupation, facilitating occupational justice[10,35,36] and promoting occupational health[57] will, I believe, be the domain of concern and field of expertise of occupational therapy within this transdisciplinary approach.

Sustainability and evaluation

Sustainability means the extent to which an activity can maintain itself without external inputs (usually economic or technical).[3] Evaluation is the use of monitoring and research data to determine program effectiveness and efficiency. Effectiveness is defined as the extent to which activities have an impact and work toward achieving goals and objectives. Efficiency is the cost of implementing activities in terms of their effectiveness as compared to alternative ways of achieving the same goals or objectives.[3]

The need for evidence-based CBR is urgent. CBR activities need to be evaluated to prove or disprove their effectiveness and efficiency. Sustainability in the sense of becoming financially independent may, unfortunately, not be attainable in the short term and is not an appropriate or ethical objective in many contexts. If sustainability in the short term becomes a prerequisite for starting a program, many programs will never start, and many people will never be assisted. Health care and disability care may have to be proved cost-effective in the developed world, but these measures, based on market-related principles, are not applicable where people die or live in extreme poverty, because they do not have access to any care at all. In developing countries the economic costs of the existence of disability will be significant, given the number of people affected by disability. The benefits in terms of social impact may provide a balance to these costs, rooted in values of dignity and humanization.[3] This does not imply that projects should not be evaluated on effectiveness and efficiency, especially given the already limited resources.

If the vision for rehabilitation is 'care and not cure', and an approach to disability and handicap from a development perspective goes beyond care, focusing on enablement and participation, it is evident that short-term programs set up for just 2 or 3 years are doomed not to succeed in progressing significantly in the direction of the objectives of inclusion, community participation, and ownership. These short-term programs may create hope in the lives of people with disabilities, but if they are discontinued too soon, frustration and despair will result due to the inability of the community to meet the needs without external assistance.

Defining a measurable outcome is not a simple matter. In order to measure something one must first define clearly what is being measured, then find a reliable and valid instrument or procedure by which it can be measured, and finally, place a correct interpretation on the results. Program implementation should be evaluated in relation to the goals set. But who is the one to set the goals?

Austin and Clark[58] wrote: 'Each perspective will yield different priorities ... in brief, the patient values subjective qualitative measures that summarize personal experiences, the manager requires reliable quantitative measures that summarize collective experiences, and the therapists need both types of measures.' In CBR all the stakeholders need to be involved and need both types of measures. The goals for the program need to be defined in collaboration with all the stakeholders, based on the priorities for development set by those who will benefit from such services. Then, attaining the defined goals may become a criterion for the success of the program, valuing and evaluating not only outcomes but also the processes.

Occupational therapy uses assessment instruments, such as the pediatric evaluation of disability inventory (PEDI)[59] and the Canadian Occupational Performance Measure (COPM),[60] as a basis for goal setting with clients. Although community settings are not excluded, the focus of these instruments is mainly on occupational performance and its meaning for individual clients. The usefulness of these tools as technical instruments in CBR practice must be questioned and their fit to this particular situation approached with even more caution, given the fact that the underlying models and theories are not grounded in the specific socio-economic and cultural-political-historical context of developing countries.

Progress in CBR is a collaborative result of the combined efforts of people with disabilities, professionals, and the community. This constitutes a strong argument for the use of participatory evaluation strategies and participatory action research in order to develop appropriate outcome measures (see Ch. 33). A barrier is that community workers and related professionals have only scarce time and resources, which are seldom invested in evaluation but above all are devoted directly to the people in need. However, it is vital that monitoring and evaluation are included in CBR programs and their funding procedures (time, resources, and training/expertise) in order to influence long-term development and sustainability.[55]

Power relationships and collaborative partnerships

CBR emphasizes the power of the people with disabilities and their communities, and de-emphasizes the influence of the professional.[8]

Practice, generally speaking, often depicts the opposite, due to the inherent contradiction of the concept of CBR being introduced mainly by professionals. The emphasis should be on the power of people with disabilities and their communities, rather than on the prescription of interventions and targets by workers. This is a self-generating process which starts in the community itself.[20] It is a grass roots approach, with a bottom-up orientation, in contrast to the centralized top-down organization of most institutional services. Empowerment and inclusion are the impelling forces in this model.[24] These constructs have to be accurately understood and their limits also fully acknowledged, otherwise the theoretical model becomes only rhetoric and loses its practical values. The Brazilian educationalist Freire is generally known as the father of empowerment. He emphasizes dialogue (involving respect and working with each other) and informed action (developing consciousness and hope in order to have the power to transform daily reality), situating the educational activity in the lived experience of the participants.[61] Empowerment is a basic construct in the Canadian Model of Occupational Performance (CMOP). It is defined as 'personal and social processes that transform visible and invisible relationships so that power is shared more equally.'[45] The concept of power is related to inequalities and conflicts.[24] Paradoxically, the CBR concept embraces collaboration in the center of its strategy in order to insure that people with disabilities are empowered. Indeed, empowerment is a process that one cannot 'do' for someone else, although it can be facilitated or hindered. Collaboration in which competition, individuality, and control are present not alone, but along with connectedness and interdependence, may, I believe, better facilitate cooperation and communion. This follows Miles[51] in his conviction that substantial contradictions exist between a European 'rights-based' approach for the disabled individual, and a 'community-based' approach to disability services in, for example, Asian societies where community and individuality are understood very differently (see Ch. 10). People with disabilities may require control and choice over their lives but they also require expert assistance and connectedness, and these constructs are not mutually exclusive.

Communication with all stakeholders is crucial in order to address the needs and interests of people with disabilities, their families, and their community organizations (e.g. schools), but also in order to insure that partners understand what the program and professional perspectives are. In this mutual exchange understanding and negotiation can take place, and a collaborative partnership is built up. Occupational therapy professionals, ideally, have an enabling role as catalysts and facilitators in supporting, and in identifying needs and aspirations. They can sometimes help create a favorable climate and enable development. Occupational therapists have to be actors, enabling and encouraging empowerment, using their professional expertise to serve this process, not to drive it.

CHALLENGES FOR THE OCCUPATIONAL THERAPY PROFESSION

A part of the secret of continuing development is the discovery that difference can be the source of strength rather than of weakness.[1]

Occupational therapy's central focus on occupation as the main domain of concern has valuable potential in CBR. Occupational therapists should be actors in these programs and should further engage as enablers in occupational development. Occupational development, the process component of development from an occupational perspective, may be addressed in individual and family settings or in the broader arena of the larger community. It should be a subject for study in occupational science.[62] All the features of CBR need to be addressed by the occupational therapy community through training, education, debate, and research in order to develop new guidelines. The potential establishment of a CBR project team is a concrete initiative already taken in this direction.[45] Participatory action research and participatory evaluation also need to be implemented (see Ch. 9 and Ch. 33).[46,52,63,64,65]

CBR's central focus on collaboration and partnership with the beneficiaries points to its fundamental participatory process. For this, a fundamental belief that multiple truths exist, and that what is true is related to how, why, and by whom this knowledge is generated is a prerequisite. Professionals need to understand the depth of others' knowledge in order to be able to respect and relate to that knowing. They must also understand that, although driven by the normative vision on human rights and health for all (invisible process), the daily reality of people with disabilities living in low-income countries requires very practical and concrete actions responding to the basic needs of survival, dignity, and quality of life (visible products).

This basic commitment to human rights leads to guidelines for program implementation at all stages, calling for participatory strategies with the beneficiaries. These strategies tie in with the CBR approach and with the core value of occupational therapy which views human beings as active subjects, able to co-shape their daily lives.

The problematical themes of cultural compatibility, community participation, sustainability and evaluation, and power relationships and collaborative partnerships emerge as being intertwined and interact on the conceptual and the practical levels. The development of attitudes conducive to reflective practice is recommended as being more useful than the prescription of 'recipes'. The learning process of CBR requires creativity and flexibility, including the art of improvisation, that are especially sensitive to context, interaction, and response. Furthermore, management skills such as program design, monitoring and evaluation, and the strengthening of sociopolitical and communication skills need to be explicitly addressed in educational settings, as presented in the *Revised Minimum Standards for the Education of Occupational Therapists*.[40] A special module on CBR and the opportunity to do fieldwork in an existing CBR program may encourage and reinforce occupational therapists' initiatives.[10] Engagement in research and scholarship related to the effectiveness of CBR and of occupational therapy's contribution to it should be promoted.

Occupational therapists are called upon to develop their agency in CBR programs and to continue critical development of the knowledge base, attitudes, and skills from an occupational perspective in the areas of:

- community development and community centered approaches, including participatory evaluation and research

- cultural competency and the cultural grounding of models

- workable definitions of the constructs of empowerment and inclusion, connectedness and interdependence, and quality of life related to real life contexts.

In the short term, useful actions may be:

- to embrace diversity and include occupational therapists from cultures other than the still dominating Western professional one, in order to develop further occupational therapy's potential to benefit every particular context;

- to network and organize sessions where research facilitators assist less experienced occupational therapists in the daily practice of CBR, including planning, education, and training in participatory strategies;

- to collect and accumulate 'occupational therapy in CBR stories';

- to collect data and build a literature base for ongoing evaluation of CBR and its significant features in order to develop a research base for evidence-based practice;

- to develop process models that come from CBR practice in order to bridge the gap between theoretical models and the reality of everyday practice;

- to establish funding for occupational therapists who engage in development studies and CBR training courses for research at master and doctorate level;

- to publish and discuss beyond the borders of occupational therapy, in interdisciplinary journals, in order to become better known as possible transformers of occupational disadvantage and enablers of occupational justice.

In closing, spare a thought for the efforts of the many millions of people with disabilities and their family members in developing countries not mentioned in this discussion, who live with and take care of each other as best they can, without the help of any official CBR program. Occupational therapists should learn from their experiences and build upon these existing strengths, offering messages of hope and propositions for positive change, and building resources and opportunities for inclusive development. In this chapter I have focused on occupational therapy and CBR in the specific context of the developing world, but it may be that the developed world also has a rich contribution to make to the concepts, the experiences, and the problematical issues addressed here. That discussion will be continued elsewhere.

Acknowledgements

I would like to thank Debbie Kramer-Roy, Karin Murk and Rachel Thibeault for their comments on earlier drafts and the editors of this book for their engagement in the discussions, which have contributed significantly to the shaping of this chapter.

References

1. Bateson MC. Composing a life. New York: Grove Press; 1989.
2. Flinkenflügel H. 'Community-based rehabilitation': *een inleiding met kanttekeningen*. Bewegen & Hulpverlening 1991; 3:199–213.
3. Krefting D. Understanding community approaches to handicap in development (CAHD). Collection Handicap and Development. Lyon: Handicap International; 2001.
4. Krefting L, Krefting D. Community approaches to handicap in development (CAHD): the next generation of CBR programs. Selected readings in CBR. Series 2. Bangalore, India: National Printing Press; 2002:100–110. (Occasional publication of the Asia Pacific Disability Rehabilitation Journal.)
5. World Health Organization. International Consultation on Reviewing Community Based Rehabilitation (CBR). Theme paper. 2003. Online. Available: www.aifo.it/cbr/HELSINKI%THEME% 20PAPER.pdf
6. Center for Disability in Development. Implementing CBR: community approaches to handicap and

disability (CAHD). Dhaka, Bangladesh: Center for Disability in Development (CDD); 1998.

7. World Health Organization. Declaration of Alma Ata. 1978. Online. Available: www.who.int/hpr/NPH/docs/DeclarationAlmaAta.pdf

8. ILO, UNESCO, UNICEF, WHO. Community based rehabilitation with and for people with disabilities. Joint position paper 2002. Online. Available: www.aifo.it/ild_sito/cbr/Joint%20Position%20paper%20Final%20Document.doc

9. IDDC CBR Task Group. Reflection Paper on CBR. International Disability and Development Consortium. 2002. Online. Available: www.iddc.org.uk/dis_dev/strategies/cbr_reflect.pdf

10. Kronenberg F, et al. Position paper on CBR for the international consultation on reviewing CBR. World Federation of Occupational Therapists; 2003. Online. Available: www.aifo.it/old_sito/cbr/WFOT%20/Position%20Paper%20on%20CBR.doc

11. Thibeault R, Hebert MA. A congruent model for health promotion in occupational therapy. Occup Ther Int 1997; 4(4):271–293.

12. United Nations Social Development Division. Understanding community-based rehabilitation. ESCAP; 1997. Online. Available: www.unescap.org/decade/cbr.htm

13. United Nations. Report of the United Nations High Commissioner for Human Rights. Human rights of persons with disabilities. Geneva: United Nations Publications; 2002. Online. Available: www.unhchr.ch/disability/study.htm.

14. UNICEF. Relief and rehabilitation of traumatised children in war situations. Paper submitted for the World Summit on children. 1990.

15. United Nations Social Development Division. Hidden sisters: women and girls with disabilities in the Asian and Pacific region. Geneva: United Nations Publications; 1995. Online. Available: www.unescap.org/decade/wwd1.htm

16. Quinn G, Degener T. Human rights and disability. The current use and future potential of UN human rights instruments in the context of disability. New York: UN; 2002. Online. Available: www.unchchr.ch/html/menu6/2/disability

17. Vanneste G. Current status of CBR in Africa; a review. Selected readings in CBR. Series 1. Bangalore, India: National Printing Press; 2000. (Occasional publication of the Asia Pacific Disability Rehabilitation Journal.)

18. World Bank. World development indicators database. 2003. Online. Available: www.worldbank.org/data

19. United Nations Development Program. Human Development Report. Millennium development goals. A compact among nations to end human poverty. United Nations Publications; 2003.

20. Kortman DC. Getting to the 21st century: voluntary action and the global agenda. West Hardford: Kumaniarian Press; 1991.

21. Coleridge P. Disability and culture. Selected readings in CBR. Series 1. Bangalore, India: National Printing Press; 2000. (Occasional publication of the Asia Pacific Disability Rehabilitation Journal.)

22. Chambers R. Poverty and livelihoods. Whose reality counts? University of Sussex; 1995.

23. Boyce W, Lysack C. Community participation: uncovering its meanings in CBR. Selected readings in CBR. Series 1. Bangalore, India: National Printing Press; 2000. (Occasional publication of the Asia Pacific Disability Rehabilitation Journal.)

24. Kendall E, Buys N, Larner J. Community-based service delivery in rehabilitation: the promise and the paradox. Disability and Rehabilitation 2000; 22(10):435–445.

25. Murk K, Kramer D. *Ergotherapie in Pakistan: een uitdagende ontwikkeling.* Ned Tijdschr Ergotherap 1993; 21(6):195–198.

26. Ying Yin Chui D. What is CBR: an implication of the roles of community OT in Hong Kong. Occup Ther Health Care 1998; 11(3):79–97.

27. Tan E. A Malaysian experience of occupational therapy in the community. WFOT Bulletin 1999; 43:21–28.

28. Nanyongo J. A specialized community-based rehabilitation in rural Uganda. BJTR 1998; 5(6):311–314.

29. Packer TL, Yaohua H, Xiaping Y. Families can make a difference: a family-based rehabilitation project in China. WFOT Bulletin 1999; 43:39–43.

30. Wirz S, Chalker P. Training issues in CBR in South Asia. Selected readings in CBR. Series 2. Bangalore, India: National Printing Press; 2002:111–127. (Occasional publication of the Asia Pacific Disability Rehabilitation Journal.)

31. Twible R, Henley E. Preparing occupational therapists and physiotherapists for community based rehabilitation. Selected readings in CBR. Series 1. Bangalore, India: National Printing Press; 2000. (Occasional publication of the Asia Pacific Disability Rehabilitation Journal.)

32. Lysack CL. Community participation and community-based rehabilitation: an Indonesian case study. Occup Ther Int 1995; 2:149–165.

33. Townsend E. Occupational therapy's social vision. Muriel Driver Lecture. Can J Occup Ther 1993; 55:69–74.

34. Grady AP. Building inclusive community: a challenge for occupational therapy. Am J Occup Ther 1995; 49:300–310.

35. Wilcock A, Townsend E. Occupational terminology interactive dialogue. JOS 2000; 7(2):84–86.

36. Townsend E, Wilcock A. Occupational justice. In: Christiansen C, Townsend E. Introduction to occupation: the art and science of living. Thorofare, NJ: Prentice Hall; 2003:243–273.

37. World Health Organization. International classification of functioning, disability and health (ICF). Geneva: WHO; 2001. Online. Available: www.who.int/icidh

38. Fransen H. Mastering daily life occupations: experience and meaning in two families of children with special needs. Master's thesis. Amsterdam: Institute for Occupational Therapy; 2002.

39. Disabled Peoples International. Position paper on CBR. Disabled Peoples International; 2003. Online. Available: www.aifo.it/old_sito/cbr/reviewofcbr.htm

40. Hocking C, Ness N. Revised minimum standards for the education of occupational therapists. Forrestfield, Australia: WFOT secretariat; 2003.

41. Kronenberg F. In search of the political nature of occupational therapy. MSc OT paper (unpublished). Sweden: Linkoping University; 2003.

42. Lang R. The role of NGOs in the process of empowerment and social transformation of people with disabilities. Selected readings in CBR. Series 1. Bangalore, India: National Printing Press; 2000. (Occasional publication of the Asia Pacific Disability Rehabilitation Journal.)

43. Townsend E. Enabling occupation. An occupational therapy perspective. Ottawa: CAOT; 1997.

44. WFOT Representation – meeting report on the WHO International Consultation on Reviewing Community Based Rehabilitation. 2003. Online. Available: www.who.int.ncd/disability

45. WFOT Meeting attendance report on the WHO International Consultation on Reviewing Community Based Rehabilitation. 2003. Online. Available: www.wfot.org

46. Stineman MG. Guiding principles for evaluating and reporting on worldwide CBR rehabilitation programs. 2002. Online. Available: www.aifo.it/cbr/HELSINKI

47. McGruder J. Culture, race, ethnicity, and other forms of human diversity in occupational therapy. In: Crepeau EB, Cohn ES, Boyt Schell B, eds. Willard and Spackman's occupational therapy. Philadelphia: Lippincott; 2003; 81–110.

48. Kinebanian A, Stomp M. Cross-cultural occupational therapy: a critical reflection. Am J Occup Ther 1992; 6(8):751–761.

49. Ramukumba A. Keynote speech 13th WFOT Congress. Living in two worlds. WFOT Bulletin 2002; 46:40–46.

50. Fitzgerald MH, Mullavey-O'Byrne C, Climson L. Cultural issues from practice. Aust Occup Ther J 1997; 44:1–21.

51. Miles M. Community and individual responses to disablement in South Asian histories: old traditions, new myths? Selected readings in CBR. Series 2. Bangalore, India: National Printing Press; 2002:1–16. (Occasional publication of the Asia Pacific Disability Rehabilitation Journal.)

52. Feuerstein MT. Partners in evaluation. Evaluating development and community programs with participants. London: Macmillan; 1986.

53. Moore A. The band community: synchronizing human activity cycles for group cooperation. In: Zemke R, Clark F, eds. Occupational science: the evolving discipline. Philadelphia: FA Davis; 1996: 95–106.

54. Townsend E. Inclusiveness: a community dimension of spirituality. Can J Occup Ther 1997; 64:146–155.

55. UNESCO. Our creative diversity. Report of the world commission on culture and development. Geneva: UNESCO; 1996.

56. Miles M. International strategies for disability-related work in developing countries: historical and critical reflections. Zeitschrift Behinderung und Dritte Welt 2003; 14(3):96–106.

57. Wilcock A. An occupational perspective on health. Thorofare, NJ: Slack; 1998.

58. Austin C, Clark C. Measure of outcome: for whom? Br J Occup Ther 1993; 54(8):305–307.

59. Haley S, Coster W, et al. Pediatric evaluation of disability inventory (PEDI). Version 1.0. Development, standardization and administration manual. Boston: New England Medical Center Hospitals; 1992.

60. Law M, et al. The Canadian occupational performance measure. Ottawa: CAOT; 1991.

61. Freire P. Pedagogy of hope. Reliving pedagogy of the oppressed. New York: Continuum; 1995.

62. Yerxa E, Clark F, Frank G. An introduction to occupational science. A foundation for occupational therapy in the 21st century. OT in Health Care 1990; 6:1–17.

63. Price P, Kuipers P. CBR action research – current status and future trends. Selected readings in CBR. Series 1. Bangalore, India: National Printing Press;

2000. (Occasional publication of the Asia Pacific Disability Rehabilitation Journal.)

64. Cockburn L, Trentham B. Participatory action research: integrating community occupational therapy practice and research. Can J Occup Ther 2002; 69(1):20–30.

65. Boyce W, Ballantyne S. Developing CBR through evaluation. Selected readings in CBR. Series 1. Bangalore, India: National Printing Press; 2000. (Occasional publication of the Asia Pacific Disability Rehabilitation Journal.)

Further reading

Helander E. Prejudice and dignity: an introduction to community-based rehabilitation. New York: United Nations Development Program; 1992.

Helander E. Sharing opportunities – a guide to disabled people's participation in sustainable human development. Geneva: United Nations Development Program Disability Action Group; 1996.

Peat M. Community based rehabilitation. London: Saunders; 1997.

Thomas M, Thomas MJ, eds. Selected readings in community based rehabilitation. Series 1 and 2. CBR in transition. Bangalore, India: 2000. (Occasional publication of the APDRJ.)

United Nations. Standard rules on the equalization of opportunities for persons with disabilities. Resolution 48/96. United Nations Publications; 1993.

Werner D. Disabled village children: a guide for community health workers, rehabilitation workers and families. 2nd edn. Berkeley: The Hesperian Foundation; 1999.

Werner D. Nothing about us without us: developing innovative technologies for, by and with disabled persons. Palo Alto, USA: Healthwrights; 1998.

Werner D. Helping health workers learn. Berkeley: The Hesperian Foundation; 2001.

Chapter 14

The Model of Human Occupation as a conceptual tool for understanding and addressing occupational apartheid

Judith Abelenda, Gary Kielhofner, Yolanda Suarez-Balcazar, Kimberly Kielhofner

---

OVERVIEW

In this chapter, we will use an occupational therapy model, the Model of Human Occupation (MOHO), to understand the contextual interaction between individuals' occupations and their environments in conditions of occupational apartheid. In such circumstances, individuals and communities are denied access to occupations that bring them satisfaction, actualization, and dignity. We will examine the concepts of MOHO in relation to issues of occupational apartheid and how these concepts can be used to guide the practice of occupational therapists engaged in social action. We will also use research examples to illustrate how three interrelated phenomena – volition, habituation, and performance capacity – play a role in the conceptualization of human occupation and social justice. Finally, the chapter will close with a case study illustrating how one occupational therapist used the MOHO to understand the situation of oppression as well as to address occupational apartheid for a particular family.

INTRODUCTION

The Model of Human Occupation[1] (MOHO) is the product of three decades of conceptualization, research, and practical application. It was designed to guide practice with people whose impairments interfere with their participation in occupations. MOHO was not originally developed to understand or address occupational problems resulting from social inequities, due to the fact that social change has not been within the scope of occupational therapy. However, recent studies have highlighted the potential role that occupational therapists can play in promoting social change at the individual, group, or organizational level.[2]

Similarly, occupational therapists who have become involved with populations whose occupational circumstances have been affected by war or economic and social injustice seem to have found in MOHO a framework well suited to their practice. MOHO has also been used as part of empowerment-oriented services that aim to overcome social forces of prejudice and discrimination directed toward persons because of their disability and/or racial/ethnic status.[3,4,5]

While most of the practice examples provided throughout this book and in this chapter come from the so-called underdeveloped countries, this does not mean that there is not a need for MOHO to be applied to the issues of occupational justice in the United States, where it was created. We have to remember that in the United States it was only in the 1960s that people of color gained basic civil rights and began receiving equal treatment and consideration for jobs and other opportunities. Moreover, issues of social injustice are still very prevalent in the United States. Unemployment for minority groups remains as high as 20%, and for people with disabilities as high as 77%.[6] 24.4% of children with disabilities[7] and 16% of all US children live in poverty.[8]

Given that MOHO is a comprehensive theory of human occupation that leads to an understanding of the interaction between people's occupations and their environment, it seems natural that therapists have tacitly acknowledged its utility. They have used it to guide interventions that address occupational deprivation resulting from social conditions, examples of which are related elsewhere in this book. None the less, the reasons why MOHO can be a useful tool for understanding occupational problems stemming from social inequity have never been explicitly discussed. In this chapter, we will take one step beyond MOHO's original purpose and examine its concepts in relationship to issues of occupational apartheid and how these concepts may guide practice directed at social action. We will try to understand and explain human occupation in the context of social injustice. By doing this, we will engage in knowledge generating systems and will use an existing validated model to understand the contextual interaction between individuals' occupations and their environment in conditions where they have no power or control over their occupations.

We know that there are challenges and limitations involved in this task. An occupational therapy model alone will not be enough to explain and address such complex social, economic, and political problems. However, we believe that MOHO has a great deal to contribute to furthering the practice of occupational therapists in contexts in which attention to oppressive social and political forces is especially relevant and where a broader understanding of the situation is needed. There are several reasons for this:

1. MOHO was one of the first models in occupational therapy to acknowledge the importance of the environment in occupational life. At a time when most other models were focused exclusively on impairment, this model emphasized that it was not only the individual's characteristics but the conditions in the environment that influenced occupational adaptation. As a consequence, there is a long history of research and application of MOHO that emphasizes environmental factors in a person's occupation and how to address them.

2. The dual focus of this model on both personal and environmental factors that influence occupation is important, because oppression is often internalized[9] or, as Freire[10] observed, feelings of hopelessness and a sense of powerlessness are internalized, when living under oppressive circumstances. This means that while the source of the occupational apartheid is in society, its consequences often end up being reflected in the self-conception, roles, and habits of the oppressed person. Consequently, addressing occupational apartheid requires that both personal and environmental issues are addressed.

3. Persons who are oppressed deserve the best resources available. MOHO is a well-researched model that involves both assessment tools and intervention strategies that have been empirically tested. These assessments and interventions have been systematically examined with persons who have been socially and economically disadvantaged.

4. MOHO is one of the few models that have been and are being examined through *participatory research*.[11] Participatory research approaches seek to empower people.[12] The cutting edge applications of MOHO all emphasize how persons who receive occupational therapy services can be empowered through both personal and environmental strategies.

While MOHO brings a number of important strengths for addressing occupational apartheid, we expect that a dialogue with the practitioners and their partners in the social arena will identify areas in which the model can be improved.[13.] In fact, as this chapter is being written, there is a project under way to broaden the environmental aspects of the model in order to address more explicitly the economic, cultural, and social factors that negatively impact persons with disabilities. Those applying MOHO have always emphasized the importance of this model being able to change and develop in response to research, new ideas, and experiences when it is applied to diverse populations.

OCCUPATIONAL APARTHEID

The constraint of occupational engagement due to social injustice has been labeled *occupational apartheid*.[14,15] Occupational apartheid is a form of oppression, i.e. it involves the 'monopoly over options available to one group at the expense of one or more vulnerable groups'.[16] Oppression entails the unequal distribution of resources and opportunities.[17] In the case of occupational apartheid, it is the resources and opportunities for choosing and engaging in occupations that are unevenly distributed. Those oppressed by occupational apartheid are denied access to occupations and/or what they do is dictated by survival needs and imposed by others who hold power status. Such oppression perpetuates ignorance, and may leave people unaware of their potentials and convinced they cannot shape their environments.[18]

A central tenet of MOHO is that people's identities and lives are shaped by what they do.[1] As people engage in daily routines of work, self-care, and leisure occupations, they create an occupational landscape that, to a very large extent, defines who they are and where they are headed. Having control over their lives, people realize their potential, enhance their quality of life, and generate personal resources through their daily rhythms and routines of doing. However, when this doing is constrained, people are robbed of actualization, life quality, resources, and identity. By highlighting the centrality of doing in human life, MOHO illuminates the ways in which occupational apartheid denies human potential and experience.

Since all forms of apartheid come from oppressive environmental conditions, we begin with an examination of how the environment influences people's occupational lives according to MOHO. This model begins with the premise that all forms of doing are inseparable from the environments in which they take place.[1] People adapt and thrive when engaged in a positive dialogue with the environment. This means that they are both influenced by and have some measure of power to choose and shape their own environments.[19]

When disenfranchised by occupational apartheid, people do not have the power to choose how to interact with or to shape their environment. Rather, they are subjected to the dictates and pressures created by those in power.[20] In some cases, occupational apartheid is imposed directly by the oppressors, as in the case of third world workers employed in subhuman conditions by multinational companies to increase their profits. In other cases, occupational apartheid is created indirectly by the social structure, which is maintained by those in power. Take, for instance, the plight of many rural women who have migrated to cities in the so-called underdeveloped countries. After failed attempts to find jobs, they barely survive by selling flowers, candy, and other goods on street corners, with their children in tow. Earning a subsistence salary, they receive no work benefits.

In the case of both groups of workers, their needs for survival and safety completely constrain what they do. Under these circumstances, the workers have few or no opportunities to shape their environments or derive pride and satisfaction from their occupations.

ENVIRONMENTAL FACTORS CREATING OCCUPATIONAL APARTHEID

According to MOHO, conditions in the social environment (groups of people and the things they do) and physical environment (objects and spaces) create demands, constraints, opportunities, and resources that impact each individual.[1] We can consider how these conditions create occupational apartheid. Most oppressed people belong to one or more disenfranchised groups (e.g. refugees, squatters in barrios, migrant laborers, opposition political parties, impoverished minorities, and/or people with disabilities). By virtue of their group membership they are often constrained from accessing social contexts such as schools and workers' unions, and are often barred from resources and opportunities.

On the other hand, these very same groups develop and sustain certain know-how (e.g. techniques for the production of local goods, or locating naturally occurring resources such as spices, food sources, and medicinal plants) that can be a resource to their members. Increasingly, however, powerful groups such as the upper classes, political parties in power, multinational corporations, or international organizations increase the isolation and powerlessness of disenfranchised groups while plundering their resources. This has become increasingly the case under the forces of globalization and concomitant trade liberalization. The following paragraph gives an example.

In West Africa women have for generations gathered a native berry and used it to sweeten food.[21] After learning about this native practice, corporate researchers identified within the berry a protein that is 500 times sweeter than sugar. The Trade Related Intellectual Property Rights agreement, a multinational policy generated under trade liberalization, allows plant and human genetics to be patented to transnational corporations. These corporations can then own and profit from indigenous knowledge. Using this policy, the corporate researchers obtained a patent on this protein and developed techniques for producing it in the laboratory, thereby eliminating the need for it to be collected or grown commercially in its native region. As a result, the West African women were deprived of an occupation that gave them an income and a valued social role in their communities.

People's occupational lives are also influenced by the kinds of spaces and objects to which they have access. Such access is routinely restricted to oppressed people. Examples abound across nations throughout history. Among them are all men's clubs that exclude women, banning from restaurants or churches on the basis of race, and internment in refugee or concentration camps on the basis of nationality or race. A more subtle discrimination of access occurs where cost is involved for travel or admission to a particular space or where capital resources are required to rent or purchase space or objects. One example is the circumstance of landless peasants. In many of the so-called underdeveloped countries large rural areas that are privately or state owned lie idle, while great numbers of peasants are denied the opportunity to engage in agriculture. Restriction of access to physical space, objects, resources, and opportunities is associated with poverty, as illustrated in the above example.

Imbedded in MOHO is the recognition that the same environment will have a different impact on individuals, depending on their own inner make-up. Individuals may be affected differently by adverse conditions such as poverty and discrimination. These individual differences are a function of how internal characteristics in conjunction with external supports predispose people to be more or less likely to feel and act helpless in the face of oppression. Person-related characteristics are in constant interplay with social and environmental factors.

Foucault[9] points out that individuals are more susceptible to social control when they internalize the watchful gaze and threats of the social environment, thereby monitoring and assuring their own domestication to the social agenda. Similarly, Kundera[22,23] illustrates in his novelistic writings that oppression operates by breaking people's spirit and will. Recognizing that people can learn not to accede to oppression, Freire[18] developed an educational method designed to overcome oppression, based on the process of developing critical consciousness. His work illustrates that individuals can be empowered and learn to attenuate the impact of their oppressive environments.

At the global level, oppression must be fought by efforts to change the social, political, and economic order. However, the primary option at the local level is to empower individuals and small groups, i.e. to facilitate the process by which they may gain access to resources and decisions that impact their lives.[24] MOHO is most useful in conceptualizing this empowerment process.

THE CONCEPTUALIZATION OF INDIVIDUALS WITHIN MOHO

Within MOHO, humans are conceptualized as being made up of three interrelated phenomena: volition, habituation, and performance capacity. Volition refers to the motivation for occupation. Habituation refers to the process by which occupation is organized into patterns or routines. Performance capacity refers to the physical and mental abilities that underlie skilled occupational performance.

Volition

As people engage in occupations, they generate thoughts and feelings about their own abilities and effectiveness, what holds importance and meaning for them, and what they find pleasurable and satisfying to do. These three elements, referred to as personal causation, values, and interests, make up each person's volition and contribute to shaping how the person, given the opportunity, will make choices about doing things.

Personal causation, values, and interests

Personal causation refers to the awareness of one's abilities and one's effectiveness in using those abilities to accomplish what one desires. When constrained by powerful social, political, and/or economic forces people may have few opportunities to engage in occupations where they can develop a sense of personal capacity and power. For example, in the context of refugee camps and facilities for persons with disabilities, people may have limited opportunity to experience a sense of ability, and may be likely to develop a sense of self-doubt, inefficacy, or hopelessness. Moreover, oppressive systems that blame the consequences of oppression on their victims[25] (e.g. labeling the poor as ignorant and lazy) may lead people to internalize negative attitudes of their own capacities. Not surprisingly, oppressed individuals often feel unable to produce any impact on their circumstances, predisposing them to fatalistic acceptance of unjust life conditions.[26]

Values are personal and collective convictions about how the world is and what good is worth pursuing in that world. People feel a sense of obligation to behave according to these convictions. While values are personal, they are strongly influenced by the surrounding culture and social conditions. Gender, social class, and ethnicity expose people to particular sets of values.[27] These values sometimes lead people to accept their oppressed status as their birthright. Oppressed groups may also internalize the values of their oppressors or of the dominant culture, thereby being unaware of their oppression and unwittingly participating in perpetuating oppression.[26] Becoming aware that one has internalized the oppressor's values is the first step toward change.[20]

Interests are those things people feel attracted to, and prefer to do, because they experience pleasure and satisfaction in doing them. In situations of occupational apartheid, people are typically denied opportunities to develop interests. When their basic needs are not met, people may see pleasure and satisfaction in doing as superfluous and irrelevant. The media may also instil in people interests that are not available to them, creating suffering and frustration.

Habituation

Many daily occupations are organized into roles. Roles provide people with a general outline of what to do in a given environment, and as people internalize them, the roles grant a sense of identity. Habits organize most of people's routine behavior. This stable construction of routine, which makes up very much of what is perceived as a lifestyle, is developed over time, through a process of repetition and selection.

People living in situations of oppression lack the choice and control that others have over establishing their roles and habits. Changes in habits and roles can also be imposed by environmental changes. For example, a group of women in Costa Rica were forced to create new roles for themselves when hundreds of men in the pacific town of Golfito became unemployed when a multinational banana company decided to move their operations to another town after months of strike.[28] Women, united by their common predicament (depressed, unemployed husbands at home), decided to start a salmon-canning factory. The new role included a thorough change in habits and routines, such as working outside their homes and learning new skills in order to transform their economic and social conditions. While this example demonstrates that oppressed persons can find means to develop new roles, it also demonstrates the extent to which they must often do so in response to social and environmental conditions created by others in situations of power.

Performance capacity and skills

While performance capacity is more closely linked to the innate abilities of persons, the skills that people develop for occupational performance are a function of learning opportunities and experiences. For the same reasons that persons who live in oppression may face restrictions in acquiring habits and roles, they are also routinely deprived of the opportunity to develop skills that would allow them to achieve more control over their life circumstances. In a study conducted in Honduras, researchers evaluated the impact of a comprehensive child survival community intervention in which low-income women were taught how to weigh their babies and keep monthly records of their weight in order to identify early on cases of weight loss due to malnutrition or disease.[29] However, women who couldn't read or write at a 3rd grade level were not able to acquire the skill of maintaining their child's progress. This example illustrates how individuals living in conditions of oppression are deprived of the opportunity to acquire new skills.

CONSIDERATIONS FOR USING MOHO IN INSTANCES OF OCCUPATIONAL APARTHEID

Oppression can only be totally eliminated by social, political, and economic changes that result in a more just situation for all who are marginalized, disenfranchised, or disadvantaged in some way. However, too often systemic change is stymied or proceeds at a pace too slow to affect individual lives.

The following are considerations which need to be taken into account when using MOHO in circumstances of occupational apartheid:

1. MOHO emphasizes changes at the individual level through occupational therapy skills that are best directed at empowering individuals and groups to make changes in their immediate circumstances, even while supporting and contributing to a higher order change in their sociopolitical environment. The gamut of these skills is broad and could range from learning to identify goals and develop timelines for action collectively, to learning how to build a fuel-saving mud stove for the preparation of community meals. Most importantly, skills need to be directly tied to the community's evaluation of its needs and current situation.

2. By giving a voice to those who are disenfranchised, and because its interventions and strategies are based on the partners' identified issues, concerns, and ideas of what culturally sensitive interventions might work, practice based on MOHO seeks to understand and support their values, interests, personal causation, habits, roles and performance.

3. The relationship established between occupational therapists and the groups and individuals they work with needs to be 'horizontal and equal'.[13] Seeking a term that more accurately describes the nature of this relationship, we use the word 'partner' throughout this chapter. The scientific and practice knowledge brought in by occupational therapists and the experiential knowledge brought in by the partners are different, but equally necessary. Therapists must form collaborative partnerships, assuming the role of facilitators, educators, mentors, or learners, as needed. Special sensitivity to the process of empowerment is required when professionals work in collaboration with victims of occupational apartheid. Such situations may occur in any social, welfare, health, or political system in which one group exerts power or control over another one. As health professionals, we belong to a system that has played its part in the oppression of minority groups, be they disabled, disowned, or marginalized persons.[30] In the professional culture, health professionals typically hold significant power over the people to whom they provide services,[31,32] and because professionals learn their values in this context, it may sometimes be difficult to discriminate these values from universal truths.

4. In situations of oppression, intervention must initially aim at helping individuals better understand their circumstances and recognize their own oppression. Together, occupational therapists and their partners should develop such understanding in terms that are satisfactory for all the parties. Afterwards they can collaboratively explore possible avenues for change, analyze their internal and external resources, select the course of action they deem most appropriate, put the plan into practice, and finally evaluate together the outcomes of their actions.[19] Otherwise, occupational therapists would be offering one more assistance program in which the community would be only a passive recipient of services.

5. Therapists should make a special effort to develop cultural competence in order to avoid reproducing colonialist models in our practice.[33] Developing cultural competence begins by increasing our personal and cultural awareness. This entails a deep, honest exploration of our own heritage of values and beliefs, and being able to acknowledge their relativity. One needs to develop a critical view of one's own cultural values, and to be able to put them to one side while working in the field, to avoid imposing them on our partners. This is an ongoing process that requires constant reflection, honest self-criticism, and the acknowledgement of one's ignorance of other cultures.[33] From this first beginning one can move into acknowledging and respecting the fact that people have the right to be different.

LINKING THEORY TO PRACTICE

Working with MOHO, the coming together of experiential knowledge (brought in by the partner) and scientific knowledge (theory- and research-based) is critical in linking theory and practice. As mentioned above, an important guiding principle of partner-centered practice is to develop an understanding of our partners from their own perspective. In community practice, no matter if the partner is an individual person, a family, an organization, or the entire community, our first goal remains the same.[34] Box 14.1 offers a four-phase framework for relating theoretical concepts to the life circumstances of our partners and collaboratively establishing goals for personal empowerment.[1]

This process allows for the development of what Freire[18] calls 'cultural action', an approach for developing awareness and critical consciousness. 'Cultural action' links theory and praxis to help individuals modify their relationship with the world. This approach as cited by Balcazar,[35] involves a process of 'conscientization' in which a person makes the transfer from 'naïve awareness' to 'critical awareness'. Naïve awareness doesn't deal with the problem, gives too much value to the past, and tends to accept mythical explanations. A critical awareness delves into problems, is open to new ideas, replaces magical explanations with real causes, and encourages dialogue. As disenfranchised groups gain critical consciousness and awareness, they become more free and committed to the transforming of themselves and society.[36]

Box 14.1   Four phase framework

Phase 1

In the first phase, we begin by formulating theory-based questions to guide our understanding of the person, community, or organization we are working with. The following are examples of possible questions:

Questions related to the partner's volition
- What are the values and beliefs/interests of this partner?
- What is the sense this partner has of their individual/collective capacities, and how confident do they feel about the possibility of using them to produce a change in their own circumstances or environment?
- How are choices made, and by whom?
- What behaviors and actions are culturally acceptable for the partner?
- Where do they want to go as an individual/group?

Questions related to the partner's habituation
- What are the roles of this person/group within this community/organization?
- How does this partner organize daily activities?

Questions related to the partner's performance capacity and skills
- What skills does this partner rely on to accomplish goals?

Questions related to the partner's environment
- What are the spaces, objects, occupational forms, and groups available to this partner?
- How does the social/physical environment in which they perform impact their occupations?

Questions related to the partner's present and past occupations and challenges
- What is the nature of this partner's participation in occupations? What do they do?
- What are the current occupational challenges/needs identified by this partner?
- What kind of individual/collective experiences do they have in the face of catastrophic changes/challenges?
- What resources, internal and external, do they have to deal with challenges?

Therapists working in cooperation with their community partners need to customize questions so that they are relevant to different partners'

characteristics and situations. Additionally, more precise questions will emerge as the relationship progresses.

Phase 2

In the second phase, one uses the questions formulated in the first phase as guidelines to gather information. At this stage, one may want to observe the person, community, or organization in a variety of situations, but first and foremost, one should talk with them, and listen to what they have to say. In some cases (as illustrated later in this chapter), formal instruments developed for use with MOHO in more health-oriented contexts are still appropriate to use. In other instances, therapists may need to use more informal assessments or procedures adapted from existing assessments to suit the local situation.

Phase 3

In the third phase, one reflects on the information gathered and uses it to generate an explanation of the situation of the person or community, which is based on theory. One should aim to understand the relationship between: how cultural and environmental circumstances impact this person/community; what the process of making choices looks like for this specific person/community; what roles and habits and skills characterize the person/community. Most importantly, one should also seek to understand the main problems and challenges faced by the person/community from their own perspective, and what resources might be available to address them.

Phase 4

In the fourth phase, the therapists and the partners develop mutual understanding and consensus through a process of feedback. By doing this, the therapists validate their understanding of the partners' concepts, ideas, values, and their situation. Sharing and co-developing knowledge helps democratize interventions as it provides partners with tools for independently understanding and dealing with their issues in the future. As a result of this exchange of ideas, the appreciation of the partners' situation will be refined, modified, and will become more accurate. Once one is assured that one's partners feel adequately understood, one can collaboratively define the goals for cooperative interaction, setting priorities and a course of action.

Thus far only a very broad overview has been provided of how MOHO might be used to guide work with victims of occupational apartheid. Case study 14.1 provides one example of a MOHO-based intervention in such a context.

Poverty and disability often combine to influence negatively people's ability to exercise key occupational roles, such as parenthood. The following case study describes how an occupational therapist used MOHO in a legal context to protect the rights of parents with a disability.[3]

CASE STUDY 14.1

In 1996 a Juvenile Court judge removed three children from the custody of an extremely impoverished couple in the province of Santa Fe, Argentina. The couple had 12 children. The judge had concluded that because both parents had mental retardation and lived in poverty, they were not capable of properly exercising their role as parents. Ironically, the judge had removed three children who were identified as 'normal' while leaving in the parents' custody a child identified as developmentally disabled.

The couple approached the Ecumenical Movement for Human Rights (EMHR) asking for legal advice. The EMHR met with the neighborhood association and together decided to mobilize community resources to prevent the institutionalization of the children and their separation from the parents. Two main strategies were designed.

First, they would present a temporary proposal to the court suggesting that a family from the neighborhood would take care of the children. The family would allow the parents to be in contact with the children. Second, an occupational therapist would carry out an evaluation of the couple's occupational performance of their role as parents.

The occupational therapist had the goal of clarifying the capacity of the parents for enacting their parental roles with their children. The court decision was based on a professional's identification of their learning disabilities, but no one had examined their ability to fulfill the daily requirements as parents.

Thus, the occupational therapist engaged in the first phase of the process that links theory to practice, by formulating theory-based questions. In order to answer those questions, she used the occupational performance history interview (OPHI),[37] the role checklist,[38] and systematic observation. The process of evaluation was designed not to interfere with the couple's daily routines, and was carried out over a period of 2 months. The therapist accompanied the couple across all the environments of their occupational performance to identify their skills more accurately and to gain an understanding of the parents' perspective on their life roles.

Based on the results of her evaluation, the therapist generated the following explanation of the family's situation. The life of this couple had been marked by constant adaptations to avoid their children being taken away from them. They worked as traveling street vendors. In the past, they went out selling with all the children in their cart. They stopped taking the children with them after some of the children were taken into custody by the state under the pretext that the parents made their children work and eat garbage. The parents then began to go out to work alone, leaving the younger children under the care of the older ones. Other children were then taken away under the pretext that they were left alone all day. Since then, they had begun to work alternating shifts to insure that one of them was always with the remaining children.

Furthermore, the occupational therapist discovered that the parents took good care of the health of their children, routinely visiting the local medical center for check-ups. The symptoms of their 9-year-old girl with epilepsy were well controlled with medication, and the couple showed good knowledge of the illness and of factors that contributed to preventing relapses. The couple expressed awareness that not only was medical care necessary to maintain the girl's health, but that also love and understanding were needed.

This girl attended school, and the parents organized their routines in such a way that they could take her to and pick her up from school every day. The couple were autonomous in all their daily living activities. The basic family needs of food and shelter were met. The couple valued their role as parents and workers as the most important they fulfilled, and their interests revolved around the care of the home and the children. Both parents showed a high level of confidence in their capacity to educate, feed, and care for their children. They had plans for the future, such as improving their quality of life by getting running water and buying new beds for the kids.

The therapist concluded that their mental retardation did not interfere in their performance of their role as parents, and that the couple's lifestyle was consistent with their cultural environment, history, and origins. In contrast, the pressures from the environment in the form of governmental intervention and the belief that they were not able to be good parents because of their disability were a source of distress and anguish that they had been suffering for 12 years. This was the real problem experienced by this family.

The occupational therapist presented this analysis to the Court of Appeals, which overturned the original decision, and the children were returned to the custody of their parents. This case created a legal precedent in the province. In this case, the use of MOHO as a theoretical guide by the profession of occupational therapy, together with the mobilization of neighbors, friends, and human rights organizations, made it possible to win a battle against occupational apartheid. Importantly, because the therapist used a well-developed model with established and researched tools, she was able to gain credence in the legal system. This underscores one of the points made early in this chapter – namely that oppressed persons have a right to the best resources available and this includes the best theoretical and intervention tools.

CONCLUSION

This chapter has discussed how one might use the Model of Human Occupation as a conceptual tool to understand and address occupational apartheid. We argue that individuals and groups in situations of oppression and marginalization, such as low-income families and people with disabilities, are victims of occupational apartheid. Individuals and communities are denied access to occupations that bring them satisfaction, actualization, and dignity. Furthermore, environmental factors that create occupational apartheid, such as issues of power and control, lack of opportunities, and the denial of access to physical space, objects, resources, and opportunities associated with one's occupation, are critical in the analysis of social justice and human occupation. We have used research examples to illustrate how three interrelated phenomena – volition, habituation, and performance capacity – play a role in the conceptualization of human occupation and social justice. We closed the chapter with a case study, which illustrates how one occupational therapist used the MOHO to understand the situation of oppression as well as to address occupational apartheid for that particular partner and their family. By understanding and being aware of partners' situations of marginalization and oppression, therapists might be in a better position to formulate interventions that facilitate social change. We are aware that to understand fully the complex social, economic, and political phenomenon that is occupational apartheid, we need to consider a multidisciplinary approach to social systems. This would enable an analysis of economic and political change and power relationships that is beyond the scope of this paper. However, as we noted, MOHO has always been an evolving model that has remained at the cutting edge of ideological, research, and practice developments. Those working with the model have been and always will be encouraged to feel that this model is a truly open approach that grows and changes in concert with the needs of those to whom it is applied.

References

1. Kielhofner G. Model of Human Occupation: theory and application. 3rd edn. Baltimore, MD: Lippincott Williams & Wilkins; 2002.

2. Robertson SC, Ramsay D. Principles of consultation: occupational therapy in community programs. Conference abstracts and resources; 1995:25–26.

3. Demiryi M. *El derecho a tener derechos*. Materia Prima 1998; 47:14–17.

4. Simó Algado S, Rodríguez Gregory JM, Egan M. Spirituality in a refugee camp. Can J Occup Ther 1997; 64(3):138–145.

5. de las Heras CG. *Manual de educación para familiares y monitores: aplicación de estrategias de rehabilitación basadas en el modelo de la ocupación humana*. Santiago de Chile: Reencuentros; 1998.

6. Zea MC, Quezada T, Belgrave, FZ. Latino cultural values and their role in adjustment to disability. J Soc Behav Per 1994; 9(2):185–200.

7. Fujiura G, Yamaki K, Czechowicz S. Disability among ethnic and racial minorities in the United States. J Disabil Policy Stud 1998; 9(2):111–129.

8. Proctor BD, Dalaker J. Poverty in the United States: 2001. Washington DC: United States Government Printing Office; 2002.

9. Foucault M. Discipline and punish: the birth of prison. New York: Vintage; 1995.

10. Freire P. Education for critical consciousness. New York: Seabury; 1973.

11. Kielhofner G, Braveman B, Finlayson M, et al. Outcomes of a vocational program for persons with AIDS. Am J Occup Ther 2004; 58:64–72.

12. Balcazar FE, Taylor RR, Kielhofner G, et al. Participatory action research (PAR): general principles and a study with chronic fatigue syndrome. In: Jason LA, Keys CB, Suarez-Balcazar Y, et al, eds. Participatory community research: theories and methods in action. Washington DC; American Psychological Association; 2004.

13. Montero M. New horizons for knowledge: the influence of citizen participation. In: Jason L, Keys C, Suarez-Balcazar Y, et al, eds. Participatory community research: theories and methods in action. Washington DC: American Psychological Association; 2004:251–262.

14. Kronenberg F. Street children: being and becoming. Research report. Heerlen, The Netherlands: Hogeschool Limburg; 1999.

15. Simó Algado S, Mehta N, Kronenberg F. Occupational therapy intervention with children survivors of war in Kosovo. Can J Occup Ther 2002; 69(4):205–217.

16. Moss J. Hurling oppression: overcoming anomie and self-hatred. In: Browser B, ed. Black male adolescents: parenting and education in community context. Lanham, MD: University Press America; 1991:98–115.

17. Watts R. Oppression and socio-political development. Community Psychol 1994; 27(2):24–29.

18. Freire P. Education for critical consciousness. New York: Continuum; 1990.

19. Vidal S. *Ecología de la acción*. Buenos Aires: Espacio Editorial; 1993.

20. Freire P. Pedagogy of the oppressed. New York: Continuum; 2000.

21. Kaihuzi M. LDC's in a globalizing world: a strategy for gender-balanced sustainable development. Geneva, Switzerland: UNCTAD; 1999.

22. Kundera M. The unbearable lightness of being. New York: Harper Perennial; 1999.

23. Kundera M. The joke. New York: Harper Collins; 1993.

24. Zimmerman M. Empowerment theory: Psychological, organizational and community levels of analysis. In: Rappaport J, Seidman E, eds.

Handbook of community psychology. New York: Kluwer Academics; 2000.

25. Ryan G. Blaming the victim. New York: Vintage; 1976.

26. Fanon F. The wretched of the earth. New York: Grove Press; 1968.

27. Stanfield II JH. Ethnic modelling in qualitative research. In: Denzin N, Lincoln Y, eds. The landscape of qualitative research. Thousand Oaks: Sage; 1998:333–358.

28. Suárez-Balcazar Y, Balcazar F, Quiroz M, et al. A case study of international cooperation for community development in Costa Rica. Prev Hum Serv 1995; 12(1):3–23.

29. Suarez-Balcazar Y, Balcazar F, Villalobos C. *Participación de la comunidad en un programa de vigilancia del crecimiento en Honduras.* (Community participation in a child growth program in Honduras.) In: Balcazar F, Montero M, Newbrough B, eds. *Modelos de psicologia comunitaria.* (Models of community psychology.) Washington, DC: Organización Mundial de la Salud; 2002.

30. Menéndez E. *Cura y control: la apropiación de lo social por la practica psiquiátrica.* México DF: Nueva Imagen; 1978.

31. Kielhofner G. Functional assessment: toward a dialectical view of person–environment relations. Am J Occup Ther 1993; 47:248–251.

32. Townsend E. Good intentions overruled: a critique of empowerment in the routine organization of mental health services. Toronto: University of Toronto Press; 1998.

33. May J. Working with diverse families: building culturally competent systems and health care delivery. J Rheumatol 1992; 33:43–38.

34. Scaffa M. Occupational therapy in community-based practice settings. Philadelphia: F A Davies; 2001.

35. Balcazar F. Lessons from liberation theology. Community Psychol 1999; 32(3):19–24.

36. Gutierrez G. The power of the poor in history. New York: Orbis; 1984.

37. Kielhofner G, Mallinson T, Crawford C, et al. A user's guide to the occupational performance history interview-II (OPHI-II) (version 2.0). Chicago: MOHO Clearinghouse; 1998.

38. Oakley F, Kielhofner G, Barris R, et al. The role checklist: development and empirical assessment of reliability. Occ Ther J Res 1986; 6:157–170.

Chapter 15

Countering disability-related marginalization using three Canadian models

Mary Egan, Elizabeth Townsend

OVERVIEW

Canadian guidelines for the client-centered process of enabling occupation have captured the imagination of occupational therapists world-wide. In this chapter we review the process of enabling occupation of individuals using the Occupational Performance Process,[1,2] with the Canadian Model of Occupational Performance,[3,4] and the Person–Environment–Occupation model.[5,6] We provide examples of questions occupational therapists can use with individuals to help them begin to reason through each step. At the end of the chapter, we describe an example of the use of these models.

Throughout, we propose questions that, we hope, will stimulate readers to reflect and make suggestions that can develop further. We also invite the reader to reflect on critical questions that highlight the cultural construction of these models.

INTRODUCTION

The process of enabling occupation using the Occupational Performance Process (OPP),[1,2] the Canadian Model of Occupational Performance (CMOP),[3,4] and the Person–Environment–Occupation model (PEO)[5,6] is imbedded in a social paradigm. Simply stated, a social paradigm guides us to recognize that the social environment is important in promoting and maintaining health.[7] Occupational therapists work *with* people toward the goal of insuring their participation in chosen daily life activities. Such daily activities, or 'occupations' are viewed as occurring within a social setting; it is impossible to examine occupation without considering this social setting.

In the present chapter, we consider the process of working with individuals that begins with these individuals reflecting on what they want to do or need to do. (In this chapter, the term individual could also refer to a group such as a family.) In the course of the process, changes may be made to the environment that will ultimately benefit others. In Chapter 9, Townsend and Whiteford outline how occupational therapists might work with populations. The choice of approach will depend on the situation of the persons with whom the therapist is working and the therapist's mandate within that context.

CMOP, PEO, AND OPP AS MODELS

The CMOP is a model outlining the factors important in creating occupation (see Fig. 15.1). The PEO is a model reflecting the optimal conditions under which occupation is created (see Fig. 15.2). The two models are similar, in that both focus on occupation and the impacts of persons and environments on occupations. The models differ in their graphic representation, in the CMOP's inclusion of spirituality, and in their philosophic grounding, points which are open for discussion in another context beyond this chapter. The OPP is a model of seven processes for enabling occupation, when an individual is having difficulty initiating or continuing occupations that are personally important (see Fig. 15.3).

We all have experience using models in some aspect of our lives. As school children, many of us learned to draw and describe a model of the atom, the living cell, or a flowering plant. We learned that models could help us understand things. Using models we were able to identify quickly the major components of an object or process. Our models also helped us explain how these things functioned, how each of the parts worked together.

As we grew, we learned that real life is much more complex than life pictured in models. We also learned that some of our models were

Figure 15.1 Canadian model of occupational performance (from Canadian Association of Occupational Therapists 2002 Enabling Occupation: An Occupational Therapy Perspective. CAOT publications,[3] with permission).

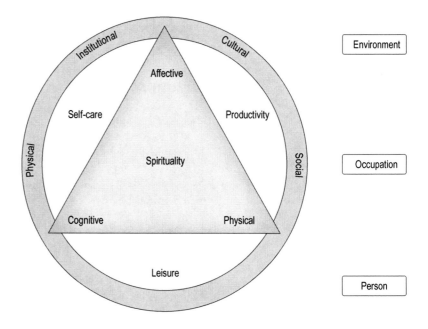

inaccurate; they may have left out important concepts or deflected our attention from other ideas that may have provided us with a better understanding. Other models proved to be relatively robust, but details regarding the relationships between concepts became better understood over time. We believe that the CMOP, PEO, and OPP are part of this latter group of models. That is, their overall structure has wide applicability for enabling occupation, but there is room for better understanding of

Figure 15.2 An illustration of changes to occupational performance as a consequence of variations in person, environment, and occupational fit (from Law et al 1996 The person–environment–occupation model: a transactive approach to occupational performance. Canadian Journal of Occupational Therapy 63(1): 9–23,[5] with permission).

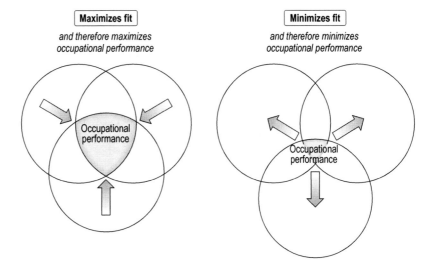

Figure 15.3 Occupational performance process model (adapted from Canadian Association of Occupational Therapists 2002 Enabling Occupation: An Occupational Therapy Perspective. CAOT publications,[3] with permission).

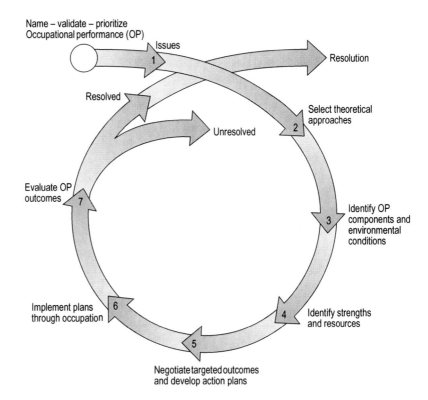

how the parts work together. In consistency with the social paradigm, we invite you to reflect and join in the discussion of what works well, what requires further elaboration, and what could be viewed differently from other perspectives.

Following a brief introduction, we will present each stage of the OPP. Within these short descriptions of the seven OPP stages, we provide a list of questions. These are designed to help occupational therapists begin reflective discussions with individuals to obtain client-centered information at each stage. In addition, within the description of the OPP stages, we elaborate on the components of the CMOP and the tenets of the PEO. At the end of the chapter we present an example of the use of the OPP, CMOP, and PEO with an individual who risks marginalization as a result of a traumatic injury.

This chapter makes use of the authors' backgrounds of providing, examining, and teaching about occupational therapy with individuals in Canada who have been marginalized as much by their disability as by other situational factors (e.g. displacement, poverty). The primary story we tell to illustrate use of the models is not based in a refugee camp or a marginalized community, but in a comfortable public school. We invite readers to reflect critically in order to determine further questions that need to be considered in their own settings.

Occupational performance as focus

When working with individuals using the OPP, CMOP, and PEO, the focus is on occupational performance. Occupational performance is defined as 'the ability to choose, organize, and satisfactorily perform meaningful occupations that are culturally defined and age appropriate for looking after oneself, enjoying life, and contributing to the social and economic fabric of a community.'[3] (p. 181) Kronenberg[8] points out that 'opportunity' to choose, organize, and satisfactorily perform an occupation is equally important, and we enthusiastically support this addition.

The therapist begins by gathering information about what the individual needs to do and wants to do (see Box 15.1, Stage 1: Name, validate and prioritize occupational performance issues). This may be done formally, using the Canadian occupational performance measure (COPM).[9] It could also be done informally, through chatting with individuals and those closest to them. In situations where it is difficult for an individual to identify desired occupations (e.g. when the individual is depressed), or otherwise envision a future including occupation, reflection on the individual's valued occupations to date may be extremely helpful.[10]

Box 15.1   OPP Stage 1: Name, validate and prioritize occupational performance issues

- What do you want to do?
- What do you need to do?
- Which activities are most meaningful to you?
- What do you dream about doing?

While stage 1 of the OPP may sound fairly straightforward, an important cultural issue arises immediately: who determines which occupations *can* be considered for enabling? From a Western perspective, we often believe that commitment to client-centered practice answers this question: i.e. the client alone, or in a decision-making group such as the family or community, in consultation with the occupational therapist determines which occupation will be pursued. Yet, in any context, the dominant social groups tend to place, explicitly or implicitly, some occupations off-limits. For example, when the authors received their entry-level education, it was not uncommon for occupational therapists to work toward the goal of returning women who had been hospitalized for depression to their role as full-time homemakers. For many such women, the repetitive, isolating, and menial activities involved, unrelieved by any forms of intellectual stimulation, may have actually contributed to the depressive illness. However, homemaking was seen as the desirable occupation for married women; dreams of other occupations were actively or passively discouraged.

The overarching issue is this: do we work to aid people to fulfill their occupational goals, when such goals are at odds with pervading beliefs of the dominant culture? For example, do we work toward the occupational aspirations of women, when the dominant cultural forces restrict women's occupations? Do we work toward the occupational ambitions of people whose goals we do not understand? Occupational desires clearly may clash with prevailing cultural norms and we need to have a clear idea first, in our own minds, about what we think are desirable occupations, and how this may limit our vision of what an individual might do in the future. Also, we must listen and observe carefully in order to reflect on our professional power and the tendency for that privileged position to silence people who feel vulnerable when they are unsure of their rights related to our services. What may assist us to avoid the tendency to restrict (consciously or unconsciously) the occupations that will be considered for enabling to those deemed appropriate by the dominant culture, is to recognize and support the idea of occupational dreams.[11]

Occupational dreams consist of what we hope to be doing. Surprisingly, while the values and beliefs articulated in *Enabling Occupation*[3,4] include that occupation is an important determinant of health and wellbeing, and that humans are occupational beings with intrinsic dignity and worth, they stop short at stating outright that people have the right to pursue their occupational dreams. We appreciate that this is an extremely controversial notion. However, failure to support the dreams of the individuals we work with limits the choice of occupations that can be enabled with occupational therapy input to those that are defined by others.

Supporting occupational dreams does not mean being unrealistic about what we as occupational therapists can offer toward the fulfillment of this dream. In stage 5, a targeted outcome, or 'dream with a deadline' is defined.[11] We carefully listen to dreams and visions in this first stage, to insure that we do not limit the individual's hope and potential.[12,13]

Once the occupational dream has been identified, theory is selected to guide reasoning in future phases (see Box 15.2, Stage 2: Select theoretical

---

Box 15.2   OPP Stage 2: Select theoretical approaches

- How do you see this problem?
- What approaches have you tried? What was your experience?
- What approach do you believe will be helpful?
- Let me tell you about an approach I think might be helpful. What do you think?

Box 15.3   OPP Stage 3: Identify occupational performance components and environmental conditions

- What do you feel you need to be able to do to complete this activity?
- What kinds of changes to the environment or task might help you complete this activity?
- I think this aspect of your performance, the environment, or the task may be making it harder for you to do this activity. Could we take a closer look at this?

---

approaches). This remains a less-developed stage in the process, although efforts have been made to categorize theory for consideration.[14] For the sake of clarity, we will use the CMOP and PEO as the sole guiding theoretical frameworks. CMOP defines the aspects of the person, the environment, and the occupation that will be considered in the process of enabling occupation and PEO states that maximizing the fit between the person, the environment, and the occupation, through modification of any of these elements, optimizes occupational performance.

In a client-centered practice, the selection of theories needs to be an open discussion in which clients' own theories are integral. For example, where clients are committed to community or non-medical healing processes, the occupational therapist needs to listen to the client, and determine how occupational theories can be aligned with these processes. An imposition of professional theories without attention to client theories and client understanding of the professional theories could result in the client dismissing occupational therapy approaches either directly or through silence.

In the next steps of the OPP (Box 15.3, Stage 3: Identify occupational performance components and environmental conditions and Box 15.4, Stage 4: Identify strengths and resources), the occupational therapist and individual client reflect on aspects of the person, the environment, the occupation and the therapist that may either hinder or facilitate the realization of the occupational dream.

The person

Spirituality

Within CMOP, people are depicted as having a *spiritual* core. Discussions in Canada include that this spiritual core is the essence of the person. A shared occupational therapy spiritually-informed value is that each person is unique and is entitled to respect from fellow human beings. This, along with other spiritual values and beliefs held dear by individuals and

> **Box 15.4   OPP Stage 4: Identify strengths and resources**
>
> - Have you dealt with similar challenges in the past? What has helped you with these? (e.g. skills, attitudes)
> - What other strengths do you bring to this challenge?
> - Are there people in your life that could help you in accomplishing this activity?
> - Are there other resources that may be helpful? (e.g. financial, community support etc.)
> - Here are the community resources that I know of that may be helpful. Would these be helpful to you?
> - Here are some skills that I have that might be helpful. What do you think?

their communities, should be considered in the process of therapy. Occupational therapists would also consider how or if individuals experience connectedness, belonging, and inclusion in their geographic, cultural, or other communities.[15] Occupational therapists learn about individuals' spirituality through a gentle process of observing and listening to what is most important to that person. They are also alert for signs of suffering, supportive of the individual's uniqueness, and aware of both the power and limitations of the therapeutic relationship.[16]

Performance components   Under CMOP, physical, cognitive, and emotional characteristics are viewed as 'performance components' that may present potential barriers or resources for enabling occupation. Physical aspects of the person include all sensory and motor functions, including such things as sensation, vision, strength, balance, range of motion, and perceptual functioning. Affective aspects include emotional and psychological functioning and social skills, such as the ability to experience and interpret a range of emotions and to read social signals. Cognitive aspects include thinking aspects such as memory, reasoning, and literacy.

Occupational therapists generally refer to the components listed in activity or occupational analysis guidelines (see, for example, Fidler[17] and Crepeau[18]), supplemented by their developing knowledge of these components through study of current findings in these areas. For example, occupational therapists working with individuals who have experienced stroke review current knowledge regarding perceptual, cognitive, affective, and physical effects of stroke.

When evaluating occupational performance issues, the occupational therapist observes, listens to, and measures the performance of natural or specially structured occupations for signs of problems in specific personal capacity areas. The therapist provides an expert opinion regarding the impacts on performance of features of the environment and the occupation. Through knowledge of activity or occupational analysis, anatomy, physiology, human kinetics, psychology, development, aging, and the course of human illnesses, the occupational therapist provides an opinion as to the possibility of changing this component and the impact that this would have on occupational performance. For example, an occupational therapist might conclude that an individual recovering from depression could move toward the goal of working as a teacher if the person's capacity to manage in the classroom and at home was improved, and that this could be done through reading, participation in a support group, and/or meditation.

Alternatively, an occupational therapist might form the opinion that, while problems with a performance component are limiting attainment of an occupational dream, change in this component may be extremely difficult to accomplish. Rather, changes in the environment or the occupation may be more effective. The occupational therapist shares these beliefs about performance components with the individual.

The occupational therapist also seeks out and considers the individual's beliefs regarding the malleability of these performance components and the desirability of promoting such change. This is done both out of respect for client-centered principles and in the belief that individuals have privileged knowledge regarding their health.[19] A key feature for occupational therapists is to determine whether change is desired at all, and what changes are relevant to those involved.

Consideration of the cultural specificity of our beliefs about the relationship between performance components and occupation is itself important, but not something we have traditionally been educated to do. However, when we come face to face with another way of developing or doing, it becomes easier to see that ideas of physical, mental, and emotional fitness in each of these domains are not universal. When the authors' grandmothers were born, a mainstream belief in Canadian society was that women did not possess adequate cognitive or emotional capacities to allow them to vote or hold public office. While Canadians no longer believe this, we still hold questionable ideas about fitness for certain daily activities. It is challenging but necessary to consider which areas of function are truly restricting realization of an occupational dream, and which just don't sit very well with us as individuals with a particular cultural background. Which pronouncements do we make about personal characteristics and the potential to participate in activities of daily life that are really just artefacts of our own cultures? For example, we may have culturally formed ideas that people with paraplegia cannot safely play rugby or that blind individuals cannot be occupational therapists. However, experience demonstrates this is untrue.[20,21] We must be vigilant that our ideas of how things can be done do not limit the occupational dreams of others.

The environment

When using the CMOP and PEO, the assumption is made that the environment has as big an impact on the attainment of the occupational dream as have the individual's capacities.[22]

Physical aspects of the environment

Occupational therapists have long been aware of the influence of physical environment characteristics on occupational performance, particularly the impact of architectural barriers on the participation of individuals who use wheelchairs for mobility.[23] Occupational therapists are trained to assess and alter aspects of the built environment that facilitate or restrict participation in daily activities. Included in this area are any conditions of the physical environment that enhance sensory processing. In this area, the occupational therapist considers such things as the effects of noise in a crowded classroom on a child who has attention problems trying to complete deskwork.

One often-overlooked aspect of the physical environment is the natural environment. For example, in many parts of the world when snowfall is heavy the mobility and occupations of elders may be severely limited. Occupational therapists can help insure that communities provide adaptations (e.g. snow clearing on sidewalks and at bus stops), rather than seeing such things as expendable budget items.

Considerations of *how* one can physically alter the environment to enable occupation will require technical expertise. Implementing such changes in the service of occupational dreams will require skill in working with community members and decision makers to insure that power and resources are shared so that physical environments are accessible places for all to participate in daily activity.

Social aspects of the environment

Social aspects of the environment have a subtler but none the less powerful impact on occupational performance. Social aspects of the environment relate to the people around us and our relationships with them. While health professionals have traditionally focused on the effect of formal, health professional–patient relationships and their impact on health, increasingly occupational therapists are coming to value the powerful effect of informal relationships on one's potential to carry out meaningful activity.[24] Rather than promoting an 'us and them' mentality regarding formal and informal supports, occupational therapists are challenged to incorporate the knowledge and skills of informal caregivers.[25]

Our increasing awareness of the value of social relationships calls us to consider these resources when enabling occupation. The interesting question remains of what we do when these resources may appear somewhat lacking. Do we consider the social environment something like the body and intervene to strengthen what we can? How well do we need to understand the social environment before we can intervene in a way that insures no harm is done, particularly when the social setting is new to us? How might we gain such an understanding? Assertive community treatment, or social network therapy may be tools that offer important insights for occupational therapists as we attempt to mobilize this important aspect of the environment.[26]

Cultural aspects of the environment

In a similar way to the effects of the social environment, the impact of cultural aspects of the environment is often less easily apparent to occupational therapists, but remains extremely important in the attainment of occupational dreams. Critiques of culture as part of our environment typically make the point that culture is not about having well-defined characteristics of thought and behavior that one shares with all members of an identifiable group. These stereotypes lock people into positions of privilege or marginalization and what Kronenberg has called *occupational apartheid* (see Ch. 6). When we believe that 'Africans like to ...' or 'Canadians all believe ...' we miss the depth and richness of our own and our clients' cultural heritages.

It is preferable to consider cultural aspects of the environment as 'guidelines for behavior' or mental templates of how occupations 'should' be done.[27] Moreover, we must note that these are produced not only through the values, beliefs, and practices passed on within an ethnic heritage, but also through a unique blend of historic and present-day regional, gender, economic, and educational influences.[27] These ideal ways of doing things must therefore be explored individually. The occupational therapist asks individuals for their vision of how the occupation should be done.

The occupational therapist also helps individuals identify resources from their cultural backgrounds. For example, to meet his goal of attending hockey games, one individual who has experienced a stroke might draw on support from a large extended family but shun help offered by neighbors and professionals in a way consistent with his traditional background. Another individual, from a similar background, may not feel this way at all. He may prefer help from friends, neighbors and professionals over that from family. His values, beliefs, and practices related to support may have been formed through other influences (e.g. positive experiences of support from friends and professionals during a divorce).

Certain cultural beliefs may hinder movement toward the occupational dream. An individual may feel that occupations can only be done in particular ways, and may be reluctant to consider alternatives. For example, if the men described above have difficulty walking, and hold to a cultural ideal of men as physically strong and active, they may have difficulty in considering the use of a wheelchair to help them manage the distances between the entrance to the sports auditorium and their seats. An occupational therapist might assist these men to see that this cultural ideal is jeopardizing their occupational dream.

Institutional aspects of the environment

The fourth aspect of the environment depicted in the CMOP, institutional characteristics, refers to the administrative rules, both implicit and explicit, which govern how things are done. The power of institutional regulation over people is both culturally defined and invisibly imbedded in the typical routines of daily life within an occupational therapy department, a community health center, a city, or a country. Such rules include by-laws and other statutes, entry criteria for disability support programs, bus schedules and job descriptions. These formal and informal structures provide powerful restrictions to the occupational participation of many individuals, while they enable others to flourish in their occupations.

Institutional aspects of the environment may remain as mysterious and challenging as the social and cultural aspects of the environment. On reflection, though, these might be the aspects most powerful in supporting occupation. With regard to official rules (or what are understood as the official rules), institutional aspects of the environment generally determine who has the power to carry out particular occupations by governing how resources are used and determining whose ideas prevail.

Influencing change at the institutional level requires both knowledge and skills. On a *micro* level, the institutional environment of an occupational therapy department will likely include rules, such as how referrals are made, when and how discharge takes place, where therapist and clients may meet, which occupations are appropriate for intervention, and how departmental activities are evaluated. On a *meso* level, such as within a health care or educational system, the institutional environment determines access criteria to services, the length and breadth of associated support services, and eligibility requirements, as well as client representation on decision-making bodies. On a *macro* level, laws, policies, and the increasingly global circles of influence are the institutional environment characteristics that define what is possible.

We can uncover and become more aware of official and unofficial rules by using research methods that describe and analyze the institutional environment. An example is the use of institutional ethnography to observe, listen to, and analyze the experience of everyday occupation in the lives of our clients, or the everyday work of occupational therapists.[28,29] This is a theory and method for displaying how everyday experiences are regulated invisibly and without force through the documents of various kinds that shape the modern world – from media images to laws and economic policies. These tools can be applied formally in research projects, or less formally by individual therapists, as part of their lifelong learning strategies.

To create enabling environments, occupational therapists may draw on and increase our knowledge of participation restrictions. We can review relevant policies and laws, and the work of advocacy groups such as the Disabled Women's Network in Canada (DAWN) and Disabled Peoples' International. As filmmaker, stroke survivor, former occupational therapy client, and advocate Bonnie Sherr Klein states, 'Learn our issues, read our literature and journals.'[3] (p. x) These strategies logically culminate in working side by side with clients for desired societal changes.[30]

Examination of the effect of institutional environmental characteristics on the realization of the occupational dream begs an important question for occupational therapists: to what extent should therapists be involved in mobilizing the institutional environment in support of valued occupation? The *International Classification of Functioning, Disability and Health* (ICF)[31] has identified that participation in the environment is the highest level of social inclusion, and that health services need to address issues of injustice related to unemployment, poor housing, and other social determinants of health. The implication is that the environment needs to be an emphasis for occupational therapy practice,[32] and the social justice foundations of occupational therapy[33] need to be made more explicit.

Again though, once the institutional aspects of the environment have been examined, what issues are involved in their alteration? What is our responsibility in evaluating the risk that advocating for change within

> **Box 15.5   OPP Stage 5: Negotiate targeted outcomes, develop action plan**
>
> - What do you hope/need to be doing at the end of this process?
> - What are your priorities?
> - How much time do we have?
> - Given what we've looked at in the last two steps, what can we put in place to attain your goals?

> **Box 15.6   OPP Stage 6: Implement plans through occupation**
>
> - Which occupations will be helpful in progressive movement towards your goal?
> - What kinds of things would you like to do as you move towards your goal?

the institutional environment may hold for the people we are working with? When we are working within our own communities, such advocacy may put us personally at risk. In exploring and perhaps exposing policies that keep marginalized persons from occupational participation, we risk being seen as a threat to the established order, an order developed in the service of the non-marginalized, a group of which we as professionals are, after all, members.

Planning and evaluation

Developing an action plan

Using information and interpretations developed from Stages 1 to 4, the occupational therapist and client develop goals and an action plan (see Box 15.5). This is a 'dream with a deadline',[11] an achievable goal defined by the individual and the occupational therapist based on the information gathered in the previous stages. There is a clear definition of what success will look like when clients have obtained their occupational goals, and there is a defined timeline. This is important for two reasons. First, limitations on time for intervention, if present (e.g. due to service limitations), must be accepted or changed. Second, a known timeline makes it easier for clients to have a more complete understanding and expectation for service delivery.

Individuals, working with the occupational therapist, move towards their goals through experience, practice, reflection, and refinement as the plan is put in motion (see Box 15.6, Stage 6: Implement plans through occupation). Ideally the occupations included in this plan are 'meaningful', i.e. clearly related to the interests, goals, and real-life environments of the individual.[34] This may be challenging for occupational therapists whose traditional resources may be selected occupations in a simulated environment in a hospital.

Evaluation and follow-up

Following plan implementation, evaluation takes place (see Box 15.7, Stage 7: Evaluate occupational performance outcomes). This can be done through re-administration of the CMOP or through discussing the previously identified goals and how satisfied individuals are with their

> **Box 15.7   OPP Stage 7: Evaluate occupational performance outcomes**
>
> - Are you doing what you hoped to be doing at this point?
> - Where are you with regard to your occupational dream?
> - Can/should/do we need to continue working together?
> - What other resources may be helpful?

progress toward these. When the occupational goal has not been met, the individual and therapist review whether they can and wish to continue working together on this issue. If they do, they will determine whether they need to revisit the barriers and facilitators to the occupational goal, and revise the plan and/or the goal. Where continued collaboration is impossible (e.g. there are funding restrictions) or undesirable (e.g. the individual wishes to pursue alternative services), the occupational therapist offers to help the individual identify other services.

ILLUSTRATING USE OF THE CMOP AND THE OPP – GRANT'S STORY

This example is a combination of real and imagined scenarios. All names are fictitious. Grant is an 11-year-old boy who lives with his parents and younger brother in Ottawa, Canada's sprawling capital city of approximately 1 million people. He loves hockey, baseball, and hanging out with his friends. Late in the winter he suffered a near complete spinal cord lesion as the result of a car accident. He is about to return to elementary school for the first time following his injury. As a bright, healthy, sporty pre-teen from a middle-class Canadian family, Grant lived a life of privilege within the mainstream of society. As a person with an acquired disability, he risks marginalization and frustration of his occupational dreams.

Marc, a recently graduated occupational therapist, met with Grant prior to his return to school, to discuss his hopes and occupational dreams. Grant stated that he wanted things to be as 'normal as possible'. He wanted to go to school, hang out with friends, play sports, and do his school work. Following the theoretical framework of the CMOP, Marc and Grant talked about the CMOP and PEO, and about Grant's ideas about what would help. Together, they considered aspects of Grant's person, occupations, and environment that would hinder or facilitate his dreams. From the person aspect, Grant lacked sensation and movement in his lower extremities and part of his trunk. He had maintained excellent upper body strength. However, given his physical limitations and the continuing adjustments that his body was making to its new state, he sometimes fatigued easily. Cognitively and emotionally he had many resources, including excellent problem-solving skills, a good sense of humor and empathy.

From an environmental standpoint, many questions remained. Would his friends, the 11-year-old athletes of the school, modify their recess games to allow his continued participation (social environment)? Would the 11-year-old girls take him on as a pet project, reflecting what they thought they should be doing, unwittingly making it even more difficult for him to rejoin his buddies (cultural environment)? Would he be able to attend his neighborhood school which was not entirely wheelchair accessible (physical environment), or would school officials determine that he must move to the newer, wheelchair accessible school, where he knew no one (institutional environment)?

Marc and Grant agreed that Marc would meet with Grant's teacher. Together they worked out strategies to adapt sports and games in physical education class to include Grant. They also discussed strategies to insure that Grant would be able to direct any assistance provided by fellow students and would not be unwittingly made to seem infantile. Furthermore, they found a way to allow Marc and Grant to practice the adapted sports and games beforehand so that Grant could develop a good level of skill to impress peers with his continuing abilities.

Marc provided the school principal with examples of accessible desks that could be purchased for Grant. He also gave her specifications for modifications to the school entrance and one of the boys' washrooms to allow accessibility for Grant. The principal obtained cost estimates for modifications and presented them to the school board, the officials who make such financial decisions. They replied that, since Grant had only 1 year remaining at his present school, it was not fiscally responsible to carry out these modifications. They prepared to have him transferred to a newer, more wheelchair accessible school.

Grant, his parents, Marc and the principal called a meeting of the school parents' council. During this meeting, the parents' council committed to raising funds and the principal stated that she would meet again with school board officials to see if she could obtain a matching amount of money from them. Grant, his parents, and the school council all felt strongly that if this request was turned down, they would go to the media with their story to try to win public support. Marc agreed to be interviewed by the media concerning the importance to Grant's daily occupations of Grant remaining at his present school.

Not everyone was happy with this plan. A number of parents noted that the school was still awaiting funds for repairs to the library ceiling, and that the senior students had no science or social studies texts. Was it really fair for the requirements of one student for 1 year to take precedence over these other needs? Marc's supervisor called him and instructed him to 'be careful'. The agency for which they both worked would soon be vying for renewal of its contract to provide school services. Annoying the public or school board officials could affect everyone's future employment.

Through this process, Grant became intrigued by how decisions were made regarding improvements to school accessibility. As part of his continuing education plan, he reviewed provincial laws and school board policies regarding improving school access. He met with a parents' group to hear their concerns regarding access and to learn about methods they had found successful for 'getting things done'. He presented these findings at a staff meeting, and together the occupational therapists brainstormed regarding methods to increase their abilities to improve accessibility. They reviewed the potential impact and risk of various strategies.

CONCLUSION

Recognition of the importance of the environment and task-related factors to participation in the daily life of a society is not new or unique to occupational therapy. Acting on these factors within a healthcare context, however, is revolutionary. The OPP used with the CMOP and PEO provides a template for occupational therapy to carry out this type of radical practice, which has so much potential for demarginalizing individuals with physical, cognitive and/or emotional differences. Such practice does not come without serious reflection on assumptions regarding what is truly required to enable occupation, how power can be shared, and why occupational therapists may face the costs of an activist practice in a conservative world.

We recognize that we may be viewed as academics who are not facing the risks of practicing within conservative communities and healthcare systems. Instead, we face the risks of advocating for teaching and research resources to educate student occupational therapists in evidence-based practice. Nevertheless, we appreciate that the magnitude of change that must occur in order to realize full occupational participation for the individuals with whom we work is large. We believe that our best hope to achieve this change is to share each of our successful and not so successful movements towards this goal, while appreciating the difficulty of the task. We also trust that application of occupational therapy models, such as the CMOP, PEO, and OPP, with critical reflection at each step, will move us closer to this goal.

References

1. Fearing VG, Clark J. Individuals in context: a practical guide to client-centred practice. Thorofare NJ: Slack; 2000.
2. Fearing VG, Law M, Clark J. An occupational performance process model: fostering client and therapist alliances. Can J Occup Ther 1997; 64:7–15.
3. Canadian Association of Occupational Therapists. Enabling occupation: an occupational therapy perspective. Ottawa, ON: Canadian Association of Occupational Therapists; 1997.
4. Townsend E. Preface to Enabling occupation: an occupational therapy perspective. Ottawa, ON: Canadian Association of Occupational Therapists; 2002.
5. Law M, Cooper B, Strong S, et al. The person–environment–occupation model: a transactive approach to occupational performance. Can J Occup Ther 1996; 63(1):9–23.
6. Strong S, Rigby P, Stewart D, et al. Application of the person–environment–occupation model: a practical tool. Can J Occup Ther 1998; 66:122–133.
7. Stewart D, Law M. The environment: paradigms and practice in health. In: Letts L, Rigby P, Stewart D, eds. Using environments to enable occupational performance. Thorofare, NJ: Slack; 2003:3–15.
8. Kronenberg F. In search of the political nature of occupational therapy. MSc OT paper (unpublished). Linkoping University, Sweden. 2003.
9. Law M, Baptistes, Carswell A, McColl MA, et al. Canadian occupational performance measure. 3rd edn. Ottawa, ON: Canadian Association of Occupational Therapists; 1998.
10. Clark F, Ennevor BL, Richardson PL. A grounded theory for techniques of occupational storytelling and occupational story making. In: Zemke R, Clark F, eds. Occupational science: the evolving discipline. Philadelphia, PA: FA Davis; 1996:373–392.

11. Clark J, Bell B. Collaborating on targeted outcomes and making action plans. In: Fearing VG, Clark J, eds. Individuals in context: a practical guide to client-centred practice. Thorofare, NJ: Slack; 2000:79–89.

12. Fearing VG. Creating our own reality. Can J Occup Ther 2001; 68:208–215.

13. Clark J, Markey A, Labron B. To practice is to believe. Can J Occup Ther 2003; 70:69–71.

14. McColl MA. Selecting a theoretical approach. In: Fearing VG, Clark J, eds. Individuals in context: a practical guide to client-centred practice. Thorofare, NJ: Slack; 2000:45–53.

15. Townsend E. Inclusiveness: a community dimension of spirituality. Can J Occup Ther 1997; 64:146–155.

16. Egan M, Swedersky J. The experience of occupational therapists who consider spirituality. Am J Occup Ther 2003; 57:525–533.

17. Fidler GS. Deciphering the message: the activity analysis. In: Fidler GS, Velde BP, eds. Activities: reality and symbol. Thorofare, NJ: Slack; 1999:47–60.

18. Crepeau EB. Activity analysis: a way of thinking about occupational performance. In: Neistadt ME, Crepeau EB, eds. Willard and Spackman's occupational therapy. Philadelphia, PA: Lippincott; 1998: 373–392.

19. Canadian Association of Occupational Therapists, Association of Canadian Occupational Therapy University Programs, Association of Canadian Occupational Therapy Regulatory Organizations, President's Advisory Committee. Joint position statement on evidence-based practice. Can J Occup Ther 1999; 66:270–272.

20. Baier S, Spaulding S. The influence of rugby participation on the level of community integration of persons with spinal cord injury. 3 July 18. Proceedings of the University of Western Ontario Occupational Therapy Conference on Evidence Based Practice. London, ON; 2003.

21. Guitard P, Lirette S. An occupational therapist that cannot see. Can it be? Proceedings of the 12th Congress of the World Federation of Occupational Therapists. Montreal. 1998.

22. Letts L, Rigby P, Stewart D, eds. Using environments to enable occupational performance. Thorofare NJ: Slack; 2003.

23. Nocon A, Pleace N. Until disabled people get consulted … the role of occupational therapy in meeting housing needs. Br J Occup Ther 1997; 60:115–122.

24. McColl MA. Social support and occupational therapy. In: Christiansen C, Baum C, eds. Occupational therapy: enabling function and well-being. Thorofare, NJ: Slack; 1997:408–425.

25. Gitlin LM, Corcoran M, Leinmiller Eckhardt S. Understanding the family perspective: an ethnographic framework for providing occupational therapy in the home. Am J Occup Ther 1995; 49:802–809.

26. Wasylenki D, James S, Clark C, et al. Clinical issues in social network therapy for clients with schizophrenia. Community Ment Health J 1992; 28:427–440.

27. Krefting LH, Krefting D. Cultural influences on performance. In: Christiansen C, Baum C, eds. Occupational therapy: overcoming human performance deficits. Thorofare NJ: Slack; 1991: 100–122.

28. Townsend E, Langille L, Ripley D. Professional tensions in client-centered practice: using institutional ethnography to generate understanding and transformation. Am J Occup Ther 2003; 57:17–28.

29. Townsend E. Institutional ethnography: a method for showing how the context shapes practice. Occup Ther J Res 1996; 16:179–199.

30. Whalley Hammell K. Changing institutional environments to enable occupation among people with severe physical impairments. In: Letts L, Rigby P, Stewart D, eds. Using environments to enable occupational performance. Thorofare, NJ: Slack; 2003: 35–53.

31. World Health Organization. The international classification of functioning, disability and health. Geneva: World Health Organization; 2001.

32. Law M. The environment: a focus for occupational therapy. Can J Occup Ther 1991; 58:171–180.

33. Townsend E. Occupational therapy's social vision. Can J Occup Ther 1993; 60:174–184.

34. Pierce DE. Occupation by design. Philadelphia, PA: FA Davis; 2003.

Chapter 16

The *Kawa* (river) model
Nature, life flow, and the power of culturally relevant occupational therapy

Michael K. Iwama

OVERVIEW

Cultural borders can be transcended in occupational therapy practice when occupational therapists think creatively beyond the usual frameworks and models, with their underlying assumptions. In this chapter the author introduces and describes the *Kawa* or river model of occupational therapy, developed by a group of Japanese occupational therapists as a response to the challenge to find a culturally safe and relevant model of practice that accorded with the day-to-day realities of their clients. The model arises from the Japanese social context and uses concepts drawn from the Japanese lexicon aligned in a structure that diverges from familiar scientific and rational form. The use of a common metaphor of nature in the model allows a focus on harmony between the subject, be it person, group, community, or organization, and the context, and fits well with the East Asian worldview. The *Kawa* model offers a framework that affirms and brings forward the importance of the client's world of meaning, and shows occupational therapists the importance of recognizing and responding to cultural differences.

INTRODUCTION

The power of occupational therapy is compromised when the ideologies that propel it become culturally out of sync with people's day-to-day realities. Those of us who have learned occupational therapy from within the very social contexts that created and fostered it to its current prominence, may have never had to contemplate its possible insignificance and disempowering effect on others. These statements may seem incredible to many who carry out occupational therapy altruistically, dedicating themselves to empowering, emancipating, and enabling their clients to better states of wellbeing. However, despite such noble intentions, conventional occupational therapy constructed on Western cultural norms and universally applied to *other* cultural contexts without alteration may achieve just the opposite of its intended benefit. These possible effects need to be considered if occupational therapy, with all of its tacit cultural features, is to be practiced without borders.

As occupational therapy continues to cross cultural boundaries in the wake of unbridled technological progress and globalization, there is a pressing need to proceed beyond merely adapting its form and technologies to meet the requirements of its varied target practice contexts. Occupational therapists and the communities they serve may need to analyze imported occupational therapy ideology, epistemology, and theory critically, and to participate in building culturally safe[1] variations and approaches that reflect and meet the needs of their diverse contexts.

No longer can we proceed into cultures that are different from our own – whether they differ in ethnicity, socio-economic class, gender, sexual orientation, or political leanings, etc. – and merely tell or instruct the other how to comprehend and apply *our* truths into *their* realities. Such subordinating acts reflect a colonial attitude, not to mention how they effectively undermine the quest for client-centered occupational therapy. In reality, modal ideals familiar to Western experience and worldviews, such as autonomy, narcissism and individual determinism, rational agency, a discrete self in relation to nature, and future temporality, amongst others that are also evident in the very structure and content of existing occupational therapy theory, are not necessarily shared universally across cultures.

As with practice lacking an adequate theoretical framework to explain, guide, and predict its outcomes, a gap can appear between the ideals of occupational therapy and the worldviews of its non-mainstream clients, as well as the meanings of their day-to-day experiences. Hence there is a fundamental requirement to construct culturally safe theory[2] and models of practice, especially when we contemplate taking occupational therapy into non-conventional settings, as in situations where clients' experiences lie outside of *middle American*[3] social, cultural, and material norms.

This chapter briefly introduces the *Kawa* model,[4] which represents one attempt by a group of Japanese occupational therapists to develop a culturally relevant conceptual model of occupational therapy. This work was initiated almost 5 years ago by a Japanese Canadian occupational therapy academic in partnership with Japanese occupational therapy practitioners who were challenged to reconcile and apply imported occupational therapy theory into their day-to-day practice realities. Without meaningful theoretical guides to support their professional enterprise, many Japanese occupational therapists described having to resort to technique-oriented approaches that were based on medical and rehabilitation models. They had difficulty explaining what occupational therapy was to their clients and colleagues in a mutually meaningful way. Subsequently, they reported having a professional identity crisis, compounded by role confusion. Most of all, they felt a burden of culpability for delivering a practice informed by ideals and professional mandates that were either confounding or ran counter to their clients' culture or world of everyday meanings.

The *Kawa* model constitutes a novel addition to the progression of conventional occupational therapy theory development in several ways.

First, the model is viewed primarily as a culturally relevant and safe work, having been raised originally from the Japanese social context, using concepts drawn from the Japanese lexicon aligned in a structure that diverges from familiar scientific and rational form. *Kawa* is the Japanese word for river, and is a familiar metaphor for life. Readers may readily associate some of the model's features with Eastern philosophical elements observable in Buddhist ideologies (particularly related to but not limited to Mahayana and Zen) as well as with Confucian and Taoist ethics, but ultimately the associations will inevitably vary according to the cultural lenses of the appraisers.

Second, this is a model that was raised from the clinical practice context through naturalistic/qualitative means, involving practitioners (and their clients) who had limited postgraduate academic experience. Thus the model is grounded in and inspired by the realities of occupational therapy practice. It should be evaluated primarily according to its utility and meaning in the practice context.

Third, the inner structure and dynamics of the model also diverge from conventional quantitative theory. Explanatory frameworks that are based on mathematical and physical logic are often challenged when employed with purpose to explain universally the complexities of subjective human experience and matters of phenomenological meaning. Matters of 'being', 'occupation', or the concept of spirituality, as examples, with their complex cultural constructions, extend beyond the predictive limits of empirical theory. The *Kawa* model is devoid of explicit, rigid, universal postulates. There are no discrete boxes connected by linear, directional arrows, nor is there any reliance on rational, artificial, mechanical metaphors (such as 'systems') to explain its dynamic. The *Kawa* model's departure from conventional scientific form will likely draw criticism from empirically oriented observers, but its unconventional structure may paradoxically represent the model's strength.

Fourth, subscribing to a more natural, cosmological, and ontological base, from which the self is viewed as imbedded in the environment, rather than to a more rational construction of self in relation to the environment, the model does not subsume nor feature a discrete, centrally situated self. Self is decentralized and imbedded in contexts of time and space, and within all other components of an inseparable environment. Harmony and balance in this fluid, comprehensive sense are not based on individual determinism or causation but on all the elements that form the context.

Fifth, the model is relational and appears to be equally useful whether applied to individuals or to collectives. Over the past 4 years, case studies of the model's application have been collected[5] across the spectrum from neonatal to end of life, from individuals to organizations and communities, and across the medical categories of rehabilitation and mental health.

Last, since it is culturally relevant, all universal premises of the model and its applicability are dismissed, making the model amenable to alteration by occupational therapists in conceptual and structural ways, to match the specific social and cultural contexts of their diverse clients.

Although the model may appear to favor Japanese cultural contexts, the *Kawa* model should not be viewed as culturally exclusive. The utility of this model for varying populations depends on the river metaphor's relevance to its subjects. Following the model's introduction outside of Japan,[6–13] groups of practitioners in other cultural locations spanning four continents have begun to use it, adapting it freely to suit the cultural requirements and unique features of their practice. The model should be employed as a tool to understand and appreciate better the complex occupational worlds and viewpoints of clients, and never as a universal framework brought to bear on compliant, subordinated clients.

Culturally safe conceptual models

Nursing and health scholars from Aotearoa (Maori term for New Zealand) in the last two decades have impressed upon the world the importance of cultural safety,[1,14] a framework by which power relationships between health professionals and the peoples they serve are critically considered. The present impact of historical, social, and political processes on minority health disparities in and beyond the Aotearoa context holds important implications for equity wherever the health issues of a particular group are being described, mediated, and evaluated by other people and their standards. The idea of cultural safety is especially pertinent to occupational therapists when we take our ideas and processes into new cultural domains, including into the lives of marginalized and disenfranchised people. Often the recipients are in weaker, disadvantaged positions and stand to be discriminated against further by standards and norms belonging to a different context. Further, they may lack the experience and means to examine critically the veracity, utility, and cultural safety of the material.

There are also relevant issues of cultural safety in the interface between theory construction and theory application. Theories and models are often developed in academic settings and can be far removed from the very people, situated in diverse, dynamic, and changing practice contexts, for whom they are designed. When we ask where the ideas have come from, on what realities these materials and ideas have been based, and who has participated in the production of such knowledge, we gain insight into some of the reasons for the gap that appears to exist between theory and practice, and between academics and practitioners.

Culture represents much more than the material features that distinguish people from others. Several definitions that are briefly discussed in Chapter 4, and in other places in this book, concur in seeing culture as a dynamic phenomenon, a complex interplay of meanings that represents and shapes the individual and collective lives of people. Until now, occupational therapists have not really taken their analyses of culture beyond cultural competency,[15] or considered how culture is an integral part of occupational therapy's conceptual models, theory, and epistemology. Therefore, when we ponder developing culturally relevant and safe models of occupational therapy, we can expect some fundamental continuity between the culture (shared meanings), ontology (views of truth), and epistemology (philosophy of knowledge) of the model constructors and their models.

THE *KAWA* MODEL

Centralized and decentralized self: balance, control and harmony

How one constructs the world and situates the self in relation to it has fundamental bearing on the conceptualizations and meanings of occupation. The interpretations and meanings of what people do in the world may vary according to whether the self is believed to be situated in a central privileged position in relation to a discrete, separate environment, or is believed to be merely one integrated part of a greater universe ('no less than the trees and the stars').[16] The possibility of alternative, competing worldviews in self construal challenges the universal premise of occupational therapy models. Brought into question is the adequacy of existing theoretical frameworks to explain occupational phenomena for all.

Our existing occupational therapy conceptual models are products of a particular dominant worldview and construal of self that are prevalent in Northern or Western cultures. These models assume a centrally situated self, separated from a surrounding, discrete environment that one 'occupies' through rational, purposeful action or 'doing'. Wellbeing coincides with balance between self and one's environs. Balance in this sense is not necessarily the kind of equilibrium indicated by 'zero' on a weighing scale but rather a state in which a privileged self is able to exploit the environment and exercise control over its perceived circumstances. With this particular self-agency comes a sense of entitlement to doing in the present that extends temporally into the future. We not only expect to control our immediate circumstances, but also to set future objectives in an attempt to control our own destinies. It should come as little surprise, then, to see that independence, autonomy, egalitarianism, and self-determinism are celebrated ideals that point to a common worldview and value pattern shared between mainstream occupational therapy ideology and the wider Western social context that raised it.[2]

In Chapter 10 the East Asian variation of the cosmological myth was briefly presented to illuminate the possible implications of an alternative ontology or worldview relative to the self. One remarkable difference in the Eastern version is that self is construed as one of many parts of an inseparable whole. One need not *occupy* anything because one is already *there*. Hence the self is decentralized and not accorded exclusive privilege to exercise stewardship, or unilateral control, over its environment or circumstances.

Temporal orientation tends to be in the here-and-now as neither the past nor the future are considered products of one's own making. A state of well being occurs when all elements in a frame, including the self, coexist in harmony. Disruption of this harmony hampers the collective synergy or life flow. 'Enhancing or restoring harmony' supplants 'enabling unilateral control' as the primary purpose for occupational therapy in many non-Western contexts.

The underlying ontology of the *Kawa* framework is harmony – a state of individual or collective being in which the subject, be it self or community, is in *balance* with the surrounding context. Here, the essence of such harmony is conceptualized as 'life energy' or 'life flow'. Occupational therapy's purpose is to help the subject enhance and balance this flow. In

Figure 16.1 Life is like a river, flowing from birth to end of life.

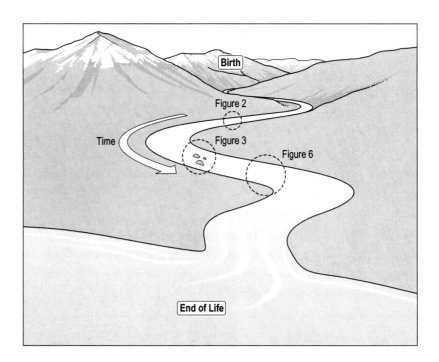

this balance, there is coexistence, a synergy between elements that affirms interdependence. How can one come to terms with one's circumstances? How can harmony between the elements, of which one is merely one part, be realized? To what extent and in what way can occupational therapy assist?

Structure and components of the *Kawa* model

This perspective of harmony in life between self and context, and its relationship to wellbeing, can be challenging to convey verbally. The dynamic might be best explained through a familiar metaphor[17] from nature. Life is a complex, profound journey that flows through time and space like a river (see Fig. 16.1). An optimal state of wellbeing in one's life or river can be portrayed metaphorically by an image of strong, deep, unimpeded flow. Certain structures and components of a river can affect its flow. Rocks (life circumstances), river walls and floor (environment), and driftwood (assets and liabilities) are all inseparable parts of a river that determine its flowing (see Fig. 16.2). Occupational therapy's purpose in this perspective, then, is to help increase and enhance life flow.

Mizu (water)

Mizu, the Japanese term for water, is the unifying concept in the *Kawa* model. Fluid, pure, spirit, filling, cleansing, and renewing are only some of the meanings and functions commonly associated with this natural element. Water is used metaphorically to represent the subject's life energy or life flow. Without water there can be no river, for it touches the rocks, walls and floor, and all other elements in its context. Water envelops, defines, and affects these other elements in a similar way to which the same elements affect the water's volume, shape, and flow rate.

Figure 16.2 A cross section view of the river can be considered at any given point along its continuum, in order to understand life's condition from the clients' vantage-point. The quality of water flow is affected by the river walls and floor, and by rocks and driftwood. Wherever there is a need to enhance life flow, there is a need for occupational therapy.

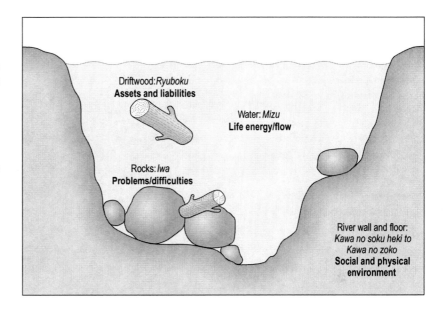

Driftwood: *Ryuboku*
Assets and liabilities

Water: *Mizu*
Life energy/flow

Rocks: *Iwa*
Problems/difficulties

River wall and floor:
*Kawa no soku heki to
Kawa no zoko*
**Social and physical
environment**

When life energy or flow weakens, the client or community can be described as unwell, or in a state of disharmony. When life energy ceases to flow altogether, blocked by life's or nature's circumstances, or when the river gives way to a vast ocean, death is signaled and the culmination of one part of a perpetual cycle is announced.

Water is fluid and takes the form of its container. Japanese people see a corollary to this in their experience and interpretation of the social context as a shaper of individual self. With a view of the cosmos that defies the rational separation of the surrounding world into discrete parts, the typical Japanese person is partial to collectives,[18] placing much greater value on the self imbedded in relationships,[19,20,18] on belonging,[20] and interdependence,[18,20] than on unilateral agency and one's own doing. Just as water in a river, at any given point, varies in flow direction, rate, volume, and clarity depending on the surrounding elements and conditions, so the self is deeply influenced and even determined by the surrounding social context at a given time and place. The driving force of one's life is interconnected with others sharing the same social frame (*ba*),[18] similar to the way in which water touches, connects, and relates all other elements of a river that have varying effects upon its form and flow.

Through the vantage-point of the *Kawa* model, a subject's state of well-being coincides with life flow. Occupational therapy's overall purpose is to enhance life flow, regardless of whether it is interpreted at the level of the individual, institution, organization, community' or society. Just as there can be many interrelated elements in a river that affect the water's flow, so a combination of circumstances and environmental structures in a life context are inextricably tied to the subject's life flow.

Kawa no soku heki (river side-wall) and Kawa no zoko (river floor)

The river's walls and floor are referred to in the Japanese lexicon respectively as *Kawa no soku heki* and *Kawa no zoko*. In the model, these elements stand for the subject's environment. The *Kawa*'s walls and floor represent

Figure 16.3 The shape and status of water, or life flow, is determined by the compounding interplay of rocks (problems), driftwood (assets/liabilities), and the river walls and floor (environment). Rocks increase in size, shape, and number, situating along a dynamic, enclosing environment, and trapping driftwood. Life flow is compromised, indicating a need for occupational therapy.

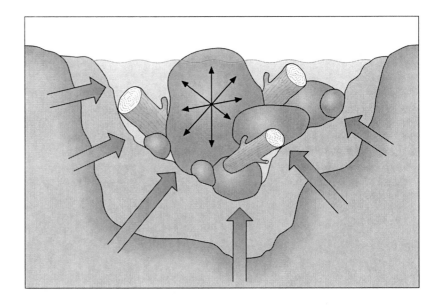

the most important determinant of the Japanese person's life flow because of the primacy that the environmental context commands in the construction of the collective-oriented Japanese self and subsequent meanings of personal action. Most often, they represent the subject's social context – mainly those people who share a direct relationship with the subject. Depending upon which social frame or *ba*[18] is perceived by the subject as being most important in a given instance and place, the river's walls and floor can represent family members, workmates, friends in a recreational club, classmates, etc. In Japan, social relationships are regarded as the central determinant[18] of individual and collective life flow.

Aspects of the surrounding social frame of the subject, such as difficult relationships, can restrict the overall flow (volume and rate) of the *Kawa*. A decrease in flow volume can precipitate a greater, compounding, negative effect on the other elements that take up space in the channel (see Fig. 16.3). If there are large rocks or other obstructions in the watercourse when the thickness of the river walls and floor are built up, the flow of the river is compromised. As we will see, the rocks in this river can directly butt up against the river walls and floor, compounding and creating larger impediments to the river's usual flow. When applying the *Kawa* model in collectivist-oriented populations, these components and the perceptions of their importance will command a large effect.

Like all other elements of the river, these features are always interpreted in relation to the whole, taking into consideration all other elements of the subject's context, and their interrelations and interdependencies.

Iwa (rocks)

Iwa is the Japanese term for large rocks or crags. In the model, they represent discrete circumstances that are considered to be impediments to one's life flow. *Iwa* represent the subject's life circumstances that are perceived to be problematic and difficult to remove. Most rivers, like people's lives, have such rocks or impediments, of varying size, shape, and number. Large rocks, by themselves or in combination with other rocks, jammed directly or indirectly against the river walls and floor can profoundly impede and obstruct flow. Their appearance may be instantaneous, as in sudden illness or injury, or it may be gradual and longstanding, such as in chronic as well as in congenital conditions. The impeding effect of *iwa* can be compounded when they are situated against, and therefore combined with, the river's walls and floor (environment). For example, the presence of functional difficulties associated with a neurological condition can be an obstacle in itself, but when these difficulties are placed in the context of work environments and/or social environments that are intolerant of people with disabilities, the barriers preventing the subject from returning to work can appear insurmountable.

Iwa are not always medically oriented problems, nor are they limited to the individual context. For example, an occupational therapy association (river) hosting an international conference might experience the sudden obstructive effect of a viral epidemic such as Sudden Acute Respiratory Syndrome (SARS) (rocks). The impeding effect of the epidemic might be compounded by suspicious attitudes and anxiety on the part of delegates (river walls and floor) who are subsequently reluctant to attend the conference. Cancelled international flights into the host country, as well as the impending quarantining of delegates on return to their home countries after the conference, represent yet other *iwa* that can further impede the flow.

Both the concepts and the contextual application of the *Kawa* model are adaptable, taking their important elements and configuration from the situation of the subject at a given time and place. The definition of problems and circumstances is broad – as broad and diverse as our clients' worlds of meanings. In turn, this particular conceptualization of people and their circumstances foreshadows the broad outlook and scope of occupational therapy interventions, when set in particular cultural contexts.

On both the individual and the collective levels, the specific *iwa*, their number, magnitude, form, and situation in the river, are determined by the subject or subjects. In collective-oriented societies like Japan, the determination of *iwa*, as with all other elements of the model, arises from either family members or a community of people connected with the issue at hand.

Ryuboku (driftwood)

Ryuboku is Japanese for driftwood. *Ryu* literally means flow, and *moku* (which changes in pronunciation to *boku* when compounded with this prefix) means wood. There is a certain implication of fate or serendipity associated with this concept. *Ryuboku* in the *Kawa* model represent the subject's personal attributes and resources, such as values (e.g. honesty, thrift), character (e.g. optimism, stubbornness), personality (e.g. reserved, outgoing), special skills (e.g. carpentry, public speaking) non-material (e.g. friendships, family relationships) and material assets (e.g. wealth, special equipment) that can positively or negatively affect the subject's circumstances and life flow. Like driftwood they are transient in nature. They can appear to be inconsequential in some situations and profoundly important in others, particularly when they lodge against and between *iwa* (rocks) and *Kawa no soku heki* and *Kawa no zoko* (river walls and bottom) to impede flow. Conversely, they may collide with the same structures to nudge obstructions out of the way. In the example used earlier of the subject desiring to return to work following a neurological injury, the subject's condition of poverty could represent a significant piece of driftwood that lodges against the other structures and further impedes the potential to overcome barriers. Having a wealthy cousin appear and lend assistance with the acquisition of specialized equipment and further remedial therapy might be like a piece of driftwood that collides against existing flow impediments and opens a greater channel for the subject's life to flow more strongly.

Ryuboku are a part of everyone's river and are the intangible components in each unique client of occupational therapy. Effective therapists pay particular attention to these components of a client's or a community's assets and circumstances, and consider their real or potential effect on the client's situation.

Sukima *(spaces between obstructions): the promise of occupational therapy*

To the occupational therapist, the *sukima* (spaces between the rocks, driftwood, and river walls and floor) are just as important as the other elements of the river when determining how to direct occupational therapy. In the *Kawa* model, these are the areas through which the client's life energy (water) continues to flow. They represent matters that the client values and deems to be worth engaging. In the most extreme sense, they are those factors that keep the client alive and hopeful of seeing a new day. For example, a space between a functional impairment such as arthritis (an *iwa* or rock) and a social group or person (represented by the river walls and floor) may represent a certain social role, such as parent, company worker, friend, etc. Water naturally coursing through these *sukima* can work to erode the *iwa* and the river walls and floor, and over time transform them into larger conduits for life flow (see Fig. 16.4). This effect reflects the latent healing potential held by each subject within the inseparable entity of self and the surrounding context. Thus occupational therapy in this perspective retains its hallmark of working with the client's abilities and assets. The model also directs occupational therapy intervention toward all elements (in this case a medically defined problem, and various aspects and levels of environment) in the context (see inner image, Fig. 16.4).

Spaces, then, represent important foci for occupational therapy. They occur throughout the context of the self and environs, between the *iwa*, *Kawa no soku heki* and *Kawa no zoko*, and the *ryuboku*. *Sukima* subsume the environment as part of the greater context of the problem and expand the scope of intervention to integrate naturally what, in the Western sense, would have been treated separately through the dualism of the internal (pertaining to self and personal attributes) and the external (environment, constructed as separate and outside of the self). *Sukima* present themselves

Figure 16.4 *Sukima* or spaces provide potential focal points for occupational therapy. Intervention can be multifaceted and may include breaking or eroding away the (medical) problem, limiting personal liabilities and/or maximizing personal assets, as well as intervening on elements of the greater environment (including the social and physical). Focusing water on these objects to erode or move them is a metaphor for clients using their own abilities or life force.

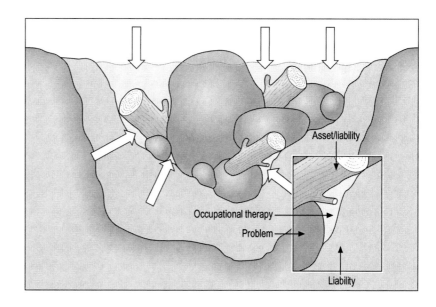

Figure 16.5 Occupational therapy helps to identify spaces where water (life force) can still flow, and focuses water through the spaces, over rocks (problems and obstacles), driftwood (resources, liabilities, and assets) and river walls and floor (environmental context), eroding the surfaces and thus increasing life flow.

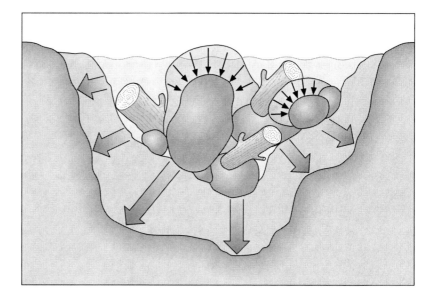

at numerous points in the client's flow, allowing client and therapist to determine multiple points and levels of intervention (see Fig. 16.5).

Rather than attempting to reduce a person's problems to discrete, isolated issues situated in a particular context, similar to the rational manner in which client problems are illuminated and discretely named or diagnosed in conventional Western health practice (i.e. focusing only on *iwa*), the *Kawa* model framework compels the occupational therapist to view and treat the person within a holistic framework, seeking to appreciate the clients' identified issues in an integrated, unified inseparable context. Occupation is regarded holistically, and includes the meaning of the activity to the self and to the community to which the individual inseparably

Figure 16.6 The power of occupational therapy is in facilitating increased life flow. All obstacles may not have been completely eliminated; some may even have remained unchanged. However, life flows more strongly, despite obstacles and challenges.

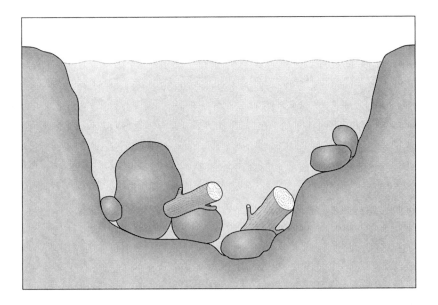

belongs, and is not just seen in terms of biomechanical components, or individual pathology and function. Life phenomena and circumstances rarely occur in isolation. In changing one aspect of the client's world, all other aspects of the person's river are also changed. The *sukima* represent opportunities to solve problems and focus therapy on positive attributes and circumstances which may have little direct relation to the person's medical condition or diagnosis.

In using this model, occupational therapists, in partnership with their clients, are directed toward stemming further obstruction of life energy or flow and can look for every opportunity to enhance it (see. Fig. 16.6).

Some considerations

This model is only as powerful as the metaphor that represents it in the cultural context in which it is being applied. Therapists applying the *Kawa* model into new or unfamiliar settings are best advised to refrain from transferring their own views of the metaphor onto the client. Rather, care should be taken to allow subjects to express their situation to the therapist, to the extent that they are capable. The therapist may want to start with: 'If your life right now was described by the image of a river, what would your river look like?' That may be augmented by: 'Here is a drawing of *my* river, and here are the structures. This is how my life is flowing at present, how about yours?' At first, clients may only be able to express a portion of their perceptions of their circumstances, but those perceptions may deepen over time as clients become more aware of their own situation and of the surrounding context.

Discussion

As occupational therapy makes its foray across new cultural frontiers, the diversity of contexts in which people define what is important and of value in daily life in relation to their states of wellbeing will only continue to broaden. War, refugee camps, political oppression, poverty, disenfranchisement, and urban shelters represent some real-world contexts for the lives of millions of people. These increasingly familiar contexts will challenge the meaning and efficacy of occupational therapy in this era. Will our existing theories and methods of application, which reflect middle-class Western-centric norms, change to meet these diverse societal needs?

Occupational therapy proceeds when clients afford occupational therapists the privilege of developing an interest in their day-to-day circumstances and worlds of meaning. To appreciate the complex dynamic between people's day-to-day realities and their contexts, and to deliver meaningful interventions that support a better state of harmony in people's lives, occupational therapists require approaches that are guided and informed by theories that are culturally relevant and safe for their clients. The *Kawa* model represents one example of the kind of theoretical material that occupational therapy may need to develop if it is to retain its relevance and effectiveness as it transcends cultural borders.

The 'ascent of man' in Western civilization, with its persistence in subjugating nature to the self and its celebration of autonomy and the ideal of independence, contrasts substantially with the ideologies and philosophical traditions of the Eastern world. Though nature can represent the greater context that envelops us, it is often passed over and frequently denied its fundamental place and power in shaping our life patterns and the meanings in what we do. Our current theories in occupational therapy reflect these leanings through their appointment of the individual to the central place of privilege as agent, distinct from the very world and circumstances that need to be brought under control. Our conceptual models appear to rationalize human experience and sometimes employ jargon and metaphors that favor contrived, mechanical forms to describe it.

The Japanese occupational therapists who raised the *Kawa* model from their day-to-day practice seek to remind their international colleagues of the primacy and importance of nature as context, and how its laws need to be more fundamentally apparent in our epistemology, theory, and practice. Despite Western man's quest to transcend and subdue nature, the earth still orbits the sun, the tides and seasons continue their turns, while birth and death continue their unremitting cycles. As long as there is a need for harmony between self and context, there is a need for occupational therapy.

There is no centralized, discrete self in the *Kawa* model. The metaphorical river, in its entirety, represents the subject, be it a person, group, community, or organization, imbedded in context. In the *Kawa* model, there is no imperative for individuals to take control of their circumstances, but rather they are directed to find a way to live in harmony with them. The idea of an omnipotent self opposing and directly engaging with barriers standing in the way of one's desired destiny gives way to an alternative perspective that seeks harmony through coexistence and cooperation. The *Kawa* model does not discourage taking direct, rational paths to a better state, but rather identifies this as just one of many possibilities. Water, like *life* force, is shared. Water slips past and around barriers, finds an equilibrium that takes into account all elements in the surrounding context, and thus is the essence of this metaphor for occupation.

Along with its acknowledgement of the primacy of nature in human experience, the *Kawa* model also serves as a prototype for a new way of regarding and employing theoretical material in our profession. In this post-modern era of recognizing cultural relativity, and variation in worldviews and interpretations of life, the notion of one rigid explanation of occupation and wellbeing is increasingly untenable. That notion would limit occupational therapy's cultural relevance and meaning for a diverse clientele. In many cases, we have grown accustomed to wielding our professional authority to require clients to abide by our own culturally bound assumptions for normal occupational performance. Occupational therapy, in an ideal sense, should be as unique as its clients, changing its form and approach according to our clients' diverse circumstances and understandings of wellbeing. To move us closer to that ideal, conceptual models and theory should be better informed, and drawn, at least in part, from the dynamic that occurs between the occupational therapist and the client.

The *Kawa* model goes only so far as to use a common metaphor of nature, of water and other elements of the river, and essentially requires clients and therapists to build relationships of trust that will affirm and bring forward the importance of the clients' worlds of meaning. The *Kawa* model shows promise as a framework to bring people and their day-to-day realities into better harmony and synchronicity. It represents a novel attempt by practice specialists to configure their occupational therapy in a manner that is culturally safe and meaningful, and powerfully beneficial for its diverse clients.

References

1. Ramsden I. *Kawa whakaruruhau* – cultural safety in nursing education in Aotearoa. Report to the Ministry of Education. Wellington: Ministry of Education; 1990.
2. Iwama M. The issue is … toward culturally relevant epistemologies in occupational therapy. Am J Occup Ther 2003; 57(5):582–588.
3. Gans H. Middle American individualism. New York: The Free Press; 1988.
4. Iwama M. Toward a culturally and clinically acceptable model of occupational therapy. Journal of the Japanese Association of Occupational Therapists 2000; 19(suppl.):516.
5. Hatsutori T, Hibino K, Iwama M, et al. Applications of the *kawa* (river) model; findings from case studies and discussions. 3rd Asia Pacific Occupational Therapy Congress. Singapore: Singapore Association of Occupational Therapists; 2003.
6. Okuda M, Iwama M, Hatsutori T, et al. 2000. A Japanese model of occupational therapy. One; the 'river model' raised from the clinical setting. Journal of the Japanese Association of Occupational Therapists 2000; 19 (suppl.):512.
7. Iwama M, Hatsutori T, Okuda M. Emerging a culturally and clinically relevant conceptual model of Japanese occupational therapy. 13th International Congress of the World Federation of Occupational Therapists. Stockholm. 2002.
8. Hibino K, Tanaka M, Iwama M, et al. Applying a new model of Japanese occupational therapy to a client case of depression. 13th International Congress of the World Federation of Occupational Therapists. Stockholm. 2002.
9. Yoshimura N, Hibino K, Iwama M. The Japanese 'kawa' model of occupational therapy in the context of mental health. 13th International Congress of the

World Federation of Occupational Therapists. Stockholm. 2002.

10. Fujimoto H, Yoshimura N, Iwama M. The *kawa* (river) model workshop – addressing diversity of culture in occupational therapy. 3rd Asia Pacific Occupational Therapy Congress. Singapore: Singapore Association of Occupational Therapists; 2003.

11. Okuda M, Kataoka N, Takahashi H, et al. The *kawa* (river) model: reflections on our culture. 3rd Asia Pacific Occupational Therapy Congress. Singapore: Singapore Association of Occupational Therapists; 2003.

12. Iwama M. Global identity; toward culturally diverse knowledge and theory in occupational therapy/ Invited Core Theme. 3rd Asia Pacific Occupational Therapy Congress. Singapore: Singapore Association of Occupational Therapists; 2003.

13. Iwama M, Fujimoto H. How does your river flow? Using a culturally relevant model of occupational therapy to break through occupational barriers. Oak Island: Occupational Therapy Atlantic; 2003.

14. Jungerson K. Culture, theory and the practice of occupational therapy in New Zealand/Aotearoa. Am J Occup Ther 1992; 46:745–750.

15. Fitzgerald M, Mullavey-O'Byrne C, Clemson L. Cultural issues from practice. Australian Occupational Therapy Journal 1997; 44:1–21.

16. Ehrmann M. *Desiderata*. Los Angeles: Brooke House;1972.

17. Lakoff G, Johnson M. Metaphors we live by. Chicago: University of Chicago Press; 1980.

18. Nakane C. *Tate shakai no ningen kankei.* (Human relations in a vertical society.) Tokyo: Kodansha; 1970.

19. Doi T. The anatomy of dependence. Tokyo: Kodansha International; 1973.

20. Lebra S. Japanese patterns of behavior. Honolulu: University of Hawaii Press; 1976.

SECTION 3

Occupational therapy practice without borders

SECTION CONTENTS

INTRODUCTION

This section examines the challenges thrown up by the context in which the practice of occupational therapy is played out against situations of occupational apartheid, extremes of occupational deprivation, perhaps extremes of human experience; but perhaps not, perhaps these are normal experiences, and occupational apartheid is, itself, a normal consequence of human occupation, occurring everywhere. How can we make sense of this, and what does occupational therapy offer the survivors of war, disaster, and those crises which threaten social or personal integrity? One strong theme that threads through these chapters is that of attempting to enable meaning through occupation, attempting to enact a story, and, whether this is initiating an individual story through play activities or whether it is a community coming to terms with experiences that have disrupted it to the core, recognizing the urgency of meaning, of being through doing.

Tellingly, these experiences are from economically stable societies as well as from those where individual lives are commonly precarious. Fujimoto and Iwama's (Ch. 26) and Sandra and Brittney Grove's (in Urbanowski's Chapter 22) moving accounts of the prioritization of treatment processes to the exclusion of personal need cry out with the same urgency as Ramugondo's description (Ch. 23) of a world where children go to their deaths without having played, or Kramer-Roy's call (Ch. 24) for the instillation of inclusive practice in education. Perhaps some of the most difficult arenas in which to develop these initiatives are the environments of street children, whose situations constrict them to thinking only of the immediate. Kronenberg (Ch. 19) describes lessons from a process of stretching occupational therapy within the profession's discourse and fields of intervention to encompass practice with such street children. This required entering and navigating the troubled waters of international cooperation and creating occupational opportunities in Guatemala to engage the children and youths and enable them to connect with strong enough goals to confront the occupational apartheid they experienced.

However, occupational apartheid is not something that just happens to people 'over there', but is a product of the unforeseen deficiencies and the unpredicted cruelties inherent as much in systems of care as in the deliberate enactment of the policies of exclusion that necessitated the work described by Simó Algado and Estuardo Cardona (Ch. 25), or evoked the responses to the bloody conflicts described by Thibeault (Ch. 17) and Simó Algado and Burgman (Ch. 18). Thibeault, especially, underlines the need for practice to be sustainable, to have continuity, and offers a set of principles through which occupational therapists can address community needs for empowerment through working with community strengths. In many cases – in many of the examples here – occupational therapists have not lived through the same experiences as the people with whom they are working, and we are often a mobile resource whose participation in a community is temporary. It is essential, therefore, to find agreed and culturally appropriate solutions that take account of diverse knowledge bases and understandings.

If occupational therapy can be described as applied common sense, then the reflective element of the profession may provide some means of overcoming the problems of a lack of imagination or forethought in others. It will not be enough to say, 'I'm sorry, I never imagined for a moment that this would be a problem.' Occupational therapists, with the concern demonstrated here for exercising the creative spirit, the essence of doing in order to be and become, show themselves to be passionate advocates for the imagination, exponents of the possible. However, the profession does not carry out this work alone. The chapter by Pollard, Smart, and the Voices Talk and Hands Write Group (Ch. 21) explores a creative process which is handed over to and then led by people with learning difficulties.

In war, disaster, aid agency work, or any experience of practice that challenges an individual's previous experience (not merely as a therapist, but all their social and personal experience) there is no 'correct' professional response. The authors have merely sought to do their best, to rely on their training and to honestly acknowledge, as Simmond (Ch. 20) does, the 'enormously scary' course of their journey beyond occupational therapy's borders. It is in the spirit of this learning experience that Simmond charts the negotiation of her practice with a Vietnamese boy, and it is to offer support to therapists confronting the issues of uncharted areas of practice that Newton and Fuller (Ch. 27) have developed the Occupational Therapy International Outreach Network (OTION), the invaluable resource they describe which will provide a vehicle for the exchange and development of occupational therapy actions. Throughout this section the authors clearly acknowledge the contribution to the development of practice made by the people with whom the process is negotiated. In an occupational therapy without borders, learning does not come so much from 'case studies', as from participation, collaboration, and action through occupation.

Chapter 17

Connecting health and social justice
A Lebanese experience

Rachel Thibeault

OVERVIEW

This chapter will describe a project developed in Lebanon with a community-based approach. The principles of intervention were integration of service, social inclusion, community participation, and long-term sustainability. Similarities between occupational therapy values and goals and sound community development will be underlined and explored, along with the role of occupational therapy in such a non-traditional context.

PROLOGUE

The road leading from Beirut to Marjeyoun, last town before the Israeli–Lebanese border, meanders dangerously between bald crests eroded by fierce winds. The moon-like landscape unfolds under a scorching sun and my colleague drives as if there was no tomorrow. It is a hair-raising roller-coaster ride in a gigantic oven. The queasiness I first felt as we left the suburbs turns into unmistakeable nausea and I beg T to stop for a few minutes.

'Can't. Setting foot off the narrow road could mean death, here. The whole region is mined and we have no clue as to the location of the mines.'

A few kilometers away, we pass a de-mining team; bearing antiquated equipment, five or six men cautiously move about the place. It is believed that over 90% of South Lebanon harbors mines but only a minute area has been de-mined. The pace is excruciatingly slow, for lack of funds. After a short while, my colleague takes a sharp right on a secondary road.

'I prefer driving through here. On the other slope, the bodies of six people belonging to the same family are strewn about a field. They'd tried to rescue each other and, one after the other, they were blown up by mines. We had to restrain other relatives who wanted to intervene: some of the victims were still alive and crying for help. We could only watch them die. And now, there is no point in risking more lives to recover the dead.'

The reality of war, so easily forgotten in sophisticated Beirut, has caught up with us. In a few moments, other victims, the survivors, will greet us in Marjeyoun.

Straddling the border, the town embodies all the contradictions of the Middle East conflict. At Fatima Gate, the Hezbollah's green and yellow banners call to vengeance against Israel while the loud-speakers chant the long lament of the martyrs' names. But behind this seemingly united front, mistrust rules; relations are tense between Muslims and Christians. And discord even infiltrates the heart of each of the religious groups: Maronite Christians fight the Greek Orthodox and the Shi'ite Muslims battle the Druze. Insidious and fatal, intolerance festers like gangrene.

BACKGROUND

For over 60 years, Lebanon has endured many a war, both internal and external. Proclaimed an independent republic in 1943, the country has seen since many conflicts involving the US, Israel, Palestine, Syria, and a variety of local religious factions, creating one of the most complex geopolitical situations in modern history. This high and long-standing instability has resulted in thousands of war victims, few means to provide them with support, and the ever looming threat of land mines. Even though Lebanon now enjoys relative peace, mines still routinely claim lives. Since 1980, the total number of victims (killed or maimed) is estimated at over 3000. In 2000 alone, 114 new victims were reported, 15 of whom were killed and 99 maimed.[1] Because the mines were laid over a long period of time by different and often enemy armies (Syrian, Israeli, Lebanese), no record of their position exists. De-mining is therefore slow and extremely precarious. To answer the needs of the survivors, several international non-governmental organizations (NGOs) have established themselves in Lebanon. Among the first was the World Rehabilitation Fund (WRF), an American NGO whose initial mandate focused on prosthetics and orthotics. With time, experience, and availability of resources, WRF eventually opened a local office in Beirut in 1987 and expanded its services to include an orphan program and an emergency rehabilitation program addressing mental health issues in children and offering community-based rehabilitation. Over the years, income generating projects were added along with land mine awareness programs and training efforts.[2]

In order to reach as many beneficiaries as possible, WRF has also called upon other local NGOs and, more specifically, on the Contact and Resource Center (CRC). The CRC was founded in Beirut in 1978, after the civil war, and has developed into the leading organization for social rehabilitation of physically disabled people in Lebanon. The CRC has long been known for its reconciliation work, bringing together, in workshops or service delivery, Muslims and Christians, disabled and able-bodied. In keeping with its main goal of rebuilding civil society and fostering peace, the CRC supports victims from all social, political, and religious backgrounds.

To best fulfill its mandate in a still potentially explosive political context, the CRC has identified early on fundamental guidelines to shape its own internal functioning.[3]

First, with social justice as its core value, the CRC constantly monitors its own governance, insuring judicious and ethical use of funds that equally benefits the target populations involved. Great care is taken to distribute resources fairly across the religious and political spectrum and prevent biases leading to further hostility.

Second, the CRC maintains absolute political and religious neutrality in all stages of intervention, from planning to service delivery and follow-up. Even though the CRC receives some funding from the Lutheran Church of America, all forms, reports, and training material focus on the war victims' issues and wellbeing without reference to religious content. No pressure is ever exerted and proselytizing is strictly prohibited.

Third, the CRC constantly reassesses the relevance of its chosen target groups and programs to prevent a duplication of services that is all too frequent in post-war reconstruction. Through a well developed network, it inquires about new programs being implemented and future developments being considered, and keeps abreast of the changes, recharting its course if required in order to remain as closely connected to community needs as possible.

Fourth, the CRC carefully assesses the social and environmental consequences of its programs. Past experience has clearly demonstrated that post-war reconstruction or economic development in poor countries can be carried out in a haphazard fashion where anti-pollution and labor laws are relaxed to make way for heavy industry.[4] The CRC supports the reactivating of local economy but within parameters respectful of environment and social equity.

Fifth, the CRC remains mindful of any impact on women's burden. The bulk of the war victims' rehabilitation and support is often added to the already extensive responsibilities of women, ultimately inducing exhaustion and disengagement.[5]

The five principles developed by the CRC for the purpose of internal audit are remarkably complementary to those adopted by WRF in 2001 for guiding comprehensive interventions in war zones. These principles were initially formulated in collaboration with another NGO, the Forum of African Women Educationists (FAWE), through its Sierra Leone chapter. First implemented in Freetown, they helped structure programs for bush wives, those young girls kidnapped during the civil war and forced into slavery, sexual slavery, or combat. (The Sierra Leone experience has been described in the Journal of Occupational Science.[6]) These same principles will now constitute the conceptual framework for analyzing the CRC's programs. These programs address a wide range of needs for people with physical, intellectual, or psychosocial disabilities: the CRC offers independent living apartments, physical therapy for the disabled, psychosocial intervention, vocational training and counseling, a specialized nursery school program, a telephone ministry for those in crisis, computer workshops for people with disabilities, and even a driver training facility for disabled persons. A community-based rehabilitation program for people with physical disabilities, that will include land mine victims, is under way. As a matter of principle, the CRC does not discriminate between war victims and other people with disabilities: inclusion criteria revolve strictly around need.

VALUE FIT WITH OCCUPATIONAL THERAPY

Even though the principles defined by the CRC arose strictly from reflection and experience, they share a striking similarity with occupational therapy basic values as presented in the Canadian Model of Occupational Performance.[7] Indeed, the CRC's approach embodies our core beliefs of *human dignity* and *potential for change*. It addresses all aspects of the individual, be they personal, social, or spiritual, and stresses the role of occupation in the healing process of people with disabilities and their war-torn countries. For the CRC, as for true client-centered practice, the notion of client often transcends the individual to encompass entire communities. And, in doing so, it speaks of social justice and the necessity for participation and inclusion.

IDENTIFYING THE CONCEPTUAL FRAMEWORK FOR INTERVENTION WITH THE TARGET POPULATIONS

Drawing from these principles so close to our occupational therapy roots, both the WRF and the CRC intervened extensively in settings where resources are few while needs are overwhelming. However, they eventually felt a need for a format that would operationalize the concepts within their specific context and thus turned to community-based rehabilitation (CBR). CBR was initially developed by the World Health Organization in 1979 and fosters local empowerment and capacity building.[8-10] Conceptually, a great deal of overlap is found between the tenets of CBR as defined by Helander[8] or Werner,[11] the principles elaborated by FAWE, and occupational therapy core values. Both Fransen (see Ch. 13) and Kronenberg and colleagues[12] have underlined the compatibility and congruence that exist between CBR and occupational therapy practice. As a result, there is a definite *goodness of fit* between the CRC's work, the 10 guiding principles, and occupational therapy philosophy.

Principle 1 – Programs must be carried in local languages and respect local culture and values

Neglecting cultural relevance in international development has been documented extensively and still constitutes the most frequent oversight when providing health care.[13,14] Occupational therapists are no exception and must remain vigilant.[10] To counterbalance this tendency, the CRC adapts to local reality.

Even though Arabic is the unifying language of Lebanon, regional differences do exist and the CRC makes a point of hiring local workers who can relate to the war victims in their particular idiom. But beyond language, the CRC also strives to respect regional culture and traditions.

When dealing, for example, with the sequelae of post-traumatic shock syndrome (PTSD), attempts are made to create a supportive setting where safe sharing can take place and where informal self-help groups can play a role. Since the use of the Western individual, psychoanalytical approach has proved only moderately effective,[14] other therapeutic means, closer to the victims' cultural roots, are given precedence. As a result, attendance increases and therapeutic outcomes are enhanced.

In occupational therapy, Kinebanian,[15] Krefting,[16] Paul[17] and Simo Algado et al[18] have already documented this phenomenon and stressed its importance. They have demonstrated that occupational therapy is best practiced in a context where specific cultural environments are understood and respected, even if this translates into service delivery that is almost entirely defined and controlled by local stakeholders.

Principle 2 – Community sensitization, mobilization, and participation are essential for successful reintegration

The CRC staff quickly realized that community reintegration is a major challenge and needs to be initiated in the earliest stages of rehabilitation. The extent of trauma experienced by some local communities in Lebanon was so extreme that it still translates into spontaneous mistrust, and some communities will object to welcoming back any individual connected with the war. Peace is fragile and reminders of a harsh past are obliterated whenever possible. As a rule, in such situations, the NGOs must then turn massively to educating local populations.[19,20] The CRC has taken a gentler approach; it makes frequent but brief sensitization visits to local leaders such as mayors, school principals, and members of government, and gradually readies local institutions eventually to receive the people with disabilities undergoing rehabilitation. A typical visit would consist in describing the legitimate needs for integration of people with disabilities and in highlighting the fact that much can be done at minimal cost with the help of numerous local volunteers. Through formal and informal channels, the CRC creates networks that will ultimately facilitate reintegration.

This choice closely reflects Grady's[21] position on inclusive communities and Townsend's[22] social vision for occupational therapy, where clients cannot be divorced from their backgrounds and where the word client often refers to an entire community. Furthermore, like the CRC, Townsend elaborates on the necessity for social inclusion and participation if we are to achieve any gains with and for people with disabilities.

Principle 3 – Sustainability is achieved mostly through local capacity building, not through punctual international aid

Previous models of aid have often failed for lack of local linkages.[23] Programs were often designed by expatriates, and strictly limited to the period of conflict without extending into the post-war phase where reconstruction occurs and requires support.[24] Results were limited and short-lived because initial interventions were not adapted to the local context and did not include significant follow-up.

With the CRC, the issues of linkages and sustainability are answered. As a national organization, it is well connected to Lebanese culture and resources, and programs are closely tailored to local needs. Moreover, unlike most NGOs working with war victims, the CRC does not see itself as a temporary support for those in need but rather as an agent for social change that will be most effective in the long-term. It is an intrinsic component of Lebanese society, fostering local knowledge transfer and working toward greater justice. Its funders support local capacity building in the truest sense of the words while, in turn, the agency gives back fully to its local partners.

This notion of partnership is a central one in occupational therapy. Fearing, Law and Clark[25] have defined and articulated the workings of client–therapist alliances within the profession, and Sherr Klein[26] has also shared her views on the topic from the client's perspective. Sherr Klein strongly warned the occupational therapy community of the danger of paying only lip service to the idea of equality, an insidious and prevalent trend that sustains ingrained patterns of paternalism towards clients. This trend was also observed and decried as contrary to our professional tenets by Townsend,[22] who studied the current organization of mental health services in Canada.

Providing resources for sustainability and supporting local capacity building have eventually proved the main occupational therapy roles in the partnership with the CRC. The CRC has no need for developing a holistic vision or sufficient expertise for structuring service delivery, since these elements have been in place for the last two decades. The identified needs that are still to be met relate mostly to the securing of permanent and stable funding sources, the acquisition of wide-ranging but costlier means for community sensitization (such as media access), the dissemination of more sophisticated material for lobbying governments and granting agencies, the development of work placements leading to permanent jobs, and the training of local agents in community-based rehabilitation. These steps would all contribute to better long-term service delivery within the local context and in accordance with local priorities.

Principle 4 – Psychological shock is treated (preferably in a group setting) prior to and during training, so that mental health issues are addressed early and training is not postponed indefinitely

Western models of psychological care need considerable adapting for relevant implementation in a post-war context. In their original form, they tend to favor individual support and deny the remarkable resilience shown by war victims and especially by children in war situations.[27–31] Interestingly, several programs in post-conflict areas have been based on what Boyden[13] calls the 'apocalypse model of conflict', a common Western perspective that casts children as passive victims rather than as active survivors. In this model, traumatized children are seen as unable to learn and all efforts are focused on psychological recovery, postponing educational and vocational issues to a distant future. Intensive, individual, and long-term psychological care is presented as the favored option, while collective, short-term intervention becomes a stopgap measure.[32,33]

Even though the CRC has not specifically targeted mental health problems as an area of intervention, it deals with the issue in what could be called a most organic way. Instead of setting up professional services, the CRC has elected to create a space where normal interactions, normalizing occupations, and deep sharing can lead to healing. In a warm, home-like atmosphere, war victims and other people with disabilities seem to connect spontaneously, create self-help groups, and establish natural support networks. No formal structure is imposed but the setting is highly conducive to centeredness, and the tolerance that prevails seems to trigger a solidarity that is reinforced by the use of meaningful occupations. Despite their wounds, the residents are expected to undertake some productive activity very early, and soon they work side by side, sharing painful memories and celebrating their resilience. Counselors are available for the more complex cases, but, as a rule, a non-professional approach is favored. Again, the CRC's position is in line with occupational therapy's long-held beliefs that mental health is intimately intertwined with the physical, and that meaningful, normalizing occupations hold extensive therapeutic power.

Principle 5 – The definition of childhood is contingent to culture and situation, and Western notions should not prevail

In a study on Lebanese children's responses to trauma, Cyrulnik[34] highlighted major differences relating to the definition of childhood. The prevalent Western view of children as being vulnerable, dependent, and passive contradicts local culture and experience. Cyrulnik's results clearly indicate that the Western definition of childhood and the medicalized model of trauma do not meet Lebanese reality. Moreover, the transition between childhood and adulthood is far more nebulous than previously believed.[35,36] Indeed, children's occupational roles vary substantially across the cultural range; what is considered detrimental or unacceptable in one culture might appear desirable or tolerable in another. In Lebanon, children are expected to contribute more to their community than their North American or European counterparts and, in a post-war context, they must even at times assume adult roles. Although these shifts are not perceived as ideal, they are not seen as overly unnatural or harmful.[37]

In its work with the young, the CRC simply attempts to respect the definition of childhood held by each different cultural or religious group. More importantly, it also takes into account the war experiences that have modulated the children's development. Children who have witnessed murder or have been responsible for the survival of their siblings have moved into an adult realm that has altered their lives forever. Cyrulnik states that such events do not prevent healing, but they definitely permeate the children's perception of the world and color their personalities.[34] So, the CRC staff will be careful not to force the children back into a mold of childhood they have outgrown, but will rather support them in their atypical journies toward adulthood.

This concern for a culturally appropriate definition of childhood has been addressed in occupational therapy by Meyers[38] and Thibeault.[6] They have corroborated Cyrulnik's findings that children's occupational roles vary considerably along the cultural spectrum and are shaped by life's circumstances. For example, Thibeault[6] reports that the child soldiers and bush wives of Sierra Leone cannot resume regular childhood occupational roles after leaving the bush where they have assumed adult responsibilities for years. Thus, a careful occupational analysis at the cultural and personal levels must necessarily precede all program design and implementation.

Principle 6 – Collective trauma must find a collective resolution

With regard to the wellbeing of survivors of war, three challenges usually arise when communities engage in collective resolution.[30] First, resources must be devoted to tracing and reunifying broken families.[39] Data from ex-war zones indicate that communities heal faster when natural families are reunited, even in cases of severe internal conflicts.[40,41] Second, given the eventual return of enemy groups to their shared community of origin, a viable modus vivendi acceptable to all must be achieved. Keeping safety as a primary concern, initial contacts between both groups should be closely monitored. Finally, communities have a need for transparency; ignoring or minimizing the history of violence would hinder collective healing.

The CRC works toward peace and reconciliation using an unlikely tool: the disability itself. Without glossing over the violence that has marred the country, the CRC staff acknowledge the damage done, but emphasize the need for solidarity. Many victims from opposing camps now require similar services that are cruelly lacking, and they will obtain them only if they move beyond their hatred and join forces. Resources are too scarce; competitive behaviors are no longer accepted and must give way to collaboration and sharing. Through tactful mediation, the CRC brings previous enemies into joint lobbying and, slowly, because of common and dire needs, eradicates old conflicts. Just as Thibeault[6] observed in the post-war context of Sierra Leone, this mediation often takes the form of a meaningful collective occupation that will, in the end, contribute to the reconstruction of society as a whole. While the CRC has opted for systematic joint lobbying for services, the Sierra Leone programs have focused mainly on the actual collective rebuilding of community infrastructures, such as schools and clinics. Do Rozario[42] and Thibeault[6] also point out the crucial role of ritual occupations in the development of connectedness. Without a feeling of connectedness rooted in shared occupations that are ritual or simply functional in nature, collective living remains a precarious enterprise.

Principle 7 – Healing is closely tied in with socio-economic recovery

Efforts aimed at psychological and community reconstruction would be rendered useless in a society where unemployment and extremely low wages are widespread. In countries struggling with civil conflicts, issues of peace and development cannot be dissociated. 'A failure to achieve broad improvements in living standards would fuel social tensions and heighten the risk of renewed war – and a return to war would shatter hopes for economic revival.'[43] (p. 287) This is true of Lebanon, where the CRC aims at securing gainful employment for its trainees and decent living conditions for people with disabilities. On a larger scale, the CRC also acts as an advocate for equal rights and accessibility with governments and other major stakeholders.

Toulmin,[44] who highlighted the links between occupation, employment, and human welfare, stresses the role of employment in the genesis of a sense of personal integrity and dignity. Fostering and maintaining such integrity and dignity at the individual and collective levels constitutes a key occupational therapy goal with, ultimately, a major impact on political stability and social recovery.

Principle 8 – Healing is best maintained within a restored civil society

Most recent civil conflicts have in the main been triggered or exacerbated by blatant, and unbearable, social inequalities.[45] These inequalities have found some of their roots in market stagnation, external debt, and unfair trade. Even though these factors take a major toll on the fledgling economies, the main culprit lies not with external financial forces but with internal corruption.[46] Consequently, eradicating corruption through good governance becomes the ultimate priority. Among other solutions, Boyce and Pastor[43] advocate, as the priority, the renovation of a legal system that would closely monitor official property rights and contracts. Since the legal body is often the first to collapse in a war-torn country, auditing mechanisms should be reimplanted quickly and applied more stringently. Also, all subsequent economic development policies should be designed according to peace building needs. Revenue should be raised by increasing taxes for the wealthy, and military expenditures and other non-essential expenses should be cut drastically.

For civil society to be fully restored and conducive to collective healing, the rights of people with disabilities, internally displaced persons, and refugees must also be officially imbedded in a proper charter. From data collected in similar settings,[47,48] it becomes evident that social inclusion does not occur spontaneously, and that advocacy and lobbying are essential for bringing policies and procedures into place at the government level.

Furthermore, fundamental values such as respect and tolerance must be reinfused in the social fabric and the moral vacuum experienced by the ex-combatants must be addressed. Peace education should become an intrinsic part of rehabilitation[29] and can be approached as a collective, reconstructive occupation, where ex-combatants who have shifted away from an aggressive stance can become role models for others. As mentioned earlier, the CRC plays an important role advocating for the most vulnerable, but it is also a leader in terms of peace education. Using both didactic means and modeling, the CRC has already had a significant impact on the communities where it works. Its services reflect its philosophy: team members from a wide variety of backgrounds, often from rival groups, collaborate peacefully in the reconstruction of Lebanese civil society. Again, Townsend's[22] voice echoes the ideals of the CRC as she argues that occupational therapists must understand that healing does not end with restoring function, but rather with establishing justice for all in a society that is fiscally and politically responsible. Our role goes beyond the narrow therapeutic range into the broad social arena. As they adapt current and often unjust conditions to foster positive outcomes in the present, occupational therapists must also keep in mind the future and articulate a vision that will have a transformative influence on society and bring about better living conditions for the disadvantaged.[10]

Principle 9 – Gender equality should evolve into a pillar of the new social order

'The plight of war widows, sexually abused women, and single female-headed households created by conflicts has been overlooked in the past by the international community, partly because such victims are not socially or politically visible.'[48] (p. 23) The unfair treatment of women in war-torn countries is well documented.[49] Few countries, however, have rectified the situation in post-war reconstruction.[50] Lebanon is no exception to the rule and the CRC is very active in lobbying for women's equal opportunities for health, education, and employment, as occupational therapists, who are devoted to the protection of all society's members, should be.

Principle 10 – Health can best be maintained in adequate environments

Civil society does not refer to political or social structures alone. Environmental factors must be taken into account and contribute to health or ill-health.[50,51] In Lebanon, as in many post-war areas, the danger arises mainly from potentially unchecked development that could result in severe environmental damage and unhealthy living conditions. Although the CRC exerts little control in this area, it includes environmental awareness in its training and insures sound ecological practices in its programs.

This strategy is reminiscent of Wilcock's[52] position on the environment: she clearly states that health cannot be optimal in unhealthy environments. Best conditions must be strived for, ecologically or otherwise, to produce a society that promotes health and wellbeing. Wilcock's concept of health, exposed in *An Occupational Perspective of Health*,[52] (p. 110) explicitly links 'social integration, support, and justice, all within and as part of a sustainable ecology'. Occupational therapists can no longer ignore the greater context and must plan their interventions not only according to therapeutic outcomes, but also in terms of their social and ecological implications.

OCCUPATIONAL THERAPY ROLES

As demonstrated earlier, a natural conceptual fit occurs between occupational therapy values and the CRC's philosophy. However, given the non-traditional nature of the setting, occupational therapy roles still had to be carefully attuned to the 10 principles outlined above. In keeping with the greater goals of **sustainability and local capacity building**, specific occupational therapy roles included the following:

1. securing resources through grant applications to governmental and non-governmental agencies;
2. providing a framework for intervention, namely community-based rehabilitation;
3. monitoring, with the organization, the program planning and its evaluation in terms of process, outcomes, and impact;
4. participating in community mobilization through the design and implementation of needs assessments;
5. taking part in sensitization programs aimed at the general public and decision makers;
6. fostering knowledge transfer through staff training and the design of culturally appropriate teaching material;
7. taking part in the planning and implementation of advocacy work;
8. facilitating networking between local NGOs and other potential partners in the field;

9. enhancing the organization's visibility through publications, publicity, and public relations;
10. offering online consultation between site visits.

CONCLUSION

This chapter's aim was to highlight the connections between health, social justice, and occupational therapy values through the use of real life examples. The Lebanese experience demonstrates not only that sound development practices are conceptually related to occupational therapy core values, but also that occupational therapists make ideal partners for local NGOs whose mandates encompass health and social justice issues. Few health professionals are trained to answer both needs, but occupational therapy's vision and exceptional positioning turn us into precious allies in war zones and other similarly ravaged settings. Maybe the time has come to define our role more explicitly as agents for social change, and offer our expertise to those most in need, within and beyond the world of traditional health care.

EPILOGUE

A waves at us from the CRC porch. The stone house could use some repair but still remains a most welcoming place: the de-mined garden, carefully tended, offers flowers, fruit, and shade. A blind woman kindly asks if I want a glass of water; a man in a wheelchair rushes to get it. The common room's atmosphere is relaxed and calm despite the large number of people it holds. These war victims have known torture, land mines, and the lack of basic health care, such as immunization, brought on by the conflict. In this small space, nearly all motor and sensory deficits are found, along with the psychological sequelae they carry.

I can't hide my surprise: 'Given the lack of resources and transportation, gathering as many people in need in a single room is nothing short of a miracle.'

T retorts: 'This is not the true miracle.'

A then introduces me to the center's staff: each comes from a different religious, social, and political background and, together, they recreate the rich fabric of Lebanese society. Here, however, solidarity replaces hostility. I stand witness to A's dream: rebuilding, around the war victims' suffering, a society torn apart by its differences. If regular citizens cannot agree on political or religious issues, couldn't they push aside their divergent views and mobilize themselves to help the victims of a war they have in common? With the shared belief of social justice for all, couldn't they weave relationships imbued with tolerance and mutual support?

The answer seems to be yes. Already, the Muslim mother and the Christian father discuss the special needs of their children, both maimed by land mines. Together, the parents will lobby local authorities to obtain specialized services. And the laborer who has been ostracized for working in Israel finds a role in

> *his community as a volunteer wheelchair technician. The wall of silent hatred,*
> *still firmly erect in the towns, starts to crumble at the CRC, because here, the*
> *Other has a name and a face; the Enemy has a story ever so similar to one's*
> *own. And as you keep meeting face and story in the truth of suffering, they*
> *start to belong to a friend.*

References

1. World Rehabilitation Fund. Mine action in Lebanon. New York: WRF; 2001.
2. World Rehabilitation Fund. Fields of work. New York: WRF; 2000.
3. Dagher A, Akiki I. Personal communication. Beirut; 2001.
4. Landes DS. The wealth and poverty of nations: why some are so rich and some so poor. New York: WW Norton; 1999.
5. Sen A. Development as freedom. New York; Random House; 1999.
6. Thibeault R. Occupation and the rebuilding of civil society: notes from the war zone. J of Occup Sci 2002; 9(1):38–47.
7. Canadian Association of Occupational Therapists. Enabling occupation: an occupational therapy perspective. Ottawa: CAOT; 1997.
8. Helander E. Prejudice and dignity: an introduction to community-based rehabilitation. New York: United Nations Development Program; 1992.
9. Peat M. Community-based rehabilitation. Toronto: Saunders; 1997.
10. Thibeault R, Forget A. From snow to sand: CBR perspectives from the Arctic and Africa. Can J Rehabil 1997; 10(2):134–140.
11. Werner D. Disabled village children. 5th edn. Berkeley: Hesparian Foundation; 1999.
12. World Federation of Occupational Therapists. Position paper on community based rehabilitation. Forrestfield, Australia: World Federation of Occupational Therapists; 2004.
13. Boyden J. Children's experiences of conflict-related emergencies: some implications for relief policy and practice. Disasters 1994; 3:67–76.
14. Maynard KA. Rebuilding community: psychosocial healing, reintegration and reconciliation at the grassroots level. In: Kumar K, ed. Rebuilding civil society after civil war: critical roles for international assistance. Boulder, Colorado: Lynne Rienner; 1997.
15. Kinebanian A, Stomp M. Cross-cultural occupational therapy: a critical reflection. Am J Occup Ther 1992; 6(8):751–761.
16. Krefting D. Understanding community approaches to handicap in development (CAHD). Handicap and development collection. Lyon, France: Handicap International; 2001.
17. Paul S. Culture and its influence on occupational therapy evaluation. Can J (Occup Ther 1995; 62:554–561.
18. Simó Algado S, Rodriguez Gregori JM, Egan M. Spirituality in a refugee camp. Can J Occup Ther 1997; 64(3):118–126.
19. Apfel RJ, Bennett S. On psychosocial interventions for children: some minders and reminders. Geneva: UNICEF; 1995.
20. Blomqvist U. Community participation in a refugee emergency – focusing on community mobilization, women and youth. Stockholm: Rädda Barnen; 1995.
21. Grady AP. Occupation as a vision. Am J Occup Ther 1992; 46:1062–1065.
22. Townsend EA. Beyond our clinics: a vision for the future. Am J Occup Ther 1991; 45:871–873.
23. Boothby N, Upton P, Sultan A. Children of Mozambique: the cost of survival. Durham, NC: Institute of Policy and Public Affairs, Duke University; 1991.
24. Kumar K. The nature and focus of international assistance for rebuilding war-torn societies. In: Kumar K, ed. Rebuilding civil society after civil war: critical roles for international assistance. Boulder, Colorado: Lynne Rienner; 1997.
25. Fearing VG, Law M, Clark M. An occupational performance process model: fostering client and therapist alliance. Can J of Occup Ther 1997; 64:7–15.
26. Sherr Klein B. Reflections on … An ally as well as a partner in practice. Can J Occup Ther 1995; 62:283–285.
27. Derviskadic-Jovanovic S, Mikus-Kos A. What can we do to support children who have been through the war? Forced Migration Review 1998; 1(3):4–8.
28. Dyregroz A, Raundalen M. Children in warfare and their special needs. Bergen, Norway: Center for Crisis Psychology; 1995.
29. Evans J. Children as zones of peace: working with young children affected by armed violence.

Geneva: The Consultative Group on Early Childhood Care and Development; 1996.

30. Herbst L. Children in war: strategies for healing. New York: Save the Children Federation; 1995.

31. Petty C, Bracken PJ. Rethinking the trauma of war: a conference report. London: Free Association Books and Save the Children Fund; 1998.

32. Stallard P, Law F. The psychological effects of traumas on children. Children and Society 1994; 8(2):567–570.

33. Sterk P. Children associated with war: child soldiers in Sierra Leone. Online. Available: www.euronet.nl/p_sterk/childsold.htm.

34. Cyrulnik B. *Le murmure des fantômes.* Paris: Odile Jacob; 2003.

35. Gibbs S. Postwar social reconstruction in Mozambique: reframing children's experiences of trauma and healing. In: Kumar K, ed. Rebuilding civil society after civil war: critical roles for international assistance. Boulder, Colorado: Lynne Rienner; 1997.

36. Holland P. What is a child? Popular images of childhood. London: Virgo Press; 1992.

37. International Save the Children Alliance Working Group on Children Affected by Armed Conflict and Displacement. Promoting psychosocial well-being among children affected by armed conflict and displacement: principles and approaches. Geneva: International Save the Children Alliance; 1996.

38. Meyers C. Among children and their families: consideration of cultural influences in assessment. Am J Occup Ther 1992; 46:737–744.

39. Bonnerjea L. Family tracing and children's rights: some questions about the best interests of separated children. Disasters 1994; 3:45–56.

40. Cohen R, Deng FM. The forsaken people: case studies of the internally displaced. Washington: Brookings Institution Press; 1998.

41. Momoh T. Personal communications. Freetown; 2000, 2001.

42. Do Rozario L. Ritual, meaning and transcendence: the role of occupation in modern life. J Occup Sci 1994; 46(3):46–53.

43. Boyce JK, Pastor M. Macroeconomic policy and peace building in El Salvador. In: Kumar K, ed. Rebuilding civil society after civil war: critical roles for international assistance. Boulder, Colorado: Lynne Rienner; 1997.

44. Toulmin SE. Occupation, employment and human welfare. J Occup Sci 1995; 2:48–57.

45. Ball N. Demobilizing and reintegrating soldiers: lessons from Africa. In: Kumar K. ed. Rebuilding civil society after civil war: critical roles for international assistance. Boulder, Colorado: Lynne Rienner; 1997.

46. United Nations. The UN 2000 report on poverty. Geneva: United Nations; 2000.

47. Women's Commission for Refugee Women and Children. Untapped potential: adolescents affected by armed conflict – a review of programs and policies. New York: Women's Commission for Refugee Women and Children; 2000.

48. Kumar K. The nature and focus of international assistance for rebuilding war-torn societies. In: Kumar K, ed. Rebuilding civil society after civil war: critical roles for international assistance. Boulder, Colorado: Lynne Rienner; 1997.

49. Women's Commission for Refugee Women and Children. The children's war towards peace in Sierra Leone: a field report assessing the protection and assistance needs of Sierra Leone children and adolescents. Geneva: Women's Commission for Refugee Women and Children; 2000.

50. Raven-Roberts A, Dick B. Safe places for youth: issues of youth in conflict zones and disordered states. Oxford: Refugee Participation Network; 1997.

51. Law M. The environment: a focus for occupational therapy. Can J Occup Ther 1991; 58:171–179.

52. Wilcock AA. An occupational perspective of health. Thorofare, NJ: Slack; 1998

Chapter **18**

Occupational therapy intervention with children survivors of war

Salvador Simó Algado, Imelda Burgman

OVERVIEW

In this chapter an occupational therapy program for children survivors of war is presented. The program, focused on the secondary prevention of the occupational and psychological consequences of war, was developed for use with children survivors of war in Gjakova, Kosovo by two occupational therapists, Nina Mehta and Salvador Simó Algado, and lasted 4 months.

The art of the project was based on a community-centered approach, developing a humanistic, holistic, and transcultural philosophy,[1-6] where meaningful occupation is the soul of the intervention. The science was based on the Model of Human Occupation[7] and the Canadian Occupational Performance Process Model.[8]

Through meaningful occupations, children were able to travel from a place of war, where they were victims, toward a more beautiful place, where they realized that they were survivors. Occupational therapy is about becoming.[9]

This chapter emphasizes the impact of war on children's spirituality and how to articulate spirituality in an intervention project, thereby developing spiritual resilience.[10]

All the children's words in this chapter are from the sessions we developed with teachers and children during our project in Gjakova. (see p. 253 below).

INTRODUCTION

My dear friend …
I do not know if the black Serbians gave you a last wish before killing you, but I know that before dying you saw a light, the light of freedom, and I know now you are an angel of peace.

When I listen to these words of a child survivor, my professional ego is listening to the voice of a 'patient', a 'victim', a traumatized child whom

I will label and attempt to heal. But the reality is that I am listening to the voice of a teacher, the voice of a survivor. If I listen carefully, removing the indifferent layer that surrounds my soul and heart, I will hear the voice of suffering and a call for action, but also the voice of the human spirit, the voice of hope.

THE CONTEXT: WAR IN GJAKOVA, KOSOVO

War is the saddest word that I can pronounce. It is a bad bird that never rests. It is the bird of death that destroys houses and steals our infancy. War is the evil bird that converts the world into hell. (Maida, 12 years)[11]

War is a short word, with a meaning that cannot truly be comprehended or even imagined in academic texts.

This story says even the sun and the clouds are crying for destroyed Kosovo, all in blood. (Besart, 11 years)

Gjakova, originally green land surrounding a mosque in the sixteenth century, is a town of 60 000 people located in the southwest region of Kosovo. Before the war, 90% of its inhabitants were ethnic Albanians and 10% were Serbians. Milosevic's new government marked the beginning of 10 years of Serbian oppression. Albanian culture, social expression, and political involvement were completely suppressed. When the North Atlantic Treaty Organization (NATO) started its military campaign in 1999, the people of Gjakova underwent 3 months of intense adversity. Jeta and Fjolla, 12-year-old children, recall that time in these words: 'the robberies, evacuations, massacres, and torture, were our daily bread' (Jeta) and 'Serb occupiers killed people and burnt houses. They killed children and pregnant women, and they made us leave. There was a river of blood. My cousin was killed with three other girls in the basement.' (Fjolla)

During the war 40% of the city was completely burned down and 20% was left partially destroyed. Gjakova was a prime target for ethnic cleansing. It is important to note that 60% of the population did not abandon Gjakova but for 3 months remained hidden in their basements, waiting their turn to die: 'At five in the morning we came out of our basement. I had fear in my heart because I thought it was our turn to die.' (Kaltrina, 12 years)

In understanding trauma, the victims' proximity to it and its frequency and duration have been documented as important factors to consider,[12] and we should not forget new sources of trauma, such as the status of prisoners. More than 1600 boys and men from Gjakova were missing. Mass graves were discovered every day:

Now we have freedom and we should be happy like the rest of the world, but this is not happening here because when they left the Serbians took 1600 hostages from my city Gjakova. This worries us a lot. We are waiting for their release. (Elza, 13 years)

The harsh winter, a lack of adequate housing, and poverty were sources of additional trauma. Land mines are eternal sentinels, which killed and maimed children: 'I am drawing a house in fire and flowers; underneath there are mines, so we must be careful when we play.' (Arjona, 8 years)

A further source of trauma was the political situation. The Albanian population believed that they had finally won their independence, giving meaning to their suffering: 'Our hands are waiting for freedom, but you can not win freedom without blood.'(Gembiana, 11 years) However, this has not been realized and Kosovo is still part of Serbia.

WAR AND THE CHILD

In war children are lost, separated from their families, abandoned, orphaned, tortured, mutilated, sexually abused, kidnapped, die of famine, are forced to become soldiers, are obligated to kill, or live by the thousands in refugee camps, with their traumatic memories. One in every two victims of world-wide conflicts is a child. Some mines are specifically designed to harm children. Particular harm is directed toward girls through sexual abuse, sometimes resulting in having to bear a child for the enemy. The consequences of war, such as hunger and the disappearance of medical services, kill 20 times more people than war itself. UNICEF confirms that every day between 35 000 and 40 000 children die due to a lack of basic care.[13] In 2000 several reports showed that in 24 of the 32 ongoing conflicts world wide, children under 15 years of age were recruited.[14] In the 10 years following the drawing up of the International Convention on the Rights of the Child in 1989, more than 2 million boys and girls were murdered by warfare, over 6 million children were wounded or left handicapped, 12 million lost their homes, and more than 10 million were left with emotional trauma because of the violence they suffered or witnessed. More than 30 million children were forced to move from the area where they lived.[15] Behind all these figures, there are children's lives, hopes, and dreams.

Trauma

In this picture I have presented crimes carried out by the Serbians: killings and massacres, burning houses, shops and mosques destroyed. I was so worried about this, and there is a big hole in my heart. (Arta, 11 years)

Fraenkel and Tallant[16] state that children who have suffered from trauma 'harbor intense feelings of fear, anger and insecurity which, when suppressed, often lead to maladaptive behavioral responses' (p.59). When left unexpressed, childhood traumatic experiences can manifest themselves later in life as psychological conditions such as depression, personality disorders, post-traumatic stress disorder, and maladaptive behavior.[13, 16–19] These maladaptive responses can be manifested through physical aggression toward peers and siblings, sleeplessness, withdrawal, anxiety, fear, and silence. Children lose their interest in play experiences and tend to suppress even the more elementary feelings, such as love for their parents.

Gavrilovic et al[18] reported that childhood trauma is a risk factor that predisposes the individual to development of mental health problems. Similarly, Valent[20] studied testimonies from holocaust survivors and found that post-traumatic responses can affect the trauma survivor's personality, morality, and existential meanings. Finally, Driver and Beltran[17] reported that children with trauma from war and displacement showed poor school performance, problematic social interactions, and difficulties with gross motor activities, such as sports.

The political nature of human occupation

Conflicts are often stirred by outside powers, with their insatiable appetite for land and natural resources.[15] Ninety percent of the weapons used are sold by industrialized countries.[13] The biggest land mine producers, such as the USA, have not ratified the Ottawa Convention for the banning of land mines. When we work in a rehabilitation center with a child who has stepped on a land mine, we should become social activists and be aware of, denounce, and combat the hidden sociopolitical conditions.[21] I believe we cannot ignore them, as we are an active part of the problem. The wellbeing of Western societies is based on the exploitation of the so-called developing countries. The globalization process, based on a market economy and on neglecting human values, can be seen as the new face of colonialism.

Spirituality

Spirit[22] is a powerful, mysterious word; its meanings spread like an invisible web through every level of existence. It is air, it is breath, and by extension it is life and speech. It is the power of divine creation, moving over the waters, and it is the divinity itself – the Great Spirit, the Holy Spirit, the Lord of All. Spirituality is knowledge of the sacred, the holy, the divine.

As human beings we have a spiritual essence. The spirit is our true self that we try to express in all our activities,[23] but 'diverse spiritual expressions and meanings are culturally and ethically grounded in different value systems, so there is no single definition of experience which can be named spirituality'.[24] (p. 3) However, two basic dimensions related to spirituality are meaning and connection.

Urbanowski and Vargo[25] define spirituality as 'the experience of meaning in everyday life'. This premise is based on three classical notions: existence, *dasein* (being in the world right here and now), and the social construction of meaning.[10]

The capacity to find meaning in traumatic experiences is a key dimension for human resilience.[26,27] Resilience is the capacity of a human being to confront trauma and to develop a meaningful life. Resilience and spirituality are linked. Ramugondo (see Ch. 23) argues that it is through resilience that we can find our own spirituality, and that spirituality in turn strengthens our ability to be resilient. Urbanowski[10] introduces the term *spiritual resiliency* and defines it as 'the successful completion and entrenchment of meaningful occupations that one engaged in prior to a life changing event occurring, or to engage in new occupations to create a post-event trajectory'(p. 102). He identifies protective factors for spiritual wellbeing: personal factors such as insight or creativity; social factors such as familial and community relationships; and cultural factors such as ethnicity, race, or gender. He distinguishes between generalized risk factors such as poverty or disability, and specific and developmental risk factors.

Individuals can experience spirituality as a feeling of belonging and connection.[28] Spirituality refers to our connection with ourselves, with our values and feelings, with the rest of humanity, and with the universe itself.[29] For one to hope, one needs to have some understanding of how we are connected to the universe (see Ch. 23). Interconnected communities are characterized by interdependence, where reciprocity and mutuality and the foundations of life are shared.[30] The power of the community connection liberates healing resources that link people and integrate those who are outside the healing circles.[31]

The Canadian Association of Occupational Therapists' definition of spirituality integrates both dimensions: 'it is a pervasive life force, manifestation of a higher self, source of will and self determination, and a sense of meaning, purpose and connectedness that people experience in the context of their environment.'[8] (p. 182)

Impact of war on children's spirituality

Experiencing war affects the essence, the soul of the child. The child may experience life as without meaning, making it difficult to develop or sustain resilience. It is extremely hard for children to understand the reality that confronts them, to connect with their own feelings, when they are suffering emotionally and their values are in crisis. War confronts children with the dark side of life:

> *In this picture I tried to draw Serbians without spirits. I do not think that anybody in the world will survive after seeing how criminal they are. [I saw] children without heads, they killed babies in their mothers' bodies, and forced their sisters to drink the blood. Killing parents in front of their children, raping daughters in front of their parents, those things are not what human beings do. This massacre was so terrible. Serbians took my aunt's sons and we have not heard anything from them. The hate in our heart was so big.* (Orjeta, 13 years)

The basic human need and capacity to connect with others is also at risk. Montagu[32] asserts that the human infant requires, beyond all else, a great deal of tender loving care. The infant's need for love is critical, and its satisfaction necessary if the infant is to grow and develop. Through being loved, power is released in the infant to love others. This is a critically important lesson, that as human beings we need to understand and learn: the cultivation of the development of love in the child should be his or her natural birthright.[33] Cirulnik[26] affirms that these emotional foundations are another foundation for resilience. War is the antithesis of love.

Children may have lost their loved ones: 'I must leave you father without saying goodbye to you, and with tears in my eyes and pain in my heart. I walk through the road of sadness.' (Gjiylizare, 12 years)

Suzuki[22] speaks of rituals as a public affirmation of meaning, values, and connection. Rituals link people with their predecessors and with their place in the world. In Gjakova the community network had been broken, including traditions, rituals, and ceremonies. The occupational apartheid of disconnection from community practices endangers children's connection with the spirit of their community and with their own spirit (see Ch. 12). In Gjakova children had no access to meaningful occupations. For example, some children spent 3 months hidden in basements, waiting for their turn to die. The mosque was severely damaged during the war period, so there were no celebrations. The children had no access to the spiritual avenues of artistic expression, play, or nature, due to ongoing combat and the presence of land mines. Their ability to connect with the spirit of their community was denied.

OCCUPATIONAL THERAPY IS ABOUT BECOMING

Wilcock[9] urges occupational therapists to expand their professional roles to include the promotion of health and wellbeing in all people, especially those living under severe political and social conditions. As occupational therapists we can no longer ignore the sociopolitical dimension of human occupation. In introducing the concept of occupational apartheid (see Ch. 6), Kronenberg[34] describes access to meaningful occupations as fundamental to the human right of health and wellbeing. The role of occupational therapy is to empower members of the community to recognize their own potential through meaningful occupations and move toward occupational justice (see Ch. 9).[35]

We, the authors of this chapter, believe that occupational therapy interventions focused on prevention are critical with children survivors of war. The benefits of preventive measures, aimed at identifying risks and promoting wellbeing, are well known,[36] so in our work in Gjakova the therapists involved developed a program of secondary prevention with the children in an attempt to counteract the psychological and occupational consequences of war. Intervention with children survivors of war challenges us, confronting us with one of the biggest atrocities of our time.

THE PROJECT

The Gjakova project was developed over 4 months in 1999 by two occupational therapists, Nina Mehta and Salvador Simó Algado, working in collaboration with the NGOs Médecins Sans Frontières and Clowns without Borders and responsible for designing and implementing a preventive mental health project with the children of Gjakova. A complementary treatment program for children was also developed and children with complex problems were referred for individual treatment to a clinical psychologist, Lulezim Arapi, who was a member of the local community. A volunteer occupational therapist, Steve Johns, from Canada, continued the project.

Occupational therapy: the art and the science

The intervention was based on a community-centered approach[1-6] (see Ch. 25), developing a humanistic, transcultural,[1-6] and holistic occupational therapy program, with meaningful occupation as the core of the intervention.

The community-centered approach applies a client-centered approach[37] to communities, with empathy, authenticity, and congruency as vital qualities. The aim is to promote the sense of an inner locus of control and inner responsibility within the community. Members of the local Albanian community were encouraged to become self sufficient, independent promoters of children's mental health.

Transcultural occupational therapy goes further than simply recognizing the beauty of all cultures; it introduces culturally meaningful occupations in the intervention.

Holistic occupational therapy means understanding the human being as a physical, psychosocial, and sociopolitical being, whose essence is spiritual, and who is immersed in an ecological and cultural environment where meaningful occupation is the occupational crossroads where the needs, capacities, and the spirit of the person meet. This definition includes the spirit of the person, because the spirit is our true self that we try to express in all our activities.[23]

The Model of Human Occupation[7] (see Ch. 14) and the Canadian Occupational Performance Process Model (COPPM)[8] (Ch. 15) formed the theoretical basis of the intervention.

To understand children and to help them to express themselves we must speak their language. Play is their most essential and meaningful occupation. Play was used in the workshops, to provide support, to promote insight, and to enable the children to experience emotional catharsis, positive experiences, and success in their activities. Expressive activities using art, clay, and narratives acted as a secondary medium through which children could communicate their thoughts, emotions, feelings, and desires.[38]

Narrative theory[39] suggests that narratives give children a context in which to regain meaning and define their lives in order to make sense of their experiences. Children suffering from trauma can benefit from expressing traumatic experiences as part of the process of normalization.[16,38] During the project the children wrote their narratives as survivors.

The intervention program

The program was intended to serve children of primary school age (6–14 years) in Gjakova. The objective was to select teachers from the five public schools and train them in the following roles:

- conducting occupational therapy workshops using expressive techniques to facilitate emotional expression of traumatic experiences at a preventive level

---

Box 18.1 Topics in theoretical sessions

1. What is mental health?
   Mental health promotion
   Mental health conditions
      Depression
      Anxiety
      Phobias
2. Principles of occupational therapy
   Holistic and humanistic view of the individual
   Occupation as a therapeutic medium
   How to develop a mental health workshop through occupational therapy
3. Model of Human Occupation
4. Logotherapy
5. Secondary trauma in the therapist
6. The child
   Childhood depression and anxiety
   Self-esteem in the child
   The language of children: play
   Behavior management techniques with children
   Use of displacement techniques
      Art
      Narratives
      Puppetry
      Clay
      Drama
      Theatre
      Collage
      Mime

- detecting children with complex or specific symptoms and referring them to a specialist.

The program consisted of three phases:

- theoretical training
- practical training
- additional training on specific topics.

After the three phases, it was expected that the local mental health promoter would develop the occupational therapy workshops.

Theoretical training

The objective was to provide the teachers with knowledge of basic concepts in mental health. There were 12 training sessions, each 2 hours long. The first hour was dedicated to theory (see Box 18.1) while the second hour was practical and involved learning to use activities with a therapeutic purpose (see Box 18.2).

As all of the teachers were also suffering from post-war trauma, it was essential to address their own mental health needs during the training.

Box 18.2   Projective techniques and activities

Activities
- Individual drawing
    - colored pencils
    - pastels
    - water colors
    - markers
    - tempera
- Collective drawing
- Finger painting
- Collage
- Puppets
- Origami
- Stories
    - balloons
    - little toys
- Theatre
- Mime
- Guided fantasy
- Construction
    - clay
    - toys
    - kits
    - plasticine
- Narratives
- Bibliotherapy

Themes
- Message to the world
- Future of Gjakova
- Message to the Serbians

Practical training

The objective was to enable teachers to conduct occupational workshops independently. Workshops were held three times a week for 2 hours each. Each session consisted of two components: fun activities such as sports, games, and songs, and projective activities for emotional expression. Complementing fun activities with displacement activities provided the children with positive experiences that motivated them to return to the sessions. It was essential to find a balance between providing support and facilitating their emotional expression. The fun activities, based on play theory,[40] were also considered therapeutic, helping to channel negative emotions in a constructive manner. They were the best moments to observe the non-verbal behavior of the children.

Each session utilized one specific projective technique (see Box 18.2). The sessions always began with games, followed by the main activity, for example painting with a free theme. The children gave their creation a title and wrote a description of what they had created, why they chose it, and what they felt while creating it. Finally, teachers gave children an opportunity to present their work to the rest of the group and thus initiate discussions about various issues. The sessions usually ended with singing or sports activities.

Initial sessions were focused on helping the children to identify different feelings and making them aware of the importance of expressing them. The initial games often identified different emotions. Puppets and plush toys were used to help children visualize different feelings. For example, a clown puppet was used to identify happiness, a demon was used for hate.

Successful sessions focused on teaching the children to realize why it is important to share feelings, and facilitating discussions about difficult emotions. We created stories with the puppets. For example, if the demon is inside the heart of a child and the clown comes and knocks at the door of the heart, what will happen? Will the demon allow the clown to enter? Initially, the children resolved the situation by throwing the demon out of the heart. This led to discussion with the children on different ways of ventilating difficult feelings such as sadness, hate, or anger. In the discussions, we concentrated on making links between the feelings and emotions identified in the drawings or puppets and the personal feelings and experiences of the children.

It was emphasized repeatedly that what the children were experiencing was normal in such extreme circumstances. By normalizing reactions and by drawing similarities between individual experiences, each child felt reassured that he or she was not the only one with feelings of sadness, fear, and loss. Children with less trauma would become more aware of others' experiences and show empathy for their peers.

Additional training

Performers from Clowns without Borders conducted extra training workshops. The role of the clowns was to transfer specific techniques and skills. The clowns also performed entertainment shows for the children in the schools and for the general community.

Results

The teachers completed more than 72 hours of training over the course of 3 months. In total, 70 schoolteachers and 30 medical students participated in the training. More than 500 children attended the program in five different schools. It was expected that the teachers would be able to work with new groups of children.

Discussion

The use of play and expressive occupational workshops demonstrated the power of meaningful occupation in helping children to express and process traumatic emotions successfully. The primary reaction of the younger children was the need to express immediate images of objects from visual memory. They began drawing images of burning houses, tanks, and corpses.

Children brought into the sessions the daily events that they had witnessed. For example, the day after the eclipse some children made drawings of it. The older children (12–14 years) expressed what they had seen more symbolically, through images, and also wrote powerful narratives and poems. An evolution from darker themes to more positive thoughts was noted.

The cultural aspect was included in the form of Kosovarian poems and songs, used to begin the sessions. The children expressed themselves very passionately. All the songs referred to the massacres, providing a socialized way of expressing their pain.

Alongside other factors, such as family and community support and proper health care and education, it was important to recognize that the occupational activities were essential in preventing future consequences of trauma in children.

Children's spirituality

If we want to articulate spirituality in our daily practice, first we must develop our own spiritual essence. It is not just a case of employing definitions or models; our own spirituality is involved. We must believe in the human spirit, and we must develop trust and hope in its power and beauty. This is not easy when we are confronted with war, devastation, hate, and suffering, but we cannot transmit hope and courage when we do not feel it.

It is extremely important to take care of our own spiritual wellbeing.[41] For some this means being in close contact with nature, but this was not possible in Kosovo. It means having time to meditate, time to transcend our direct reality, to recover peace of mind and heart; time to become immersed in the ocean of prayer, where we can meet our loved ones, time to realize we are not alone, that there are many hands in our hands, that our voice speaks for many voices. Although not Muslim, I (Simó Algado) used to go to the mosque where the people still went to pray even though it had been destroyed. I sat there meditating, sharing the moment with the people. The most important source of spiritual healing was the children with whom we had the privilege to walk. We received such a beautiful lesson of courage and spiritual resilience from them, and so much love and tenderness.

During the project the occupational therapists and the teachers listened to the children with great respect. We were amazed by the wisdom that they expressed, and their understanding of the deeper realities of human life. They expressed even their saddest feelings in such a poetical way:

> *My friend Dorina*
> *I remember happy days with you*
> *Every face was happy,*
> *Now every face is sad.*
> *Oh, those black Serbians didn't spare you as a child,*
> *They didn't spare your sisters and brothers,*
> *but burnt you alive in the houses.*
> *In my school*
> *Teaching has started*
> *Your empty place*
>
> *Is searching for you.*
> *We cover it with flowers*

> *We cover it with tears*
> *For the blossom*
> *That we can never forget.* (Dielleza, 11years)

To be listened to with respect helped them to listen to themselves:[42] 'During this drawing I had special feelings; I imagined myself in a house where I could be relaxed and forget all the troubles I had received from Serbians. I thought and asked myself "Can I play freely without fear?" and the answer is finally "Yes." ' (Orjeta, 13 years) It is so important to understand the way children express themselves and to respect their rhythm; we can invite but never force their expression.[43] We needed to speak their language, play, as the soul of the intervention.

The project supported the children in recovering their daily rituals,[44–46] and in returning to their natural environment, their schools. We tried to rebuild an inclusive community, since inclusiveness is the community dimension of spirituality,[47] by promoting community awareness about the problems that the children had faced. This was done in the schools with the children and teachers, and in larger meetings with the parents. Human values such as solidarity and love were recovered. The teachers and children enacted many beautiful examples of love. The teachers developed the project as volunteers, transcending their own problems. The children themselves tenderly took care of those who had confronted more traumatic events. For example, one day the younger children were playing, performing as fashion models and applauding each other. One girl was receiving more applause than the rest. I asked one child why this should be. The reply came: 'Because now she is an orphan, and we are taking care of her.' Special attention was paid to working with the children's feelings of hate and revenge, transforming them into positive human values. One theme suggested was a letter to the Serbian soldiers who had committed the atrocities, starting a discussion about hate and how to channel it.

Through engagement in meaningful occupations the children were able to look for and find meaning in the experiences they had suffered, and to give new meaning to their daily lives.[48] All this took place in a spontaneous way, highlighting the spiritual potential of the children. They associated the massacres with the meaning of freedom, acknowledging that through the sacrifice of their loved ones, others survived: 'A mother of one Albanian soldier is crying and says: "If I could find the body of my dead son ... I would feel as if he is alive, and maybe he would say to me 'mother we got what we wanted: freedom.' " '(Saranda, 11 years)

It is difficult for children who have lived through the trauma of war to move from the present to a possible future.[49] We asked the children to draw the future of Gjakova, helping them to develop hope for the future.[50] The poet Emily Dickinson wrote: 'Hope is the thing with feathers that perches in the soul, And sings the tune without words, And never stops at all.'[51] The bird of hope sang freely again in Kosovo.

The children explored different art expressions. We could not develop occupations in nature due to the land mines, but themes related to nature were constantly in their drawings. In images of nature the children found visions to express hope, visions of the future, and of sadness: 'I am drawing a tree without leaves to express Kosovo without her children, who are dead or in jail' (Saranda, 11 years); or 'I am drawing Spring in the village. Everything is sad. There are not many flowers. The river is silent because there is no child to swim in it.' (Drenusha, 13 years) They talked about beauty, and they talked about the spirit: 'I drew the beauty of future Springs. I was relaxed because the colors of the Spring make the spirit relaxed.' (Durhata, 10 years)

Doves, symbolizing peace, and butterflies like the ones that had been found carved by children in the concentration camps during the Second World War appeared in the children's drawings. Butterflies are the symbol of a liberated soul. In discussions with the children they talked about the angels of Kosovo and about paradise: 'We can see how dearly bought our freedom was, but when we imagine them [the dead] now we can breathe freely; maybe we can confront this because the dead bodies now are angels of peace.'

CONCLUSION

The law of love will work, just as the law of gravity will work, whether we accept [it] or not ... a man who applies the law of love with scientific precision can work great wonders ... The men who discovered for us the law of love were greater scientists than any of our modern scientists ... the more I work on this love, the more I feel the delight of life, the delight in the scheme of the universe. It gives me peace and a meaning of the mysteries of nature that I have no power to describe.

(Mahatma Ghandi, quoted in Crean and Kome).[52]

McColl[53] (p. 126) says: 'it appears that occupation has the power to evoke spirit, and spirit has the power to evoke healing.' Spirituality is part of every occupational therapy session in every intervention.[10] If we consider spirituality as the essence of the human being, we need to articulate spirituality in our daily practice. This project was an attempt to do so.

It is crucial to develop our own spirituality as individuals, as a profession, and as members of the human family. Thibeault asserts that we must advance toward maturity.[21] This maturity is reflected as a path from existence to essence, from urgency to calm, from knowledge to wisdom, from self-focus to social responsibility and even activism. She suggests that there are several reasons to achieve maturity. First, we owe it to ourselves: 'by persisting in our immature ways, we sabotage our destiny and curb our authentic fulfillment. We fail ourselves and our personal future.' Second, she points out that if we keep lingering in mediocrity and incompleteness, 'we jeopardize our collective future'. And working toward this maturity is not an agonizing process: 'the required efforts are not super human and they do bring rewards. Stronger resilience, improved discernment, sharper understanding, and steadfast compassion all come with the territory, making us more capable healers.'[21] (p. 92)

There are several paths to spirituality. Work is another path, as a medium for service and contribution, for participation in a shared mission.[54] Our work can empower our own spirituality. To develop the 'spirituality' of our profession we must be true to our values and serve all populations facing occupational apartheid. This is not easy, immersed as we are in an economically centered society, but we can help to develop this 'occupational dream', contributing our gifts and knowledge, as we walk towards occupational justice.

Why should we do this? Because we are part of the human family. As Levinas has said: 'All is there, in the face',[55] the face being that of a child, a woman, a man, an elder. The faces are the next generation. We cannot neglect human suffering, because it is our suffering. As Donne said: 'And therefore never seek to know for whom the bell tolls; It tolls for *thee.*'[56]

As members of the human family, confronting world chaos, we must hold onto our hope. Marcel[57] said that hope is the medium of persistence, so we do not fall into despair. It is the decision to never give up. Hope also implies universal solidarity, and progress toward a common ideal, that of peace, justice, and love. It means not betraying others and being ready to receive others' help. All creation is called to collaborate in this undertaking.

Our partners in this heroic enterprise are the survivors. Walking through the streets of a destroyed city, smelling the burnt houses, taking care not to step on a land mine, mindful of all the suffering among the ruins of the streets, my heart silently starts to cry. Then I listen to a bird, in the form of children's laughter; I find some children playing and smiling; they embrace me; I have discovered the spirit of survivors. Who can negate the power of the spirit? Who can deny that life is stronger than death? Who can say there is no beauty? In the face of this, our hearts join the bird of hope in song.

Dedication

This chapter is dedicated to the memory of the angels of Gjakova, and especially to my soulmates, Nina and my father; both died one year after we finished the project, and I believe they are now playing together.

People of Orphalese, beauty is life, when life unveils her holy face.
But you are life and you are the veil.
The beauty is eternity gazing at itself in a mirror.
But you are eternity and you are the mirror
Because
For what is to die but to stand naked in the wind and to melt into the sun?
And what is it to cease breathing but to free the breath from its restless tides, that it may rise and expand and seek God unencumbered?
Only when you drink from the river of silence shall you indeed sing.
And when you have reached the mountain top, then you shall begin to climb.
And when the Earth shall claim your limbs, then shall you truly dance.[58]

References

1. Simó Algado S, Rodriguez Gregori JM, Egan M. Spirituality in a refugee camp. Can J Occup Ther 1994; 61:88–94.

2. Simó Algado S, Mehta N, Kronenberg F, et al. Occupational therapy intervention with children survivors of war. Can J Occup Ther 2002; 69(4):205–217.

3. Simó Algado S, Thibeault R, Urbanowski R, Kronenberg F, Pollard N. *La terapia ocupacional en el mundo penitenciario.* Terapia Ocupacional 2003; 33:10–20.

4. Simó Algado S. *El retorno del hombre de maiz, intervención desde la terapia ocupacional con una comunidad indígena maya.* Terapia Ocupacional 2002; 28:30–35.

5. Simó Algado S, Mehta N, Kronenberg F. *Niños supervivientes de conflicto bélico.* Terapia Ocupacional 2003; 31(April):26–40.

6. Simó Algado S, Kronenberg F. *Intervención con una comunidad indígena maya.* Materia Prima 2000; 5(16):28–32.

7. Kielhofner G. A model of human occupation: theory and application. 2nd edn. Baltimore, MD: Williams and Wilkins; 1995.

8. Canadian Association of Occupational Therapists. Enabling occupation: an occupational perspective. Ottawa, ON: CAOT Publications ACE; 1997.

9. Wilcock AA. Reflections on doing, being and becoming. Can J Occup Ther 1998; 65(5):248–256.

10. Urbanowski R. Spirituality in changed occupational lives. In: McColl MA. Spirituality and occupational therapy. Ottawa, ON: CAOT Publications ACE; 2003: 95–114.

11. UNICEF. *Sueño con la Paz.* FOLIO 1993; 39.

12. Agger I. Theory and practice of psychosocial projects for victims of war in Croatia and Bosnia-Herzegovina. Zagreb: European Community Task Force; 1994.

13. Monestier M. *Los niños esclavos.* Madrid, Spain: Alianza Editorial; 1999.

14. Walker G. *Los niños refugiados, os veces victimas de la violencia.* In: Sanchez G. Niños de la guerra. Barcelona: Blume; 2000.

15. Bru O. *Todas las guerras son contra los niños.* In: Sanchez G. Niños de la guerra. Barcelona: Blume; 2000.

16. Fraenkel L, Tallant B. Mostly me: a treatment approach for emotionally disturbed children. Can J Occup Ther 1987; 54(2):59–65.

17. Driver C, Beltran R. Impact of refugee trauma and children's occupational role as school students. Australian Occupational Therapy Journal 1998; 45:23–38.

18. Gavrilovic J, Lecic-Tosevski D, Jovic M. Actual symptomatology, defence mechanisms and childhood traumatic experiences in war traumatized patients. Psihijatrija Danas 1998; 30(4):509–521.

19. Hubbard JJ. Adaptive functioning and post-trauma symptoms in adolescent survivors of massive childhood trauma. Dissertation Abstracts International: The Sciences and Engineering 1998; 58(11B):6258.

20. Valent P. Documented childhood trauma (Holocaust): its sequelae and applications to other traumas. Psychiatry, Psychology and Law 1995; 2(1): 81–89.

21. Thibeault R. Experiential and philosophical considerations on occupation and the genesis of meaning and resilience. In: McColl MA. Spirituality and occupational therapy. Ottawa, ON: CAOT Publications ACE, 2003:83–94.

22. Suzuki D. The sacred balance. Vancouver/Toronto: Greystone; 2002.

23. Egan M, DeLaat D. Considering spirituality in occupational therapy practice. Can J Occup Ther 1994; 61(2):95–101.

24. Townsend E, DeLaat D, Egan M, Thibeault R, Wright WA. Spirituality in enabling occupation: a learner centered workbook. Ottawa, ON: CAOT Publications ACE, 1999.

25. Urbanowski R, Vargo J. Spirituality, daily practice and the occupational performance model. Can J Occup Ther 1994; 61:88–94.

26. Cirulnik B. *Los patitos feos.* Barcelona: Gedisa; 2002.

27. Vanistendael S. *La felicidad es posible.* Barcelona: Gedisa; 2002.

28. Freire P, transl Macedo D. The politics of education: culture, power and liberation. Boston MA: Bergin and Garvey; 1985.

29. Bellingham R, Cohen B, Jones T, Spaniol L. Connectedness: some skills for spiritual health. American Journal for Health Promotion 1989; 4: 18–31.

30. Condeluci A. Interdependence: the route to community, 2nd edn. Boca Raton, FL; Saint Lucie Press, 1995.

31. Katz R. Empowerment and synergy: expanding the community's healing resources. Prevention in Human Services 1984; 3:201–226.

32. Montagu A. The direction of human development. New York: Harper & Brothers; 1955.

33. Montagu A. Growing young. New York: McGraw Hill; 1981.

34. Kronenberg F. Street children: being and becoming. Research study. The Netherlands; Hogeschool Limburg, 1999.

35. Townsend E. Occupational therapy's social vision. Can J Occup Ther 1993; 60(4):174–184.

36. West WL. Professional responsibility in times of change. In: Llorens L, ed. Consultation in the community: occupational therapy in child health. Rockville, MD: American Association of Occupational Therapy, 1993.

37. Canadian Association of Occupational Therapists. Occupational therapy guidelines for client-centered practice. Toronto, ON: CAOT Publications ACE; 1991.

38. Ainscough K. The therapeutic value of activity in child psychiatry. B J Occup Ther 1998; 61(5):223–226.

39. Mattingly S. Clinical reasoning forms of inquiry in a therapeutic practice. Philadelphia, PA: FA Davis; 1994.

40. Morrison CD, Metzger PA, Pratt PN. Play. In: Case-Smith J, Allen AS, Pratt PN, eds. Occupational therapy for children. 4th edn. St Louis, MO: Mosby; 2000: 504–523.

41. Moore T. Care of the soul. New York: HarperCollins; 1992.

42. Rogers CR. Client-centered therapy. Its current practice, implications, and theory. Boston, MA: Houghton Mifflin; 1951.

43. Moustakas CE. Psychotherapy with children. New York: Harper & Rowe; 1959.

44. Coles R. The moral life of children. New York: Atlantic Monthly Press; 1986.

45. Fazel M, Stein A. The mental health of refugee children. Arch Dis Child 2002; 87(5):366–370.

46. Weine S, Becker DF, McGlashan TH, et al. Adolescent survivors of 'ethnic cleansing': observations on the first year in America. J Am Acad Child Adolesc Psychiatry 1995; 34(9):1153–1159.

47. Townsend E. Inclusiveness: a community dimension of spirituality. Can J Occup Ther 1997; June 64(3): 146–155.

48. Egan M, DeLaat MD. Considering spirituality in occupational therapy practice. Can J Occup Ther 1994; 61(2):95–101.

49. Yahne CA, Miller WR. Evoking hope. In: Miller WR, ed. Integrating spirituality into treatment. Resources for practitioners. Washington DC: American Psychological Association; 1999:217–234.

50. Neuhaus BE. Including hope in occupational therapy practice: a pilot study. Am J Occup Ther 1997; 51(3):228–234.

51. Dickinson E. Collected poems. Philadelphia, PA: Running Press; 1991.

52. Crean P, Kome P, eds. A dream unfolding. Toronto: Lester & Orpen Dennys; 1986.

53. McColl MA. Toward a conceptual model for spirituality in occupational therapy. In: McColl MA, Spirituality and occupational therapy. Ottawa, ON: CAOT Publications ACE; 2003.

54. McColl MA. Toward a model of practice for spirituality in occupational therapy. In: McColl MA. Spirituality and occupational therapy. Ottawa, ON: CAOT Publications ACE: 2003:133–144.

55. Levinas E. *Etica e infinito*. Madrid: Editorial Visor; 1991.

56. Donne J. Devotions upon emergent occasions. In: Complete poetry and selected prose. New York: Random House; 1929.

57. Marcel G. *El hombre problemático*. Buenos Aires: Editorial Sudamericana; 1956.

58. Gibran K. El profeta. Madrid: Edimat Libros; 1995.

Chapter 19

Occupational therapy with street children

Frank Kronenberg

OVERVIEW

Street children are among the most vulnerable citizens of the world and have been described as 'the extreme manifestation of deteriorating social capital and social exclusion'.[1] Occupational therapists have a mandate to respond to the complex occupational needs and rights of this population.[2,3]

This chapter shares the author's experiences of occupational therapy with street children in Mexico[2] and Guatemala.[4] These interventions encountered and overcame challenges at different levels, three of which have been selected and are addressed in terms of conflict and cooperation situations (see Chapter 6), experiences of crossing the 'borders' of conventional occupational therapy:

- thinking, to encompass practice with street children
- practice contexts, the field of international cooperation
- populations, street children confronting occupational apartheid.

In the paragraphs below, each situation of conflict and cooperation is described, including identification of key elements, and then illustrated and discussed.

Based on these preliminary experiences, I propose that occupational therapy can help organizations to enable street children to leave the streets and transform their lives. How? Through engagement in rightful occupations that are meaningful and relevant to their own unfolding life stories. It is recommended that these children need to be treated as subjects with human rights having a political drama of their own.

... It was a day for celebrating tolerance, and street children, delinquents, cannot serve as role models for our youngsters ...

Representative of former Guatemalan government
party at the 'Day of International Tolerance'
(see Example 1 in Chapter 6)

INTRODUCTION

It has been estimated that more than 100 million street and working children around the world are struggling to survive under harsh and often exploitative conditions. While accurate figures are elusive, there is evidence of an increase in numbers in areas undergoing economic or political transitions, such as the former Soviet countries, Africa, Central and South America (see the ENSCW website address at the end of this Chapter). Unfortunately, even the label 'street children' is demeaning in itself. It depersonalizes each child, making him or her 'a problem to be solved',[6] rather than 'persons with names and a human face',[2] and 'potentially important participants in the social struggles of their countries, representing the future of the world'.[5]

Every year children are pushed onto the street by economic need, or by problems at home, commercial exploitation, or poor access to schools. The vast majority of street-based children are neither homeless nor delinquent, but are unprotected working children who are highly vulnerable to exploitation. Their existence on the streets reduces their opportunities to form emotional connections to caring adults, or to develop the social abilities, education, or job skills necessary to lead productive and meaningful lives. They survive – if they survive at all – in the margins, losing out on childhood and on mainstream opportunities to improve their prospects for the future.[6]

My motivation to become an occupational therapist was largely inspired and fuelled by my engagement as a volunteer with street children at Casa Alianza (CA) in Mexico City back in 1992/1993. I was struck by children's extremely troubled immediate situations and histories, but also amazed by their resilience and spirit for survival. I learned a lot through our interactions and came to appreciate my own life more.

Reading about the genesis of occupational therapy at the beginning of the twentieth century provided me with a strong vision that through the profession I could make a difference with children and youth who are denied the right to live a dignified and meaningful life. My direct exposure to the gross injustices and needs of this population would not allow me to forget about them and put these experiences behind me. I felt and continue to feel compelled to do something about it and, to be honest, to serve my own experience of wellbeing, understood in terms of having found meaning and purpose in my life.

With disagreement in the literature about causes, characteristics and children's relationship with public spaces[7], an occupational therapy approach to understanding street children recognizes 'their agency, while acknowledging many potential ways in which these children may be excluded and their voices ignored, in a context in which they do not hold political, civic and economic power'.[7]

Those occupational therapists who are inspired and motivated to explore the relevance of their vision, knowledge and skills across the borders of conventional fields of practice (including education and research) are likely to meet with scepticism and/or resistance at many levels. They will be challenged by their own colleagues and other professionals, funding bodies and governments to justify the need to expand practice outside the mainstream. And of course, most importantly, the people they aspire to work with – individuals, groups and communities who experience and are fighting to overcome disabling conditions – will have to be willing to allow occupational therapists to walk with and learn from them.

STRETCHING OCCUPATIONAL THERAPY TO ENCOMPASS PRACTICE WITH STREET CHILDREN

My privileged occupational therapy education in the Netherlands (see Chapter 31) did not encourage and prepare me for practice with street children. Further, a review of international occupational therapy literature found scarce evidence of occupational therapists engaging with this population. The main professional actors in this field of work appeared to be people who were trained in education, social work, psychology and policy making.[2] Given the mandate of occupational therapy to engage with *all* people whose dignified and meaningful social participation in daily life is limited or denied due to disabling conditions that are physical, mental and/or sociopolitical,[3,8,9,10] this exclusion appears to be problematic.

How could occupational therapy's apparent lack of concept, experience and commitment with regard to sharing our profession's social responsibility for the complex and highly problematic phenomenon of street children be addressed? I used the final assignment of my professional training to carry out exploratory research, developing a case for occupational therapy with this population, for which the rehabilitation program of CA in Mexico (see CA website) served as a reference group. None of the faculty had any knowledge or experience with street children (or similar populations) and some expressed scepticism about whether or not occupational therapy had a role to play with this population, and there was no time or other resources to collect research data directly in situ.

The following illustration briefly describes the process and outcomes of this study, which aimed to conceptualize how occupational therapy could contribute to this non-traditional field of practice.

ILLUSTRATION 1

The first challenge was to convince the occupational therapy program staff at my school that these obstacles could be overcome. Fortunately, internet access had just become available at the school and this allowed the 'borders' of conventional education to be crossed. The internet enabled the collection of data (via a locally conducted interview and a written questionnaire) on occupational needs and contexts of the children within the CA programs, and also helped me to find seven occupational therapists from seven different countries (Brazil, Mexico, United States, Canada, Spain, Belgium and the Netherlands) with experience and/or a special interest in working with at-risk children and youth.

This group participated in a Delphi study, 'a qualitative method for structuring a group communication process, so that the process is effective in allowing a group of individuals, as a whole, to deal with a complex problem'.[11] also called 'sophisticated brainstorming'.[12] This 'structured communication' was accomplished using the seven stages of the Canadian Occupational Performance Process Model[13] and the Model of Human Occupation.[14] My personal work experiences with street children (1992/1993), and the information from the interview and questionnaire, informed the writing of a conceptual occupational therapy response to what the staff of CA had perceived as the most challenging occupational performance issue of this population (Box 19.1). The conceptual response was shared with and individually critiqued and refined by the Delphi participants over two rounds of feedback.[2]

The main challenge perceived by the staff of Casa Allianza Mexico was that, 'many street children are just not motivated to make the occupational transition from life on the street to a new life through participation in our rehabilitation programs.'

Viewed from an occupational *needs* and *rights* perspective, the study conceptualized this perceived challenge to be rooted in complex and severe contextual conditions that chronically deprived these children/youth of rightful and meaningful occupational experiences. There was no occupational therapy term available to define these conditions, which led to coining the notion of *occupational apartheid* (see Chapter 6). In the worst cases observed, children experienced occupational alienation; 'a sense of isolation, powerlessness, frustration, loss of control, estrangement from society or self as a result of engagement in occupations which do not satisfy inner needs'.[15,16]

Galhiego, a Delhi study participant from Brazil, said:

The choice [that] empowered the children to leave the shacks they live in, their abusive parents, the sewage that runs inside their shacks and the lack of food, and go to the streets to show how miserable life has been for them.

The occupational therapy approach to address the street children's perceived 'lack of motivation to change' was to create a variety of occupational forms,[17] that could arouse their curiosity, hold their attention, and touch them. These represented opportunities for meaningful and purposeful engagement to enable them (and us) to discover, connect with and learn about their occupational needs, strengths and talents:

- building self-confidence and a (new) sense of belonging
- learning to listen to, express and make sense of personal experiences and feelings
- learning about and confronting the real roots of the occupational apartheid they experienced
- working to establish a new structure of habits and roles that would enable them to shape their destinies.

The occupational therapy process can only enable people to transform their lives if they see meaning and relevance to their own unfolding life stories.[18] Hence, narrative reasoning[19] could offer a valuable tool 'to understand how the street children read their own reality, assess their own difficulties and present their values and beliefs'.[2] Examples of concrete occupational forms were:

- expressive therapy
- social projects
- workshops in play
- personal growing
- corporal expression
- making wooden toys and puppetry
- raising cultural awareness
- self-advocacy training
- a radio and newspaper project
- sports and vocational orientation.

Intervention modalities can be: 'music, dance, poetry, art, philosophy, myths, legends, politics, logo therapy'.[20] It was envisioned that engagement in these occupational forms could afford the children/youth with opportunities to reconnect with their sense of self (*being*), exploring who they are, what they can do, what they enjoy doing, what they would like to do (*becoming*).

> *Children and youth with deeper links to street life and drugs are often highly resistant to be engaged in traditional or formal treatment programs.*

Galheigo, Delphi participant from Brazil

Discussion

The opportunity to conduct research in the field of street children presented itself as very meaningful and purposeful, as it enabled me to reconnect with my original drive to become an occupational therapist. This motivation was crucial in overcoming initial resistance of the occupational therapy program to allowing this study to be carried out.

Since the lack of concept was identified as one of the obstacles that had to be overcome to stretch occupational therapy to encompass practice with street children, the introduction of the term *occupational apartheid* (see Chapter 6) can be considered as a key outcome of this study. It affords occupational therapists a way to identify, name and explain – from an occupational therapy perspective – everyday realities that are experienced by street children (and indeed other people living in disadvantaged situations). As Galheigo, one of the Delphi participants, emphasized:

> *If the problems related to street children are not addressed in broadly critical terms the children can be framed as being responsible for their own problems too easily – the social mechanism of 'blaming the victim'.*

It may also urge occupational therapists to critically question their own practice: with whom are they working, which populations are excluded from their services, what factors determine or influence these realities? Engaging in ongoing critical debate about these and related questions may encourage and enable occupational therapists to become more politically aware, active and effective in order to cross the 'borders' of mainstream practice, education and research when people's access to dignified and meaningful participation in daily life is restricted or denied.

ENTERING AND NAVIGATING THE TROUBLED WATERS OF INTERNATIONAL COOPERATION

Once we had introduced a concept of how occupational therapy could contribute to making a difference in the lives of street children, we needed to find an opportunity to verify its value and usefulness in practice. 'Spirit of Survivors – Occupational Therapists without Borders' (see Preface) had previously collaborated with Payasos sin Fronteras (PsF) (see Box 19.1) in a preventative mental health project in Kosovo (see Chapter 18), which learned that the art and science of occupational therapy 'without borders' and their 'humanitarian aid through the arts' had great synergy potential.

At that time, PsF had already established contact with Casa Allianza in Guatemala (see Box 19.2) because they were exploring the possibilities for working with street children and at-risk youth in Central America.

However, they lacked a conceptualization of how to go about working in this field. When they learned about the occupational therapy research,[2] we were invited to design a pilot project which employed clowns and artists to enable former street children to empower themselves, 'to develop their capacity and power to construct their own destinies'.[21] This pilot project was proposed to CA in Guatemala and this section describes some of the difficulties we experienced when trying to establish and maintain a collaboration in the context of international cooperation.

Box 19.1   Payasos sin Fronteras (PsF)

An international non-governmental humanitarian aid organization of clowns and other artists, PsF seeks to improve life in refugee camps and areas of conflict through volunteer artist performances, as well as workshops with children and with educators. PsF also seeks to raise society's awareness of affected populations and to promote a spirit of solidarity. Their motto:

No child without a smile

Box 19.2   Casa Alianza (CA)

An independent, non-profit organization dedicated to the rehabilitation and defence of street children and youth at-risk in Guatemala (1981), Honduras, Mexico (1986) and Nicaragua (1998). CA is the Latin American branch of the New York-based Covenant House. Most of the children and youth in this region have been orphaned by civil war, abused or rejected by dysfunctional and poverty-stricken families, and further traumatized by the indifference of the societies in which they live. Their motto:

The street is no place for children

Given that their profession is virtually unknown in the field of practice with street children, occupational therapists are challenged both to make the other active groups involved aware of its potential contribution and to negotiate their way into the field to demonstrate it. No single profession has all the answers to respond to the diverse and complex situations in which street children find themselves, thus cooperation between skilled people from different sectors is vital to building a stronger, more effective field of work. One way of doing this is to forge creative partnerships across sectors.[22]

How did our partnerships come about? Our partner organization PsF had worked within the rehabilitation programs of CA in 2000, based on the occupational therapy project proposal. However, CA had invited the clowns in the mistaken belief that the proposed role of the occupational therapist could be easily performed by the social workers, psychologists or educators within their programs. The project flopped, because it wasn't developed in collaboration with staff and children in the programs, and the activities had been carried out without regard to the situated meanings and needs of the local population. All of this led to many confused communications between and frustrations among the different active groups.

At the end of 2000 we asked the administration of CA for a 'second chance', and this time the project would be coordinated by an occupational therapist.

ILLUSTRATION 2

The context of conflict–cooperation situations, in which the occupational therapy pilot project 'Survivors of the Street' was to be developed, was 'Guatemala'. As a result of more than 36 years of internal armed conflict, the history of this Central American country holds many episodes of horror, violence, systematic human rights abuse, shame and hostility, distortions and terror, pain and misery.[23]

Various Guatemalan governments exercised a policy of apartheid against mostly indigenous girls, boys, youth, adults, women and men. Guatemalans experienced a war that left more than 200 000 dead, 1.5 million displaced, and a population living in the shadow of fear, death and disappearance.[23] More than half of Guatemala's 12 million citizens are children under the age of 15.

According to local authorities 60 500 people, including many street-involved children, belong to 'maras' (the Spanish term for youth gangs) in Central American countries. Guatemala, Honduras, and El Salvador have established so-called 'anti-gang' laws – repressive measures against youth gangs. These allow the arrest and detention of anyone suspected of being a member of a gang (often 'proven' by the child having a tattoo with the name of a gang) and the practice of 'social cleansing' – extra judicial executions of children and youth.[24] And yet these countries do not offer children the opportunities to which they have a right, as an alternative to involvement in these gangs.

At our first meeting with the executives of CA (March 2001), we learned that the project proposal[25] had not yet been distributed among the – at that time more than 130 – CA staff working in 12 program sites located in and around Guatemala City. We were also informed that CA was facing an institutional crisis. Its funding partners demanded evidence about the effectiveness of their services, which urged the institution to rethink its 'Modelo de Atención', the methodology used in its rehabilitation programs. A formal collaboration agreement between CA and PsF was formulated and signed, before a concrete plan of roles and responsibilities was established, which caused frustrations during the development and implementation of the pilot project. However, it was hoped that the experiences of the PsF project could contribute new perspectives and ideas to help strengthen CA's methodology.

To allow the project to be developed and implemented in tune with the lived needs and experiences of the staff within the different programs, 3-day workshops were carried out with virtually all the workers of each program: six different groups of coordinators, educators, psychologists, social workers, nurses, kitchen staff and volunteers (total 109). To establish a foundation for collaboration, these workshops aimed:

- to introduce, discuss and adapt the original project proposal in relation to the challenges within the individual programs.
- to explain what occupational therapy is, how it is complementary with social work, psychology and pedagogy and how the roles of clowns and artists were to be understood.

Discussion

If all active groups were to benefit from their involvement in the project (win–win situations), we needed to learn about the aims, motives and interests of the children, the staff of CA, the staff of PsF, and the funding partners. A critical reflection of the occupational narratives of each group (meanings and purposes; needs and interests) helped to gain insight into the political dimensions of practice within the context of international cooperation. In this dynamic, it emerged that children were hardly involved at all in the design and decision-making process that informed the development of programs that were intended to benefit them.

None of the 150-plus employees of CA (including administration, logistic support and kitchen staff) had any first-hand experience of street-living, or had passed through a CA rehabilitation program. This raised the critical question: whose interests are we serving – those of street children or our own?

Besides creating rapport between staff of CA and PsF, the workshop experiences learned that the CA rehabilitation methodology appeared to view the population as 'charitable causes' ('asistencialismo') and used an institution-centered approach. On the other hand, the occupational therapy project proposed to relate to children as 'subjects with human rights' and potential investments, using a self-empowerment approach which was to enable them to guide and inform their own process of change.

It was curious to discover that the staff of CA Guatemala framed the biggest obstacle in working with street children in the same way as did the staff of CA in Mexico, namely the 'lack of motivation to change' which resides in the children. CA also had a workers union, which was involved in its own discussion and formulation of how to strengthen the vision and methodology of CA's programs. It appeared that CA, PsF and the workers' union all lacked insight into children's own perceptions and their experiences of the institution's interventions.

The partnership between PsF and SOS-OTwB was based on a shared intent to contribute to processes of individual and social transformations in street children, through enabled engagement in occupations from the world of the arts and clowning. However, during the development of the project in situ, it became apparent at times that we possessed an insufficient understanding of each other's aims and motives. Occasionally, this led to preoccupations with our own (occupational) needs and interests, and competition in demonstrating our individual worth.

The interest of the financial partners of CA was expressed in terms of 'best practice' – providing evidence demonstrating the effectiveness of methods and programs, resulting in 'successfully rehabilitated children'. The sponsors of the PsF project appeared to be mainly interested in receiving statistical and visual evidence – numbers and pictures of workshops, (public) performances, participants and press coverage.

WHY WOULD STREET CHILDREN WANT TO ENGAGE IN OCCUPATIONAL THERAPY?

The third level of conflict concerns the engagement of street children in occupational therapy within different rehabilitation programs of CA in Guatemala. From the perspective of occupational apartheid (see Chapter 6), the children's perceived 'lack of motivation to participate in the CA rehabilitation program' was challenged by the question, 'why should they participate?'.

In order to serve the needs and interests of the children, it was fundamental to find out what those needs and interests were. Taking the position that needs and interests are culturally defined (see Chapter 10), our project proposed a rights-based approach[26] as a framework for identification of 'needs'. This can be interpreted as 'the need to access a right not yet enjoyed by the child'. However, how do we know what rights these children – 'survivors of the street' – most need and want? For us to find out, the children would have to allow us to walk with and learn from them – what it means to suffer occupational apartheid – and inform us of whether they would be interested in finding ways of cooperation to overcome their social exclusion.

To encourage departure from the street, occupational therapy needed to offer the children opportunities to connect with their interests and enable them to identify and build on their strengths. This approach aimed to occupationally enrich the regular activity programs of CA for both the children and the staff, and it was hoped that these experiences could also help guide and inform CA in its process of rethinking and strengthening its methodology, building evidence in the light of 'best practice', and cost-effectiveness in terms of numbers of children who successfully graduate from their programs.

Box 19.3   Overview of the project

Specific goals
- Increase self-esteem and a sense of belonging
- Create opportunities for children's protagonism
- Educate in getting and expressing a voice
- Address traumatic experiences
- Improve interpersonal interaction skills
- Train teenage mothers (Early Intervention)
- Raise self and public awareness
- Provide experience of fun/joy
- Promote solidarity and shared responsibility

Action plan
- Workshops with the staff
- Workshops with the children on the street and in other programs
- Public performances
- Invite maximum media coverage

Activities
- Clowning, mime, juggling, acrobatics, dance, percussion, rap, graffiti, puppetry, theatre, props-making, maquillage
- Journalism, video, photography, writing
- Early intervention, baby massage, toy-making
- Expressive therapy, image theatre
- First aid courses
- Public performances at schools and in public places

Coordinated and supervised by an occupational therapist, the PsF project team consisted of many different individuals and groups of clowns, artists and occupational therapy students from Spain, Mexico, Argentina, Venezuela and Guatemala. Some interacted with the children and the staff of CA for a couple of weeks and others for several months.

Box 19.3 offers an overview of the project's specific goals, action plan and the occupational spaces which were offered to the children and staff in the:

- street-based program
- crisis centers for boys and girls
- teenage mothers' home
- community center
- transitional and group homes in more limited ways, because the populations in these centers were already involved in school and/or vocational training.

The following illustration briefly describes some of these occupational experiences.

ILLUSTRATION 3

The street program included the 'Escuela de la Calle', a mobile school (http://www.mobileschool.org) which consisted of a number of blackboards used to invite children to engage in basic reading and math, and also offered a space for the children to have a voice and be listened to. Two clowns used a mix of acrobatics and humor to express daily life situations which the children were invited to identify and describe, including associated feelings. This fun and educational activity allowed children to learn words for, give meaning to and make sense of their experiences. It also attracted the attention of pedestrians who at times engaged in conversation with the children.

Some street-living children who made money at traffic lights by taking gasoline in their mouths and 'spitting fire' learned to juggle with torches, an activity considerably less hazardous to their health, which never the less generated an income.

Other activities included mime and role-playing on the sidewalks, acting-out violent and harassing encounters with the police or security forces, which they experienced at night. It offered children an opportunity and a medium to express their feelings, to be listened to and also to raise awareness of passers by about their lived reality on the street. Playing out the roles of street children and the police put their realities in another perspective, helping them come to understand that how they were being treated was wrong, and encouraging them to learn about children's rights.

Most activities were developed with and offered to the staff and populations of the three crisis centers for boys and girls. These were characterized by a high turnover rate of children, especially the shelter for boys in the center of the city. These children had the most 'free time' and energy available to them, but many had experienced relapses back to the street, sometimes related to drugs or gang affiliations. They lacked meaningful things to do within the program. With this project they could choose to engage in acrobatics, juggling, puppet-making and puppetry, percussion, rap, graffiti, theatre and/or dance workshops, all of which were to address a combination of specific goals (Box 19.3).

An added incentive to commit themselves to a process of learning skills and new roles through these activities was the perspective of becoming an actor in the 'Survivors of the Street' public performance group. These occupational experiences were to enable them to make the transition from 'crisis' to living together in a home with a small group of peers, going to school and learning a trade.

The occupational form journalism enabled the children to interview each other, to take pictures of life in the street, of themselves, and to write narratives. These were published as *Testimonios de Jovenes por Jovenes* ('Testimonies by Youth for Youth'), a collective diary which was edited and put together by the children from the different CA programs, including those that were still living in the street. They made use of 'write hands', through which kids who couldn't write had their stories written up by those who could. A number of children learned to operate a video-camera and filmed the performances and workshops. The recordings were later taken from program to program and watched with tremendous interest and joy. Seeing themselves perform, having fun together with others, contributed to building self-esteem and a sense of belonging.

The everyday life in the home for teenage mothers and their babies and young children was characterized by a lot of stress. Five or six days-a-week they got up at 3 or 4 o'clock in the morning to feed and take care of their babies and carry out domestic routines, prepare breakfast and then go to work at 7am, working for very low wages, mostly in sweat-shops. Lack of formal education and training and having one or more visible tattoos (the stigma of gang affiliation) limited their employment possibilities. Their children would be dropped off at a day-care center. Upon return to the home after 7pm they attended to domestic chores and to their babies and children who were craving (often crying for) attention.

The occupational needs expressed by the mothers and their infants and the staff can be summarized by the terms 'occupational deprivation', 'imbalance' and 'alienation'. To address these issues, the young mothers and their children were offered (independently and together) occupational spaces in which they were enabled to connect with themselves – with who they were, what they wished to become in relation to the tough realities that they had lived and were living. Making bamboo toys and mobiles which they gave to their children, learning early intervention skills and baby massage techniques which helped establish and improve the bonds between mothers and babies, and excursions on Sundays broke the routines of work and domestic chores.

One night, after a spontaneous 'dance party' in the home, for which all of them had dressed up and taken care with their appearance, we found one of the girls crying outside on the roof-top. When we asked her what happened, she answered, 'I didn't know that life could feel so beautiful'. The atmosphere in the home improved significantly by enriching their daily routines with chances to see their lives, their strengths and their needs in other perspectives.

The CA prevention program 'centro comunitario' was in the process of initiating support services for families in marginalized zones on the outskirts of Guatemala City. What was going on in those neighbourhoods – who could enter and who couldn't – was said to be largely controlled by 'maras' (gangs). Thus, establishing contact, trust and rapport with the people in these communities was not easy. We used the social occupational form 'espectaculos' – interactive clowns, mime, theatre and music performances – to 'break the ice' and enable this CA program to build communication and cooperation with the local schools, the church and other community organizing groups. It was amazingly powerful how humor and playful interactions helped overcome obstacles of distrust, fear and paranoia.

One mime performance by an Argentinean and a Mexican clown on a basketball court in the impoverished 'Zona 18' attracted a whole community of people – children of local schools, teachers, neighbors and 'mareros' (gang members). They were involved as a kind of *spect-actors* in forum theatre,[27] playing/acting out situations that are close to their life experiences, putting them in other perspectives by using humor, and questioning them. Building on these interactive encounters, workshops similar to those in other CA programs were offered to the children in this community.

What appeared to be the project's most powerful occupational form, in terms of enabling transformations at individual and social levels, was public performance. Collectives of (former street) children and professional clowns and artists went on road-shows to demonstrate what they had trained for, i.e. a range of circus techniques, dance, percussion and rap. These performances took place at public and private schools, market places, parks, a psychiatric hospital (the only one in all of Guatemala!), in parades, to provide 'comic relief' to a community of survivors of the hurricane Mitch, and at public events such as the International Day of Tolerance (see Chapter 6, Example 1). Besides fostering their self-esteem and sense of belonging, the kids being the principal actors, these occupational spaces also offered the children opportunities to raise public awareness about their lived realities.

Discussion

If the dominant powers' opinion of a society, in our Illustrations Guatemala and Mexico, appear to view 'street children' as 'delinquents' who are not capable of taking, or even worthy of, a chance and support to exercise their human and citizen's rights and demonstrate their true worth, then it is essential that occupational therapy with this population challenges practice at systems levels.

Many a night, after long and intense days of interaction with the extreme realities of daily life in Guatemala (where 60% of the population is under 18), we came to understand that in order to improve the lives of street-involved children, it may be more urgent and effective to engage the national security forces (police, (para)military, politicians) in clowning workshops. If their violent, prejudiced attitudes toward this population could be transformed/sensitized, then one of the biggest obstacles to building a Guatemala that affords its young a present and a future, would be removed.

CONCLUSION

The lived experiences of the research and practice projects can be described as a continuous 'conflict and cooperation dialectic' between the participating actor groups, which convincingly awakened my critical awareness about the political nature of occupational therapy (see Chapter 6).

Stretching occupational therapy to encompass practice with street children required the challenging of internal professional (and personal) 'borders', which may translate in reality into a different worldview, limited capacities, insecurities, or an inappropriate use of authority. If occupational therapy is to live up to its mandate to serve *all* people, including street children who could benefit from its attention, then its educators, researchers and practitioners are obliged to extend efforts to the limit of their abilities or talents, which seems to call for engagement in conflict and cooperation dynamics with other relevant active groups. Making optimal use of information technology allowed me to consult with an international group of occupational therapy colleagues, and through cooperation we achieved a conceptualization of a potential contribution of occupational therapy to the field of practice with street children.

The context of international cooperation (i.e. humanitarian aid, development) can be described as a minefield of (complex) conflicts between the (many) different active groups that have vested interests in this field. For occupational therapists that enter this relatively new and controversial field of practice, so-called good intentions, enthusiasm and a degree of idealism may help, but are not likely to buy them a welcome by established active groups. A strategy that may prove to be effective in negotiating their way into this field is to demonstrate their capacity to enable street children who are experiencing disabling conditions to identify and articulate their own needs and interests. This would be a prerequisite for active participation in decision-making processes that determine and influence the design, development and realization of international cooperation projects or programs from which *they* are to be the principal beneficiaries.

For about 9 months, CA and PsF invested in building relationships of trust and commitment with the children, raised expectations, and even achieved progress with some, but in the end our partnership did not last due to a number of conflicts at organizational level, which did not allow us to follow through with what we had started with the children – we were left not knowing how this affected them. Thus, a key principle to be kept in mind and advanced when entering the field of international cooperation is: first, do no harm to those you aspire to serve.

Although based on preliminary experiences, a significant number of children within the different CA programs demonstrated a motivation and commitment to 'trade' their life on the streets for prolonged participation in the project's occupational spaces. Some of them made occupational transitions from the street into CA group homes. In focus groups carried out by external reviewers,[28] children expressed that their participation was triggered by factors of meaning ('I've found a reason to live where I didn't before'), purpose ('I want to become a photographer'), and because of the non-authoritarian way in which the project staff related to them. Through the realization of public performances, a number of relations were established with children, students and adults from other social sectors, which allowed projection and improvement of the public image of street children and therefore CA.[28]

Occupational therapists (and others practicing in this field) have lots to learn from these children. Enabling them to guide and inform (our) professional contributions may help to make sure that the children are benefiting from our attention.

RECOMMENDATIONS

Occupational therapists need to increase their understanding of, and active involvement in, policy-making processes which can largely determine the occupational playground space of street children, and of their own roles as social actors. This may enable the children's self-empowerment and increase their capacity to challenge and influence the making of rules and regulations that may set unacceptable, unjustified 'borders', allowing some sections of the population to enjoy guaranteed access to power and capacity to construct their own destiny, by denying or restricting other groups. This political engagement (or activism) appears to be fundamental in confronting occupational apartheid.[29,30]

The set of 'pADL questions' (political Activities of Daily Living) that are introduced in Chapter 6 provide an analytical tool to explore the political nature of any conflict and cooperation situation. If necessary in a modified way, this tool can also be used with street children and other involved groups to gain insight into and enable the sharing of decision-making power, to determine or influence access to dignified and meaningful participation in daily life.

Guided by the concept of occupational apartheid (see Chapter 6), the following set of questions may help inform occupational therapy research and the development of its roles in the field of practice with street children:

- How are the interventions with the children formulated?
- How are they implemented?
- How are they experienced by the children; the staff; the administration; various active groups involved?
- Why are some occupational spaces more often accessed and sustainable than others?
- How do children's experiences feed back into rethinking of a project's or program's methodology and its implementation?

While this chapter may only describe a beginning, it is both my hope and promise that occupational therapists will become engaged in sharing their responsibility for the enablement of 'children on the edges of societies to find their way to the center, to achieve wellbeing within their communities, to become fully fledged participants instead of excluded onlookers'.[22] As my Guatemalan friend Cesar Melendez[31] says:

> *Dales una oportunidad … y verás cuán capaces son para cambiar el mundo junto a vos*
> 'Give them a chance … and you will see how capable they are to change the world together with you.'

Acknowledgements

With special thanks to the children actors of the project 'Survivors of the Street', the Delphi research participants, colleagues of Payasos sin Fronteras, and the administration and staff members of Casa Alianza in Mexico and Guatemala.

References

1. Volpi E. Street Children: Promising Practices and Approaches. Washington, DC; World Bank Institute: 2002; p VII.

2. Kronenberg F. Street Children: Being and Becoming. Heerlen, The Netherlands: Hogeschool Limburg; 1999.

3. World Federation of Occupational Therapists. Code of Ethics. Forrestfield, Australia: WFOT; 2004.
4. Kronenberg F. Juggling with Survivors of the Street: Occupational Therapy, Clowns and Street Children. Paper presented at the WFOT congress in Stockholm, 2002.
5. Orenstein F. Multi-cultural Celebrations: The paintings of Betty LaDuke 1972–1992. Beverly Hills, CA: Pomegranate; 1993.
6. Thomas de Benitez S. What works in Street Children Programming: The JUCONI Model. Baltimore, MD: International Youth Foundation; 2001.
7. Thomas de Benitez S. Societies Investing in Street Children: Literature Review and Research Plan for a study of social policy processes and children's experiences in Puebla City. Submission for a major review, London: London School of Economics; 2004.
8. World Federation of Occupational Therapists. Definition of occupational therapy. Forrestfield, Australia: WFOT; 2004.
9. World Federation of Occupational Therapists. Position paper on Community Based Rehabilitation. Forrestfield, Australia: WFOT; 2004.
10. World Health Organization. International Classification of Functioning, Disability and Health. Geneva: WHO; 2001.
11. Linstone HA, Turoff M. The Delphi Method, Techniques and Applications. Reading, MA: Addison-Wesley Publishing Company; 1975.
12. Van Doorn J, Van Vught F. Forecasting, methoden en technieken voor toekomst onderzoek. Amsterdam, The Netherlands: Van Gorcum; 1978.
13. Canadian Association of Occupational Therapists Enabling Occupation, An Occupational Therapy Perspective. Toronto: CAOT Publications; 1997.
14. Kielhofner G. A Model of Human Occupation, Theory and Application. Baltimore, MD: Williams & Wilkins; 1995.
15. Wilcock AA. An Occupational Perspective of Health. Thorofare, NJ: Slack; 1998.
16. Bellingham R, Cohen B, Jones T, Spaniol L. Connectedness: some skills for spiritual health. Am J Health Promot 1989; 4:18–31.
17. Nelson D. Occupation: form and performance. Am J Occup Ther 1988; 42(10):633–641.
18. Helfrich C, Kielhofner G. Volitional narratives and the meaning of therapy. Am J Occup Ther 1994, 48(4):319–326.
19. Mattingly Ch, Hayes Fleming M. Clinical Reasoning, Forms of Inquiry in a Therapeutic Practice. Philadelphia, PA: F.A. Davis Company; 1994.
20. Frankl VE. Man's Search for Meaning. Washington, DC: Washington Square Press; 1994.
21. Cardona, CE. ¿Qué es y para qué sirve la política?, Educación para la Paz. Documento interno. Edición 1. Ciudad de Guatemala: Oficina Pastoral Social Arzobispado de Guatemala OPSAG; 2001.
22. Thomas de Benitez S. Green Light for Street Children's Rights. Brussels: European Network on Street Children Worldwide; 2003.
23. Melendez Cardona C. Estudio descriptivo de 'Supervivientes de las Calles', documento de investigación y propuestal. Barcelona: Payasos sin Fronteras; 2002.
24. Casa Alianza. Inter-American commission to review war on youth gangs. Rapid-response 2004 (rapid-response@casa-alianza.org).
25. Kronenberg F, Simo Algado S, Gonzalez-Vigil A. Supervivientes de la calle, Proyecto propuesta. Barcelona: Payasos sin Fronteras; 2000.
26. United Nations. Convention on the Rights of the Child. New York: United Nations; 1989.
27. Boal A. Games for Actors and Non-Actors. London: Routledge; 1992:17–29.
28. Ordonez A, Munoz L. Informe de la evaluacion del proyecto 'Supervivientes de la Calle. Ciudad de Guatemala: Casa Alianza Guatemala and Payasos sin Fronteras; 2001.
29. Kronenberg F. In search of the political nature of occupational therapy. MSc OT paper. Sweden: Linköping University; 2003.
30. Kronenberg F. Understanding and Facing up to the Political Nature of Occupational Therapy. Paper presented at the 7th European Occupational Therapy Congress, Athens, Greece, September 2004.
31. Meléndez Cardona C. Hacia una conceptualizacion de los 'supervivientes de las calles. Barcelona: Payasos sin Fronteras; 2001.

Useful websites

Casa Alianza http://www.casa-alianza.org
Payasos Sin Fronteras http://www.clowns.org
Spirit of Survivors – Occupational Therapists without Borders http://sos-otwb.org
Mobile School http://www.mobileschool.org

World Federation of Occupational Therapists http://www.wfot.org
European Network on Street Children Worldwide http://www.enscw.org

Chapter 20

Practicing to learn
Occupational therapy with the children of Viet Nam

Melina Simmond

OVERVIEW

The information in this chapter is intended to help the reader:

- explore the possible role/s of pediatric occupational therapy with children and their caregivers in a resource-poor setting;

- begin to understand the processes one goes through while initiating an 'occupational therapy without borders' program by highlighting concrete practice examples of occupational deprivation and methods used to achieve occupational justice; and

- begin to appreciate the personal and professional challenges and joys involved in working with children in a resource-poor setting and recognize how the resilience and spirituality demonstrated by children can rise above all odds and enrich the lives of those around them.

INTRODUCTION

It all started quite innocently. During a holiday to Asia several years ago, I had the opportunity to spend some time at a local child-focused non-governmental organization (NGO) that zealously works toward eradicating poverty and improving the quality of life of Viet Nam's most marginalized children and their families. Working with children has always been my passion and immediately I was captivated by the selfless commitment and determination that characterized the organization and its employees. At the end of that year, the exhaustion of completing my thesis prompted me, on the spur of the moment, to throw a couple of t-shirts, a pile of pediatric assessments, and a stack of toys into a suitcase, bid my loved ones farewell, and board a plane returning to Viet Nam. Little was I to know, however, that this decision, anticipated as only a brief break from occupational therapy in Australia, would evolve into a life changing experience.

Despite having traveled extensively throughout South-East Asia, upon arrival in Viet Nam I found myself naïve and unprepared for many of the events that were to occur. These experiences were more demanding than practice in Australia in a myriad of ways. Instead of working within my comfort zone, I was forced to reassess and reconstruct many of my basic assumptions related to both professional and personal life. I was forced not only to recognize the beauty of different cultures, but also to look for culturally meaningful occupations that would enrich the lives the people I worked with.[1] This is the story of the challenges and joys I, an Australian-trained occupational therapist, encountered while working with the children of Viet Nam. Some of this account is focused around the story of Nghia (see Case study 20.1).

CASE STUDY 20.1 INTRODUCING NGHIA

Nghia, a much loved member of the medical center, finally reached the end of a courageous struggle and returned home after a long period in our care. Nghia arrived at the medical center in Ho Chi Minh City over a year ago with a cleft palate that had resulted in his being severely malnourished by the time he presented to our staff. He was also experiencing orthopedic problems that were limiting his ability to mobilize independently. His father, mother, and siblings live in an isolated rural area in Viet Nam where a lack of education, funds, medical resources, and basic rehabilitation services meant that his problems were left unaddressed until he was 3 years old. After several months of preoperative care with us, Nghia received the first in a succession of corrective operations. Many months of further medical intervention and intensive rehabilitation intended to remediate his feeding and walking difficulties were also to follow. However, inspiringly Nghia has fought his disabilities, and today the staff of the medical center looked on proudly as Nghia's enduring spirit and resilience enabled him to walk home with a brand new smile.

SETTING THE SCENE

It was a typical hot, humid pre-monsoon morning in Viet Nam. I had just entered the brightly painted concrete building, brimming with enthusiasm on the first day of my new life working as an occupational therapist at the NGO's medical center, a facility that over the years has provided a spectrum of child health services, ranging from emergency medical care to longer-term rehabilitation, to orphans, street children, malnourished infants, children with disabilities, and children of 'poor' families of southern Viet Nam. In the corner of the room, propped on a blue plastic chair, was a small boy of about 3 or 4 years. In one hand he was holding a small white plastic container, in the other a spoon. The boy was engaged in the most exciting game. Every time a child or nurse rounded the corner into the dining area he would fire spoonful after spoonful of yoghurt across the room toward the unsuspecting victim, splattering the walls and floors in the process. Every minute or two between firings he would raise his spoon to his mouth, but rather than swallowing the spoonful, would proceed to wipe the yoghurt across his face in a feeble attempt to disguise his cheeky grin. By the end of breakfast, the boy, the other children, the nurses and the contents of the room were covered in a layer of the sticky white dessert, and the medical center was filled with giggles and smiles.

Nghia first arrived at the medical center about a year before me. According to the Vietnamese staff, upon reaching the city Nghia's father was very distressed about his son's state of health. Nghia's mother, on the other hand, was nowhere to be seen. Despite the obvious barriers in verbal communication, using an interpreter I was able to establish that since his birth, despite always caring for her son, Nghia's mother had experienced great difficulty in forming any type of emotional attachment to him. In many parts of the developing world prejudicial attitudes against people with disabilities, attitudes that ultimately feed occupational apartheid conditions[2] among the wider community, remain prevalent.[3,4] In Viet Nam there is a significant stigma attached to having a child with an obvious physical deformity. In this case, Nghia's cleft palate was perceived as a sign of bad luck for the whole family.

Due to his occupationally deprived childhood, by the time Nghia reached the medical center many aspects of his development were delayed. Apparently, Nghia was physically tired, hungry, and irritable upon his arrival in Ho Chi Minh City. His withdrawn mood made it challenging for the staff to engage him in any purposeful activity. He was simply not interested in interacting socially on any level with the other children. Sleeping in his cot was Nghia's occupational choice. He also craved attention from the nurses, and would scream and throw tantrums in order to get what he wanted. By the time I reached Viet Nam, Nghia had come a long way. Already, one round of corrective surgery had been successfully conducted and Nghia was being fed at regular intervals by means of nasogastric tubing. He was also able to walk semi-independently and was often caught trying to escape the medical center in order to scoot round the front courtyard with the aid of his much-admired brand new red walking frame! However, many more challenges were yet to come.

SWIMMING IN THE POOL OF OCCUPATIONAL NEEDS

Being the only expatriate health professional working at the NGO, my position in the medical center held great autonomy. I had the freedom, within the boundaries of the NGO's values of course, to do whatever I wanted, whenever I wanted. This, on the one hand, was a breath of fresh air. At last I did not have an endless list of stringent rules and regulations restricting my activities. On the other hand, it was enormously scary! How could I possibly begin to tackle the complex and diverse nature of individual children's needs at the micro level, while simultaneously instigating sustainable changes to the lives of greater numbers of children at the societal or macro level?

Being a professional, I have been taught that I have the understanding and expertise to find a solution to any problem I encounter. Being a helping professional, I have a strong drive to alleviate any suffering I see. Yet, as an occupational therapist, I know that the will and drive, the motivation to act, must come from within the people with whom I am working. As occupational therapists, our goal is to facilitate the empowerment of the client's strengths and visions, not to impose our own,[5] by using a client-centered and/or community-centered approach, such as community-based rehabilitation (CBR),[1] in our practice.

However, in the developing world, all too often[6] we have seen nationals fall into a pattern of 'learned helplessness',[7] which inevitably results in an unhealthy reliance on the assistance of expatriates. As Western, 'more privileged' professionals we should in no way exert a power differential over our national colleagues. In my opinion, one of the major roles of expatriate occupational therapists is to build the capacity of our local counterparts by working in close partnership and transferring skills. I would like to highlight, however, that this process can be extremely difficult!

In establishing a process of cooperation between several and different stakeholders, as occupational therapists we must also face – as a collective challenge – the fundamental conflict of the reality that 'we' and 'they' are not equals in rights and opportunities. If as a profession we accept the emerging concept of occupational justice as 'the foundation and fundamental purpose of occupational therapy',[8] we must also accept that all people around the world should have equal human rights of access to occupational opportunities that they find meaningful and purposeful in their environment. In order for this to be made reality, the artificial borders between us, as so-called professionals, and the people we aspire to work with must be made explicit and challenged.

We also need to acknowledge that so-called Western or foreign aid to peripheral countries seems to have been offered historically, and in many ways is still offered, to perpetuate dependency. Marginalized people are not encouraged to walk on their own legs. The dominant political-economic system seems to require a large majority of the world's population to be and remain poor so the privileged minority may stay rich, or become richer. Despite all odds, however, they still manage to walk independently, even in extremely adverse conditions.

It was my aim in Viet Nam to challenge these concepts. I wanted to narrow the gap between 'us' and 'them', or at least begin the process of doing so. I wanted to empower communities I worked with to take their fate into their own hands, thus contributing to the eradication of the destructive sense of dependency in the country. Furthermore, I wanted to transfer new skills to the families and staff I worked with so that, following my departure, they could continue to create occupational opportunities that would allow their children to grow and develop to their full potential.

DOWN TO WORK – A GLIMPSE AT THE OCCUPATIONAL PROCESSES

Theoretical approaches

In my experience, all too often health professionals providing consultancy services to developing countries export Western practice models, irrespective of whether or not they complement the intricacies of the local culture. I was very conscious of not doing this. My mission, as always, was to advocate for the fundamental right of every child to engage in meaningful occupation. Occupational therapy's community-centered,[9] transcultural, and holistic[1] approach to practice was at the forefront of my mind.

I also branched out and experimented with a couple of models I had not previously used. In a country not familiar with the profession of occupational therapy, my use of jargon was inappropriate and confusing for the local staff. Therefore, not only was the ICF (the *International Classification of Functioning, Disability and Health*)[10] the acronym on everyone's lips at the time, I also found that this model provided a common language base across professions. In addition, as it focuses on healthy functioning by taking an enabling occupation approach to practice, I found the model's 'without borders' way of understanding the notions of health and disability to be a useful everyday advocacy tool in a country where people, for the greater part, tended to dwell on pathology, limitations, and inability.

In moments of confusion and frustration, I also found that the four predominant ideas of the *United Nations Convention on the Rights of the Child*,[11] (non-discrimination; best interests of the child; right to life, survival, and development; and views of the child) provided much-needed meaning, purpose, and guidance. For example, while working in the medical center I became actively involved in the discharge/community re-entry process. In this role, based on the four above-mentioned principles, I often found myself advocating to government and community health personnel the need to focus on community rather than institution-based care of children.

Prioritizing occupational therapy goals

During the process of identifying and prioritizing Nghia's occupational needs, a task left solely to myself, I found that remaining diligent at respecting the priorities of all stakeholders, such as the NGO, Nghia's parents and other health providers, while also striving for cultural safety in my approach, was, at times, most challenging. At the medical center, my choice was twofold. I could identify a few children with the most outstanding needs and work with them on an individual basis, or I could work for the betterment of all the children the center serves by conducting a range of community-based activities for the staff, parents, and general community. In the end I decided to do a bit of both.

Assessment

While child development tends to follow the same rough path for children all around the world,[12] I soon discovered that my standardized assessments, based on Western constructions of childhood,[13] were going to be of little or no use to me in Viet Nam. The children in the medical center spent a large part of their day either lying in their cots or crawling around the floor (a classic example of occupational deprivation), and while many toys had been donated to the organization, they remained lined up neatly on the shelves out of reach of eager little hands. Having never been exposed to wooden pegs, scissors, or blocks, how could these children have been accurately assessed for their developmental capabilities using assessments standardized on children from the developed world? Instead I found it far more useful to follow my clinical instincts and observe spontaneous play. So, I started by playing games with Nghia. He thrived on one-on-one attention, and I found that as my rapport with him increased, I was able to assess his developmental capabilities.

However, coming from the so-called developed world where accountability and documentation are imperative to our practice as professionals, I also decided to use a self-devised checklist-style assessment of child development. This assessment took into account the local cultural and socio-economic conditions of Viet Nam, and linked assessment not just to developmental scales but also to what the children and those who surrounded them identified as meaningful and purposeful. It also assisted me in monitoring and evaluating the efficacy of my interventions.

Intervention

Based on my informal assessments of Nghia, recognizing that there were many underlying causes contributing to his developmental delay, I then proceeded with the difficult task of deciding upon appropriate intervention strategies. The interventions I chose to implement at the medical center were varied, ranging from individual therapy focusing on the enhancement of developmental skills, the introduction of occupation-based programs (i.e. art and music) for all children in the center, the running of health education sessions for the Vietnamese nurses, provision of rehabilitation equipment, consultation regarding the day-to-day operation of the medical center, and assistance during the discharge/community re-entry process. The overall aim behind all these interventions was to enable occupation and to facilitate the people that I worked with at the center to become more empowered at both the individual and societal levels.

CHALLENGES ALONG THE WAY

Working from a medical, reductionist perspective

The medical center operated under the traditional medical approach to diagnosis and treatment of illness. In these circumstances, rarely were the social or economic factors related to a child's ill health investigated, or even acknowledged. Being an occupational therapist who practices from a holistic, occupational justice perspective, I found working in a facility operating in this manner to be undeniably frustrating. Email contact with colleagues and mentors overseas, including those registered with the Occupational Therapy International Outreach Network (OTION),[14] (see Ch. 27) became an invaluable means of frustration management and an avenue for both personal and professional support.

Balancing priorities of different stakeholders

In developed countries the usual practice for children with cleft lip and/or palate is to perform corrective surgery within the first couple of months of birth; in many parts of Viet Nam corrective surgery does not usually take place until the child is 1–2 years old, due to limited medical services. In Nghia's situation, social and economic disadvantage meant that his medical problems remained untreated until he was 3 years old. In light of this, the NGO was concerned to arrange for Nghia's corrective surgery to be conducted as soon as possible. As the NGO seeks to maximize the potential of each child in the context of the family and community, another major goal was to discharge Nghia back to the care of his family as soon as possible. Nghia's parents were, however, very anxious about their son's imminent return home. Despite loving Nghia, their feelings of uncertainty regarding their ability to adequately care for him resulted in their belief that he would be better cared for in the medical center. Balancing the priorities of these stakeholders, while simultaneously working in line with the best interests of the child, was a constant process of collaboration and negotiation.

The value of play

During the intervention stage, I often found that my good intentions and conventional Western approaches collided with reality. Initially, I had grand schemes of how I would establish gross motor groups for the children who had coordination and balance problems, open a sensory integration room, and organize recreational outings. I observed that despite play being considered the primary 'occupation' and vehicle for development for children in the developed world,[15] it seems to hold little value in Viet Nam. Perhaps this is because from an early age Vietnamese children are required to assist their parents with income-generating activities to supplement the family's income. Or perhaps this is because Vietnamese adults lacked positive and constructive play experiences themselves while they were young, and hence do not understand the need for their children to engage in play. Causation aside, the staff at the center did not see it as their role to stimulate the children through play, and hence the children would spend many hours of the day occupationally deprived, confined to the limits of their cots. I found encouraging parents and children to play communally to be a positive way to challenge this cultural norm.

The 'expert'

After seeing a string of volunteers come and go, the center's staff were quite reserved about accepting my ideas, but as the rapport-building process progressed they soon came to view me as an 'expert' on everything. Consequently, I rapidly and quite wrongly acquired the reputation of being the resident occupational therapist, physiotherapist, speech therapist, social worker, and doctor. This situation made me acutely aware of my professional and personal capacities and limitations, and the way in which the local Vietnamese people view foreign professionals, including the unrealistic expectations that come hand-in-hand with this. Rapport building and subtle challenging of stereotypes on a daily basis were the means by which I attempted to overcome this situation.

Resource limitations

Resources at the medical center were scarce and, if available, often archaic. The first level of the center consisted of little more than a couple of dozen cots lined up in a row, a changing table, and a rusty oxygen tank. Medications were minimal, and the quality of the available drugs questionable. Notwithstanding lack of resources, armed only with a therapy degree and a handful of pediatric first aid skills, I needed to look past my lack of control and utilize my knowledge and creativity, and that of the people I worked with, as best I could. In the end I discovered that a lack of resources did not hinder or compromise the achievement of the therapy goals we set.

Occupational transitions

When faced with communities that experience occupational deprivation on such a large scale, it is very easy to become overwhelmed and depressed by the situation. As expatriates working with marginalized populations, we tend to be drawn into trying to save people and change the world. Occupational transition and sustainable development are processes that are, at times, unfathomably slow. I have learnt, however, that if we can focus on achievable and effective grassroots changes, we can often have a much greater effect on the quality of life of our clients than we first anticipate. I have also come to better understand and appreciate the Brazilian sociologist Herbert de Souza's principle: 'the end is not primarily about attaining determined goals, but above all about the processes.'[16]

REFLECTIONS – PROFESSIONAL AND PERSONAL

Despite all these challenges, at the end of the day what matters is that I worked with a group of remarkably committed and compassionate people, all unconditionally dedicated to working toward the betterment of child health in Viet Nam. In addition, the children never failed to exude a contagious sense of cheerfulness and spirit, another great source of inspiration. In my view, spirituality, the true essence of the human being,[1] has a profound effect on the ability to achieve occupational performance, and I have no doubt that the shining spirit of these young survivors significantly contributed to their rapid progress in therapy. In my view, lack of a sense of hope destroys the fabric of society. Spirituality has been referred to as being at the intersection of occupation and the environment,[17] and in light of this I believe that empowering people to recover their spiritual balance is a fundamental aspect of working with marginalized populations. Despite all the challenges and frustrations my position involved, all it took was one big smile or hug to make me forget all the negatives and look forward to the next day I was to spend with the children. Never before have I leapt out of bed every morning in anticipation of a day spent at work!

Living and working in a developing country provokes a re-evaluation of life priorities. The children of Viet Nam allowed me to rediscover the intrinsic joys that accompany childhood, joys that have no cultural boundaries. In spite of all their background differences, children are still children, and the children of Viet Nam were no exception. They laughed, they cried, grabbed toys, hit each other, and chased me around the medical center. They took pleasure in the simple things that you and I as adults take for granted: the feel of the first rain of monsoon falling on their faces, watching fish dart around a small cracked fish tank, play fights during tooth brushing time. Many aspects of the human spirit transcend cultural boundaries and after working with Nghia I now appreciate more than ever the resilience and courage of children.

I strongly believe that occupational therapists possess a refreshing perspective on occupation, health, and wellbeing that can greatly enhance the lives of people from marginalized populations. However, as we are a relatively invisible and rapidly changing profession, the value of our skills is often not appreciated, or even acknowledged, by many. There is no cookbook solution for the profession in clearly defining its role when working with marginalized populations, as the needs of different communities within different countries vary so greatly. As actively involved clinicians we need to map out the roles of the various other health professions and develop our own roles so that we can be in a position to act as a 'change agent within the system'[18] rather than simply fitting into existing systems that may be perpetuating occupational apartheid. To achieve this, it is critical that we accurately assess the need for occupational therapy in the overall spheres of health care, social services, and education. We need to identify those areas in which we can most quickly and obviously have an effect. For example, health education and prevention of disability can be important spheres for occupational therapists working with marginalized populations.

We may well find that in countries where infectious diseases are not controlled, potable water is not available, and malnutrition is widespread, neither the government nor community members will understand the need for occupational therapy services. In such cases it is up to proactive therapists to adapt their roles, guided by their occupational visions, principles, and theories, to the nature and levels of needs that communities present. When asked directly, marginalized people want fair access to occupational opportunities that afford them the capacity and power to construct their own destinies.[19] Occupation is essential for life and health, and as such, occupation is a basic human right. In the world today there are communities that suffer occupational deprivation and the inevitable detrimental health consequences. As occupational therapists we have a humanitarian, moral, and professional obligation to address such cases of occupational deprivation. In sharing my experiences, I encourage the profession to come together, embrace the value of occupation, and continue to promote the value of innovative 'occupational therapy without borders' programs.

CONCLUSION

Finally, you may be wondering what has happened to little Nghia. Well, I am pleased to inform you that he is back home, living happily with his Mum, Dad and family in the hills of Viet Nam. Despite rapid globalization and the injection of considerable amounts of foreign aid in recent decades, a large proportion of Viet Nam's population continue to live below the poverty line, and many children and families continue to fall victim to occupational apartheid. Working in the medical center has enabled me to understand better the realities of life in Viet Nam through the eyes of the local children and communities, a perspective I do not feel I could fully appreciate otherwise. My experience of walking with the children of Viet Nam has given me the opportunity to witness their fighting spirit shining through time after time, offering me a comforting sense of hope and reassurance for the future. Walking with the children has taught me about love, life, and the immense power of occupation.

References

1. Simó Algado S, Mehta N, Kronenberg F, et al. Occupational therapy intervention with children survivors of war. Can J Occup Ther 2002; 69(4):205–217.
2. Kronenberg FCW. Street children: being and becoming. Research study. Heerlen, The Netherlands: Hogeschool Limburg; 1999.
3. Kohl H. Speechless occupational therapy. Br J Occup Ther 1990; 53(3):98–100.
4. Yeoman S. Occupation and disability: a role for occupational therapists in developing countries. Br J Occup Ther 1998; 61(11):523–527.
5. Canadian Association of Occupational Therapists. Enabling occupation: an occupational therapy perspective. Ottawa: CAOT Publications ACE; 1997.
6. Hancock G. Lords of poverty. London: Mandarin Paperbacks; 1991.
7. Peterson C, Maier S, Seligman MEP. Learned helplessness: a theory for the age of personal control. New York: Oxford University Press; 1993.
8. Wilcock A, Townsend E. Occupational terminology interactive dialogue. J Occup Sci 2000; 7(2):84–86.
9. Kronenberg FCW, Simó Algado S. Overcoming occupational apartheid: working towards occupational justice. Paper presented at the European Congress of Occupational Therapy. Paris. 2000.
10. World Health Organization. International classification of functioning, disability and health (ICF). Geneva: World Health Organization; 2001.
11. United Nations. United Nations convention on the rights of the child. New York: United Nations; 1991.
12. de Lemos M. Patterns of young children's development: an international comparison of development as assessed by Who Am I? Quebec: Development Canada; 2002.
13. Galheigo S. Challenging the constructions of childhood used by therapeutic models. Paper presented at the WFOT Conference. Montreal. 1998.
14. Occupational Therapy International Outreach Network. Online. Available: www.wfot.org.au/otion. 27 Oct 2003.
15. Case-Smith J, Allen A, Pratt P. Occupational therapy for children. St Louis: Mosby-Year Book; 1996.
16. Molinas Maldonado MM, Monroy Peralta JG. *Sistematizacion de experiencias: una invitacion para la accion – una propuesta para instituciones y/o programas que trabajan con el sector de la infancia.* Guatemala: Childhope; 1999.
17. Unruh A, Versnel J, Kerr N. Spirituality unplugged: a review of commonalities and contentions, and a resolution. Can J Occup Ther 2002; 69(1):5–19.
18. Wood W, Nielson C, Humphry R, et al. A curricular renaissance: graduate education centered on occupation. Am J Occup Ther 2000; 54(6):586–597.
19. Burnside J, ed. From nothing to zero. Melbourne: Lonely Planet Publications; 2003.

Chapter 21

Voices Talk and Hands Write

Nick Pollard, Pat Smart, and the Voices Talk and Hands Write group

OVERVIEW

This chapter describes writing and community publishing activities with a group of people with learning difficulties in North East Lincolnshire, an area with chronic urban and rural poverty and social exclusion issues. The project was set up as an initiative between the Federation of Worker Writers and Community Publishers (FWWCP) and North East Lincolnshire Council Social Services, with assistance from Pecket Well College, from volunteers from Grimsby Writers, and from Sheffield Hallam University. North East Lincolnshire Council agreed to fund a twelve session writing group with day center and other local service users with learning difficulties to produce publications of the participants' writing, and would, with their agreement, aim to publish the project in the health professional media. The second author of this chapter, an education worker from Pecket Well College (a self-administered adult and basic education college in West Yorkshire, and another FWWCP member) was to lead the sessions.

Using a participatory research approach, the authors explore the project's development into a cohesive writing and publishing group, producing individual publications for all the participants with learning difficulties, and encouraging individuals to realize new communication and creative abilities. All those involved have learned from the experience, which also provided educational and experiential opportunities for adult learners from the partner college, day center staff, and volunteers to become 'writing hands' (see Ch. 5) for the participants.

The account is considered against the background of the literature on therapeutic writing and community publishing and conclusions and recommendations are drawn for further developments. Since the workshops, the group has been involved in further writing and publishing activities, demonstrating longer term outcomes from the project.

WHAT IS 'THERAPEUTIC' ABOUT CREATIVE WRITING AND COMMUNITY PUBLISHING?

Publications by people with learning difficulties which aim to share their experiences with a wider audience are rare. Even amongst the first author's own collection of over 750 items of community published material, most from the UK, only a few are specifically associated with individuals with learning difficulties: an anthology of poetry from children with learning disabilities,[1] two from adults with learning difficulties,[2,3] and an inspirational publication by adult women.[4] Since the FWWCP's definition of 'publishing' includes any form of dissemination to an audience, including tape recordings and performance material, this would be missed in a search of publications in printed form. Performances are the principal vehicle for reaching an audience amongst FWWCP member groups. A proportion of adult literacy reading books may have originated from writers with learning difficulties. For example, members of Pecket Well College (see Ch. 5), which has for years supported a publishing group, would not, as a principle of empowerment, make distinctions between adult learners attending its courses.

A myth persists that people with intellectual disabilities do not have the capacity for a voice,[5] or perhaps, if their voices are heard, that they might say something which transgresses social mores on disability – for example about sex, or anger.[6] Perhaps this perception is also shared by people with experiences of learning difficulties themselves. No surprise, therefore, that Johnson,[7] (p. 186) at the end of her ethnographic study of women with 'intellectual disabilities' in a closing institution, should have a problem understanding 'who the women were ... their stories continued to escape us.' This view of people with experience of learning difficulties, which arises perhaps from a tradition of care through containment, corresponds with the experience of occupational apartheid explored in Chapter 6.

Organizing and sustaining publication activities with occupational therapy service users from an institutional base can be difficult.[8] Problems in finding a suitable space, maintaining a group with competing treatment and other activity demands, and developing a publication which is truly owned by the participants, can detrimentally affect motivation and interest over something that is a drawn out process. It is significant that, even though the print run of the combined total of the Voices Talk and Hands Write group publications will be less than half that of The Thursday Club's[4] lavish and colorful book *Our Lives, Our Group*, the participants have produced 17 booklets of their own.

Community publishing – unrealized potential

Writing by people with experiences of learning difficulties rarely occurs in print. The therapeutic potential of community publishing as an extension of the writing process has only recently begun to be explored,[9–11] especially in the field of occupational therapy,[12–17] but, with the exception of these, so far there has been little covering the practice and methodology of community publishing in relation to health and social care, let alone learning difficulties. This chapter describes a community publishing project involving people with learning difficulties in making their own publications which combines occupational therapy theory and practice with its own practices and approaches. The first and second authors of this chapter share a background in community publishing through the Federation of Worker Writers and Community Publishers (FWWCP), an organization which is concerned with the enabling and facilitation of publications by people who are marginalized (see Ch. 5).

In a therapeutic context, writing has been addressed more for the creative, expressive opportunity it offers and its narrative content than in terms of an end publishing process, but as Willinsky[18] (pp. 186–187) remarks, 'publication is the principal post-writing activity for the serious writing program; it is intended to demonstrate a regard for the students' work, treating their word as if it counted in the world.' It is equally important to address the full import of the empowerment offered by writing.[19] Whereas being enabled to read may mean being enabled to read merely in order to accept what has been written by others, the act of writing offers the potential to make one's own version of the story, to challenge truth itself, if necessary, with one's own truth. It offers a means of power to challenge occupational apartheid with weapons of mass construction, deconstruction, and/or reconstruction (see Ch. 6). With the exception of Lorenzo,[13,14] authors writing on community publishing have not considered using the processes involved as a participatory action research tool; rather, they have seen community publishing as a practical and interactive process for consciousness raising and recording history through community writing.[20–27] Of particular significance has been the combination of community publication with adult literacy to develop a 'public literacy'.[28]

Another function of creative writing can be to 're-create our past'. This can produce some of the benefits from imagined experiences and be 'a healing experience' which enables us to 'find new perspectives, new aims, freedoms and confidence'.[29] Many publications on creative writing as therapy suggest exercises which are too demanding for clients with cognitive impairments.[30] The 'therapy' word implies a perception of writing as cathartic rather than as deliberate expression. It has an awkward history in connection with FWWCP writing and publishing, having been used to dismiss the 'worker writing' for its lack of literary quality, negating its content,[20,31] and its use of dialect, and assuming an incapacity for full expression.[20,32] Indeed, some writers have felt unable to celebrate their published work at events because difficulty in signing their names will reveal that they are literacy learners or have an illness.[33]

Celebration and agency

Writers in health and social care environments and user groups are often vulnerable, and there are professional and ethical concerns concerning publication of 'the unsifted contents of a troubled mind'.[34] (p. 225). Bolton is justifiably wary of exposing therapeutic writing to the risks and false expectations of publication, but others report the value in developing creative writing with adults with learning difficulties where it may have hitherto been denied.[35,36] Sampson, while admitting Bolton's concerns, also accords with Willinsky,[18] suggesting that publishing and broadcasting have potential value in an arsenal of devices for social inclusion, where the writer with learning difficulties is taken at face value as a writer. Community publishing is a political act which involves a shift in consciousness toward making things happen in a collaborative way, based on the needs of the publication project and, as Mason[5] has identified, an interdependence.

Writing produces changing perceptions in both the writer and the audience, a personal change which Jones,[29] a nondisabled workshop facilitator, explains is not an experience reserved for an elite who have scaled the ladder of excellence, but is for everyone 'to fulfill their own need for expression and aesthetic experience'. For Jones, the key qualities in such writing are that people have been enabled to write freely and powerfully. Community publishing and the creative writing groups organized around it produce such participant reported outcomes as personal growth through creative expression, opportunities for social participation and inclusion, education and self-actualization, group structures, and vocational and voluntary roles, as well as the publications themselves (which may take many forms, performances, print, or sound recordings amongst them).[15] In Chapter 5 Pat Smart describes her own emergence through community publishing and the opportunities it has provided for facilitating others. We have decided against describing the outcomes of the project as 'therapy', since the word occludes the horizons of an activist community publishing paradigm. From the point of view of an FWWCP practitioner, the aim of writing and publishing with people with learning difficulties is the same as for everyone else, as Taylor[37] (p. 37) says, 'to be adept at making your own rules and making your own shapes with writing, and to be able to make something of a blank page – that is to start shining yourself.'

PARTICIPATORY RESEARCH, CONSCIOUSNESS RAISING, AND ETHICAL ISSUES

Community publishing groups often emerge from other projects, in response to a need to communicate a message, as well as the mutual discovery of an interest in writing.[20,29] The participatory nature of community publication and its relationship to community issues suggests a process which is not so much therapeutic as spontaneous. Even where it has not been initially generated by the participants, as with this project, once the process is in hand everyone is involved. Many of the outcomes will not have been forecast. Given the absence of control that this process needs for empowerment to be maximized, a participatory research model seemed to be the most appropriate methodology to enable outcomes to be described.

The lack of research exploring the benefits of community publishing was another factor behind the political need for the FWWCP to develop this project. In this sense there were actually several sets of participants or actors – the Voices Talk and Hands Write group, the FWWCP, Pecket Well College and Grimsby Writers members, and the local social services staff – coming together with different needs, which would be served by enabling people with learning difficulties in their capacity for expression.

Using the activities of community publishing and its concern with recording experiences to raise political consciousness and practical publishing and writing skills democratically are valuable aims in themselves for justifying a participatory process,[38,39] and although community activity in itself cannot be described as research, Letts[40] gives examples of the use of participatory research techniques to develop knowledge of an activity in process, something which cannot be achieved or adequately described using more rigid, quantitative methods.

Using a participatory research process with people with learning difficulties raises questions about genuine empowerment and the sharing of rewards,[41] particularly as in this project several levels of involvement and empowerment may have operated simultaneously, serving different needs and under different forms of contractual arrangement.[5] Whereas some actors were being paid for their participation as part of their work role, others were volunteers, and others had come to participate in a writing workshop. All of us were learning about the process we were engaged in, but clearly were working from differing levels of knowledge and difficulty in assimilating knowledge.

Financial resources were limited, and the ideas which led to the project's initiation began from the activist standpoint of a small group of actors within the FWWCP who wanted to find a means of developing community publishing with new participants, and local workers who wanted to increase the activities that could be accessed by the people they were working with. Even the involvement of those who were paid for their role depended on managers and employers allocating their time. Projects with marginalized groups are often created from gaps and margins, and rely on an activist capacity to 'wangle' opportunities (see Ch. 5).[20] The appropriate research strategy appears to be to recognize and approach the difficulties.[42,43]

Without attempts to engage marginalized groups and enable their narratives to be documented, these people remain silent; the writing process in which we hoped to involve the Voices Talk and Hands Write group would be one which aimed at developing their active consciousness and capacity for determining their needs.[44] In developing and negotiating the dissemination of the project, the authors have negotiated with the group. While this is in line with both the participatory research methodology and the Canadian Occupational Performance Process Model (COPPM)[45] it is also consistent with the approach described by the second author in Chapter 5, which derives from the practices developed by Pecket Well College. The participants have consented to the material in which they were involved being used for training purposes and for publication, and have themselves asserted the importance of sharing practice.

WRITING HANDS

The workshops began in September 2003. No specific inclusion criteria were operated, except that participants should be able to benefit from being in the group. The group eventually had 17 participants (of whom

12–14 attended regularly) and an additional group of supporters who were designated as 'writing hands'. In a program which relied on voluntary input from a range of organizations, with some individuals making 200 mile round trips to facilitate the group, and with so many participants, it was inevitable that some inconsistency would occur. Illness and competing work commitments limited the attendance of some of the writing hands. However, participants were made to feel that they were the focus of special attention and interest – it was emphasized to them that the project was work which had not been done before by the FWWCP. Furthermore, because many of the writing hands were themselves people with disabilities, the participants found that facilitators' needs also had to be accommodated in the sessions.

An initial meeting introduced support workers from social services and members from the local writing workshop to being writing hands. Moving beyond functional uses of writing, i.e. shopping lists and personal letters, into facilitating creative expression presents a challenge when the creator is not the person doing the physical writing. There is a risk that the transcription of the oral version may lack the life of the original. Pecket Well College developed the 'writing hand' as a kind of scribe who writes down only what the person they are working with wants them to (see Ch. 5). A writing hand does not interpret for the person, but takes the time to establish with the person what they mean, does not correct their grammar, respects their dialect, and writes legibly so that the piece being developed is clear. The writing hands may have to read out to others, on behalf of their partners what has been written if the partners are unable to do this themselves, a more difficult task than if they have just been writing for themselves.

An introductory exercise enabled the writing hands to discuss issues such as dealing with silences, digressions, or the interruptions in sequencing – such as jumping back and forth between periods in a life story – which occur in oral language, and resisting the temptation to adjust the written piece for the person in order to make it more logical. Writing hands don't just rely on the narrative they are being told, but also on facial expression and hand signals, especially as the person they are working with may have difficulty in verbal expression.

Plans for the sessions involving the participants were first outlined to the writing hands, in order to enable them to take on the new task of facilitation. The writing produced was to be collected at each session to build up material for publication, and individuals were to be invited to contribute their writing to the group forum during sessions. Individuals could either read this themselves or use their writing hand to read for them. Writing hands would remain after the meeting for a half an hour to an hour to discuss each session, and any specific issues that had arisen, and to plan the next.

VOICES TALK AND HANDS WRITE

The full group met at the day center for 2 hours every Friday afternoon. A flipchart was used each week to record group decisions and, over the series of activities, to refer back when necessary to previous sessions. Some activities involved role play and working in small groups with writing hands. Some participants were able to write independently – three of them kept diaries before joining the group – though most made use of writing hands or supporters to prompt them in developing their work.

Each session began with a review of the previous week's activity, and an exploration of the topic which had been decided upon for the activity that day. Participants would then work with the writing hands. Some sessions involved working with larger groups to develop short sketches. At the conclusion of each session writing was shared with the rest of the group. Initially, writing hands generally did the reading, but this pattern changed over the program. They held the work of the person they were working with, so that the participant could read it and confirm what was being shared with the rest of the group, but a significant number of participants were confident and able to read their own work. Every contribution was applauded.

The group operated as a writers' workshop might, at a social and informal level, as well as concentrating on the business of writing. The socializing that took place at the beginning, break time, and end of the group involved everyone. Some of the participants took on roles which contributed to the sessions, such as writing out name labels and sticking them on people as they came into the group, or meeting with the workshop leader and writing hands from Pecket Well as they discussed the preparation for the group in the cafe across the road. The sessions included a couple of parties, in which the participants brought contributions and assisted with putting food out or clearing up. These and other activities associated with the project might be considered as 'occupational spin-offs'[46] from the writing and publishing activities. There were often changes amongst the writing hands as not all those involved could contribute to the full program of sessions, and occasional visitors, when they came, were also drafted in as writing hands. This often added to the social interest of the group. This arrangement also meant that participants and writing hands did not form fixed groups. A significant number of the writing hands themselves had disabilities, which probably contributed to the facilitation of the sessions, particularly the discussion of experiences of disability.

Most of the participants attended throughout the program, although one died during the series. That this group of people, who might be supposed to have limited concentration, continued both in the organized program and in its subsequent continuation is evidence of the interest it held for them, and the sense of achievement they derived from it. At the conclusion of the first phase of the project a total of 17 different booklets were published, in which each author had a collection of their own writing along with the output by the rest of the group. To introduce the idea of being published, a selection of example publications from materials that the second author had produced with other groups, and also from FWWCP member organizations, were explained and distributed for the participants to examine. This was to enable them to imagine the kind of book or magazine that would be possible. In evaluating this work it is important to consider several factors. Participants had not been in a creative writing group before and had not, in many cases, been asked to produce any creative written work since school. Some, but not all, were regular readers. However, individuals produced some very imaginative writing. 'Walking talking doll'[47] was a spontaneously told and funny story in which a doll bought for a sick child rebelled against its owner. Even in the earlier stages of the group, participants were describing personal experiences and feelings.

The program

The first session explored the central topic of dreams and aspirations, and the object of publication, the range of writing forms which might be used, and the use of writing hands. Participants were informed that all decisions made by the group would be achieved through their consensus. Ground rules were elicited by asking the participants what they understood by having 'rights' and the responsibilities that go with them, e.g. the right to be independent requires that others' independence is respected. The participants were thus enabled to determine how their group would work together, agreeing on issues such as the right to speak, to free expression, not to be made fun of, and the times of breaks.

The subsequent sessions, a total of 14, two more than originally projected, explored topics which included 'favorite things', 'what job would you like to do', 'leisure and pleasure, social lives and hobbies', and 'disabilities'. The latter topic was spread over four sessions.

One objective of the first topics was to encourage the group members to open up possibilities through reflection and writing about desires and needs. At the end of the second session, participants were asked for their own suggestions for further topics. In the session in which they were asked what job they would like to do, participants were encouraged to think beyond 'working in a shop' to perhaps being the shop manager. One participant revealed that she'd previously worked with horses, but had not done so for some time, although she'd clearly derived a lot of pleasure from this. Having identified their job, participants were then asked to work out some practical steps they would have to take to achieve their 'ambition'; for example, to become a teacher it would be necessary to go to college, but participants could identify skills which they might be able to teach other people and others might need to learn. For the benefit of readers it is pertinent to point out that while this matches the steps outlined in the COPPM,[45] it is also consistent with the issues discussed by Pat Smart in Chapter 5, and derives from processes Pecket Well College devised to answer its own needs.

A second objective of these first weeks was to enable the group to find out about each other. The initial topics covered the information of social exchange, so that the group came together. Thus, by the fourth session group members were readily volunteering suggestions and one contribution would spark off another. In relating their individual accounts of hobbies and leisure pursuits, group members gave enthusiastic and sometimes animated descriptions of them to their writing hands.

In a significant development, one of the participants asked the supporters to describe *their* hobbies to the group.

Writing about Disability

Four of the sessions focused on the group's experiences of disability and the role of writing and publishing their own accounts. The group initially found this difficult and deferred their decision on whether to write about this, to give themselves time to think about it. A second session began with the group evaluating some writing by other people with disabilities in terms of positive and negative aspects of the experiences described. The subsequent discussion explored positive and negative elements of the participants' experiences of disability, issues such as being called names, obtaining physical access to accommodation, work, and social events, and several examples of how poor planning impacted on their ability to do the things they wanted. In this session in particular, the experiences of disability shared by many of the writing hands with the participants were useful in generating a more spontaneous discussion of incidents through the sharing of anecdotes. The conversation moved on from examples of discrimination to developing a local campaign group. Afterwards, some of the writers combined disability issues and description in the most personal and telling pieces produced in the whole series of meetings.

The third disability session explored 'how things should be for disabled people'. After the initial discussion the group split into two large groups, feeding back at the end with practical proposals, not only ideas for educating others but also expressions of participants' individual needs. Participants gave examples of the kind of information about themselves which they thought would give a more positive image of people with disabilities, such as the fact that some of them work, or live in their own homes and can look after themselves with support.

Finally, the group used role play to explore situations involving disability. Three situations were offered to the group: a job interview, trying to get past a doctor's receptionist for an emergency appointment, and going for a meal in a restaurant. In each of these the disabled person would encounter someone being obstructive because of their disability. Participants were asked to volunteer for the key parts, and those not actually participating in the scene were to act as observers and report back what they noticed.

This exercise produced a lot of comment and debate – participants had a lot to say about both the sketches they had just seen or been involved in, and their own experience of similar situations. For example, after the restaurant sketch one participant felt that the restaurant would have been better prepared for disabled customers had they booked in advance, and that people in wheelchairs should avoid causing obstructions and, where possible, transfer into a dining chair. Other participants suggested initiatives such as training for restaurant staff, and better organization to allow for people with disabilities. One participant was praised by the group for her persistence in getting an appointment, despite the studied ignorance which a writing hand presented as a 'receptionist'. Another, exposed to belittling questions such as 'can you write, love' in a job interview, asked to see the 'interviewer's' boss.

Personal writing

Several sessions enabled participants to produce examples of personal writing. When one of the group died, a session was set aside for writing tributes. The composition of these and their subsequent feedback was quiet and thoughtful. The activity provided an opportunity to grieve; some group members cried as they heard the pieces which had been written during the feedback.

Another considered themes such as: if you were someone else for a week, childhood memories, imagination writing (which involved subjects picked from a hat to offer suggestions), something you're not happy about (and changed or would like to change), bad box things (if you have something or somebody you'd like locked up for ever, why would you lock it up, and where would you lock it up?) produced sustained and coherent pieces. Some were imaginative and humorous.[47–49] Others confidently revealed real dreams and desires of motherhood,[50] and a hearty lifestyle.[51] These pieces take on Lewis's[6] (p. 51) disability taboo 'limitations', i.e. topics which non-disabled people feel are inappropriate: people with a learning difficulty writing about their reflections on, respectively, political power, motherhood, and drinking.

Writing about Christmas can be a difficult topic, although this had been chosen by the group. As George[52] points out, 'it's lonely when you're on your own, very', but in a group which is concerned with empowerment it is important to confront seasonal issues in a way which allows a range of options for the expression of different experiences, including those which are less happy. Not everyone chose to read or have their pieces read. However, several pieces revealed a sense of humor.[53–55] These pieces were applauded and, in view of the different feelings people might have about Christmas, left to stand by themselves.

Party time

The participants proposed that the eleventh session should be a party, to which everyone brought food to share. The entire afternoon was spent socializing. While this was not directly a writing activity, it is an important part of the writing workshop experience. Most writers' workshop members get together informally, decamping after meetings to the pub, and socializing and networking are a large and important part of any FWWCP activity. Although people join writers' workshops in order to write, there are probably many who rely on them as a social outlet.

The final session, in which everyone received a certificate of achievement, also included a surprise birthday party for one of the participants. She had previously mentioned that it would be her birthday but that she would have no one to celebrate it with. This example of isolation alone perhaps illustrates the value of situating the activity in the kind of social context those of us who represent an FWWCP experience are used to in our own groups. Combined with the presentation of certificates and a bunch of flowers, it produced a suitable ceremonial ending to the activities program, and was much enjoyed by the participants. By this time the group had clear coherency, and individuals were mixing and socializing with each other, chatting across the room in a relaxed and informal way, something that had not happened suddenly but a process that had developed gradually over the sessions.'

EVALUATION

The meaning of evaluation was explained to the group as a way of finding out whether the activity had been carried out properly, and then ideas were taken from the participants about what they would like to include in an evaluation, whether good or bad. The group was told that it was possibly the first of its kind, where a community publishing group had been set up in a day center to work with other community publishing groups, and that the FWWCP hoped to apply information from this exercise elsewhere, with other groups who ordinarily would not be involved in community publishing. We could only do this if the participants agreed.

Participants were asked to come up with advice for others setting up similar writing groups, and about what we should do with the information we had developed with the participants. Proposals came swiftly from the group about informing other people of the exercises they had undertaken. Some participants had seen a production by a local theater group which they discussed as the kind of activity they could be involved in, in the future. Participants reported that they had enjoyed the sessions, had been involved in decision making through the use of the flipchart so that they could see what they decided, had written about disability, learned a lot, learned about teamwork, and had been able to talk about their problems. Some had been surprised to be involved in role play as well as writing, and several were pleased with the work they had produced.

The writing hands also participated in the evaluation: 'At the first … meeting I wasn't sure what to expect but I've loved every minute of it … it has really opened my eyes to ideas. It has given me the opporunity to work with my people from day centers but also people I wouldn't normally get to meet … our staff, the day center staff and the people from the Fed [FWWCP], you've all gelled so well, I think it has been really relevant that you've all worked so well together.' Others commented: 'I've learned a lot … I've learned to listen', and 'I've watched people grow more confident … as they've gone on they've managed to tell us more and more about themselves.'

When the council press officer came to take a statement, Voices Talk and Hands Write decided that it would address her together, rather than just delegate a few people to meet with her. They had taken on a group identity and, with this, responsibility for the way they were to be represented, with the group spontaneously giving examples of how they had benefited from being involved. When one participant asked if there would be a photo accompanying the report in the paper, another asked for everyone to be included in the picture.

LOOKING FORWARD

The most significant outcome from the project has been that the group continues to write and publish within the broader FWWCP terms of publication: it has given performances at civic events, participated in an event with the FWWCP and Grimsby Writers, and has had radio and press coverage.[56] Print, through its permanence, remains an important medium for publication, and the idea of publishing books has been important to the participants. Together, they have exercised their right to write and to publish, producing writing that offers insights into lives about which much is assumed but whose voices are seldom heard. They have produced good, interesting writing: work which is lively, amusing, poignant, reflective; writing which, according to Jones'[29] criteria, has been produced freely and is powerful.

Writing and publishing have been developed by the group as meaningful occupations in the sense of Wilcock's 'doing, being and becoming'. For example, as well as writing, being a group member has provided other opportunities for self-expression. Not all the pieces of writing produced by individuals were collected as 'finished' pieces. Some work may have been withheld because participants were dissatisfied with it, but all submitted some writing which they thought a good enough contribution to a book which they understood would be read by others. It is not appropriate to quantify the output of the Voices Talk and Hands Write group; people have differing abilities to produce work, and the interest one person may take in reading the same piece several times, and another's production of several pieces of work to perform over the same period of time, may be of similar expressive value if taking up the chance for participation is taken as a measure.

Participants have expressed their enjoyment of the activities and the way the group has been facilitated to enable them to take part. Over the course the regular writing hands took on a more facilitative approach, leading less and giving the participants they were working with time to develop their material more. By the fifth session more of the participants were writing their own material rather than relying on the writing hands, and people who had allowed others to read their work for them were choosing to read themselves.

The individual participants showed signs of personal development in areas such as increased confidence and capacity for expression. No baseline was taken for this, but one measure might be the increasing degree of spontaneity in group discussion during the sessions. This was very evident from around the fifth meeting, during which participants were reminded that they had not settled on a name for the group. By this point participants were beginning to take more responsibility in maintaining the continuity of the group, proposing suggestions through the business part of the meeting, taking part in a convoluted voting process, and reminding the session leader to check what the group wanted to do in the following session.

Individual participants continued to express an interest in the process and the outcomes, often asking about the progress on behalf of the whole group. This reveals not only their assertiveness, but a confidence that their rights and requests will be recognized by the supporters. Participants were concerned that their group would not be used as a vehicle by other people, yet so far some of the experiences the group has had – for example with the press statements from the local council – suggest that the writing it has produced and the achievements of the group have still to be recognized as meaningful outside the group itself. The group's success has increased demand for the activity and there are new people wanting to join. The impact of this, however, has been minimal in terms of realizing external support for the group, who continue to meet and write using resources provided by one of the volunteers in lieu of proper funding. The group will require continued support from day center staff and a local writing workshop to do this, although eventually some of the people it currently facilitates, or perhaps some amongst those who join it later, may take a larger part in convening it, or acting as writing hands, just as has been modeled by some of the supporters from Pecket Well College.

A key initiating factor in the project was the activism of the FWWCP in seeking out potential new members. Occupational therapists seeking to develop similar projects need to work collaboratively, something which the Department of Health's paper *Valuing People*[57] has suggested. This may require finding the means outside existing service arrangements, and in the process, as happened with this project, giving the lead to people with experience of disabling conditions in order to bring out the group's full occupational potential. This does not mean that occupational therapy is superseded; instead, it is enabled, as part of a collaboration which strengthens the doing, being, and becoming of everyone involved. As we have noted, occupational therapy approaches such as COPPM[45] can complement and dovetail in with those needs-centered strategies which have been devised by other participant actors, enabling them to assist in project development through the identification of outcomes and occupational spin-offs. Occupational therapists need to recognize connections between approaches that have arisen from marginalized groups in answer to their own needs, and are here applied to others, and the tools that have been devised for clinical settings, and exchange practice in order to enhance the resources of the communities in which they share.

It seems appropriate to re-emphasize the words of Sean Taylor[37] reflecting on working with the group of adult writers with learning difficulties known as the Chatshow Writers: 'To be adept at making your own rules and making your own shapes with writing, and to be able to make something of a blank page – that is to start shining yourself.' However, a group like this requires continued input to see how far it can develop. The Voices Talk and Hands Write group and its supporters are on a learning process of finding out where local sources of financial and practical help reside.

Acknowledgements

Thanks are due to the following: June Baxendale, Matthew Blastard, Mandy Carpenter, Vicky Caster, Claire Clayton, Natalie Davidson, Tim Diggles, Helen Elige, Jayne Fletcher, Sally Fox, Gary Gant, Iris Garrity, Trevor George, Michael Hardaker, Brian Haughie, Amanda Ives, Ellen

Jebsen, Elaine Johnson, Kenny Money, Corinna Mundy, Sandra O'Brien, Trevor Parkinson, Iris Reeder, Diane Robinson, Heather Seward, John Smart, Kim Stowe, Erica Turner, Lauren Viszniewski, Keith Watson, Jim White, Maggie Winsnip.

References

1. Milsom S, Gadd D. My new glasses: an anthology of poetry by children with learning difficulties. Hebden Bridge: Alice Publications; 1990.
2. Taylor S, ed. Cheese and chips are related to the moon. London: Eastside Books; 1991.
3. Fullman J, ed. Flower from Brazil. London: Eastside Books; 1996.
4. The Thursday Club. Our lives our group. Sheffield: The Thursday Club; 2002.
5. Mason M. Incurably human. London: wORking Press; 2002.
6. Lewis JJ. Signs of protest. In: Ott G, ed. No restraints. An anthology of disability and culture in Philadelphia. Philadelphia: New City Press; 2002:47–57.
7. Johnson K. Deinstitutionalising women. Cambridge: Cambridge University Press; 1998.
8. Pollard N. Creative writing and publishing with enduring mental health clients. Work based learning project towards MSc in Occupational Therapy. Sheffield Hallam University, College of Occupational Therapists Library; 2001.
9. Harthill G, Low J, Moran S, et al. A case study: the Kingfisher Project. In: Sampson F, ed. Creative writing in health and social care. London: Jessica Kingsley Publishers; 2004:92–116.
10. Smith A, Burgieres M. National jamboree '96 report. London: Survivors' Press; 1996.
11. Sampson F. The healing word: a practical guide to poetry and personal development activities. Milton Keynes: The Poetry Society; 1999.
12. Lorenzo T, Saunders L, January M, Mdlokolo P. On the road of hope: stories told by disabled women in Khayelitsha. Cape Town: Disabled People South Africa, Zanepilo Disability Project, University of Cape Town; 2002.
13. Lorenzo T. No African renaissance without disabled women: a communal approach to human development in Cape Town, South Africa. Disability and Society 2003; 18(6):759–778.
14. Lorenzo T. Equalizing opportunities for occupational engagement: disabled women's stories. In: Watson R, Swartz L, eds. Transformation through occupation. London: Whurr; 2004:85–102.
15. Pollard N, Bryer M. Community publishing and rehabilitation: stories of ordinary lives. RED Journal 2002; Winter:6–10.
16. Pollard N, Krónenberg F, Simó Algado S. Community-based rehabilitation – a role for worker writers and community publishers. Federation 2004; 27:12–14.
17. Pollard N. Notes towards a therapeutic use for creative writing in occupational therapy. In: Sampson F, ed. Creative writing in health and social care. London: Jessica Kingsley Publishers; 2004: 189–206.
18. Willinsky J. The new literacy: redefining reading and writing in the schools. New York: Routledge; 1990.
19. Taylor P. The texts of Paulo Friere. Buckingham: Open University Press; 1993.
20. Morley D, Worpole K, eds. The republic of letters: working class writing and local publishing. London: Comedia/MPG; 1982.
21. Worpole K. Reading by numbers: contemporary publishing and popular fiction. London: Comedia/MPG; 1984.
22. Thompson P. The voice of the past. Oxford: Oxford University Press; 1988.
23. Bornat J. Oral history as a social movement. Oral History 1989; 17(2):16–20.
24. Shohet L. Community writing, connecting literacy and the literary. Federation 2000; 19:18–19.
25. Pollard N. DIY publishing – part 1. Federation Magazine 2003; 26:27–30.
26. Pollard N. DIY publishing – part 2. Federation Magazine 2004; 27:28–29.
27. Pollard N. DIY publishing – part 3. Federation Magazine; 28:27–30.
28. Mace J. Introduction. In: Mace J, ed. Literacy, language and community publishing: essays in adult education. Clevedon: Multilingual Matters; 1995: ix–xx.
29. Jones L. Good writing – powerful writing. In: Griffiths S, Jones L, Mackrell K, et al, eds. From circle to spiral. Brighton: QueenSpark; 1995:4–9.
30. Philips D, Linington L, Penman D. Writing well: creative writing and mental health. London: Jessica Kingsley Publishers; 1999.

31. Courtman S. Frierian liberation, cultural transaction and writing from 'the working class and the spades'. The Society for Caribbean Studies annual conference papers. 2000. Online. Available: http://www.scsonline.freeserve.co.uk/olv1p6.pdf 28 March 2004.

32. Harris R. Disappearing language: fragments and fractures between speech and writing. In: Mace J, ed. Literacy, language and community publishing: essays in adult education. Clevedon: Multilingual Matters; 1995:118–144.

33. Fitzpatrick S. Sailing out from safe harbors: writing for publication in adult basic education. In: Mace J, ed. Literacy, language and community publishing: essays in adult education. Clevedon: Multilingual Matters; 1995:1–22.

34. Bolton G. The therapeutic potential of creative writing: writing myself. London: Jessica Kingsley Publishers; 1999.

35. McDowell A. Creative writing: how it is viewed by adults with learning disabilities. British Journal of Therapy and Rehabilitation 1998; 5(9):465–467.

36. Sampson F. 'Men wearing pyjamas'; using creative writing with people with learning disabilities. In: Hunt C, Sampson F, eds. The self on the page: theory and practice of creative writing in personal development. London: Jessica Kingsley Publishers; 1998:63–77.

37. Taylor S. Improving on the blank page. In: Mace J, ed. Literacy, language and community publishing: essays in adult education. Clevedon: Multilingual Matters; 1995.

38. Hammersley M. The politics of social research. London: Sage; 1995.

39. Marshall C, Rossman GB. Designing qualitative research, 3rd ed. Thousand Oaks: Sage; 1999.

40. Letts L. Occupational therapy and participatory research: a partnership worth pursuing. American Journal of Occupational Therapy 2003; 57(1):77–87.

41. Stanfield JH. Ethnic modelling in qualitative research. In: Denzin NK, Lincoln YS, eds. The landscape of qualitative research. Thousand Oaks: Sage; 1998:333–358.

42. Beazley S, Moore M, Benzie D. Involving disabled people in research. In: Barnes C, Mercer G. Doing disability research. Leeds: The Disability Press; 1997.

43. Olesen V. Feminisms and models of qualitative research. In: Denzin NK, Lincoln YS, eds. The landscape of qualitative research. Thousand Oaks: Sage; 1998:300–332.

44. Mies M. Towards a methodology for feminist research. In: Hammersley M, ed. Social research: philosophy, politics and practice. London: Sage; 1993:64–82.

45. Fearing VC, Law M, Clark J. An occupational performance process model: fostering client and therapist alliances. Can J Occup Ther 1997; 64(1):7–15.

46. Rebeiro K. Occupational spin-off. Occupational therapy interactive dialogue. Journal of Occupational Science 2001; 8(1):33–34.

47. Turner E. Walking talking doll. In: Turner E. Voices Talk and Hands Write group. Pecket Well, UK: FWWCP & Pecket Well College; 2004.

48. Garrity I. What I'd do, what I'd really, really do. In: Garrity I. Voices Talk and Hands Write group. Pecket Well, UK: FWWCP & Pecket Well College; 2004.

49. Fox S. Green door. In: Fox S. Voices Talk and Hands Write group. Pecket Well, UK: FWWCP & Pecket Well College; 2004.

50. Stowe K. A mum. In: Stowe K. Voices Talk and Hands Write group. Pecket Well, UK: FWWCP & Pecket Well College; 2004.

51. Blastard M. Big roast dinner. In: Blastard M. Voices Talk and Hands Write group. Pecket Well, UK: FWWCP & Pecket Well College; 2004.

52. George T. My ideal Christmas. In: George T. Voices Talk and Hands Write group. Pecket Well, UK: FWWCP & Pecket Well College; 2004.

53. Blastard M. for Christmas Time. In: Blastard M. Voices Talk and Hands Write group. Pecket Well, UK: FWWCP & Pecket Well College; 2004.

54. Turner E. What would I really like for Christmas. In: Turner E. Voices Talk and Hands Write group. Pecket Well, UK: FWWCP & Pecket Well College; 2004.

55. Watson K. Sort Christmas Day out on my own. In: Watson K. Voices Talk and Hands Write group. Pecket Well, UK: FWWCP & Pecket Well College; 2004.

56. White J. Grimsby project update. Federation Magazine 28:28.

57. Department of Health. Valuing people: a new strategy for learning disability in the 21st century. London: HMSO; 2001.

Chapter 22

Transcending practice borders through perspective transformation

Reg Urbanowski

With contributions from Hank Brewer, Heather Ivany, Kerry Hicks, Sandra Groves, Brittney Groves and Nancy Rushford

OVERVIEW

The purpose of this chapter is to describe the process of meaning and worldview transformation that people undergo when faced with the new realities imposed by a life-changing event. It is concerned with the transformations that occur when occupational therapists are able to shed the blinders associated with systemic barriers and understand the contexts in which their clients are situated. This chapter also highlights the transformative processes that some marginalized people undergo and the way the relationship between a person and an occupational therapist affects the occupational therapist. These transformative processes are concerned with changes in worldview and subsequent changes in the meaning of occupations in daily life.[1,2] The term transformation is taken from the literature on transformative learning developed by Mezirow.[3] Contributors to this chapter have provided glimpses of their worldviews. By understanding the interplay between meaning and worldview transformation in the people occupational therapists work with, therapists will be better able to meet the needs of people by transcending borders imposed by the very systems they work in. This chapter describes Canadian experiences, but it may well apply to occupational therapists working with people across other political, cultural, and national borders.

ESSENTIAL CONCEPTS

All theory, dear friend, is grey; but the precious tree of life is green.[4]

The effective strength of a model lies in its ability to enhance the capacity of the occupational therapist to meet the needs of the people served, therefore it is vital that models identify the systemic barriers that prevent people from attaining a meaningful life premised on notions of positive health. Being able to practice without borders means being able to understand and act on the marginalization forces that affect occupational therapy service recipients. The road to understanding their marginalization is littered with discarded models as well as those which impose a hegemonic pattern of conditioning in the minds of occupational therapists. For that reason no particular model will be utilized in this chapter.

A collection of concepts from occupational therapy (occupational justice, occupational apartheid, spirituality, enablement) and social science (empowerment, meaning, marginalization) will be used to develop the discussion in this chapter. Leaving the concepts free from the entanglements of a particular model will enable readers to socially construct relationships between the concepts in a way that pertains to their situated context.

Marginalization refers to the pushing of people to the periphery of society.[5] People on the margins of society are not accorded the rights and privileges of people in the mainstream. The concept of *occupational apartheid* (see Ch. 6) refers to chronic (established) environmental conditions that deny marginalized people access to rightful, meaningful occupations, thus jeopardizing their health and wellbeing. This concept defines health and wellbeing as fundamental human rights in accessing meaningful occupations.[6] The environmental conditions may include the organization and delivery of occupational services. For example, the creation of specific access and exit criteria may be forms of occupational apartheid. The necessity of a physician prescription to access occupational therapy services may exclude people from these services, because physicians may lack awareness of what occupational therapy is and/or the value that it has. Even more insidious, and potentially more damaging, is when occupational therapists negate, deny, or refute the implication of systemic barriers in the daily lives of those they serve. In these instances, the occupational therapist acts as a marginalizing agent rather than an agent of enlightenment, enablement, or empowerment. For example, a woman in chronic poverty may be assigned characteristics associated with lack of training, lack of life skills, poor motivation, or a host of psychosocial factors that prevent her from accessing employment. This form of prejudice may preclude the occupational therapist from understanding that there may be systemic barriers preventing this person from accessing suitable employment. Lack of adequate day care or lack of substantial financial support to prevent the person from slipping into chronic poverty may all play a part. In order to be able to practice without borders the therapist must become aware of the forces of marginalization and must also be involved in advocacy and activism at an individual and social level.

A current definition of *occupational justice* (see Ch. 9) refers to the rights, responsibilities, and liberties of enablement.[7] *Enablement* is providing a person with the means to develop and maintain an occupational life trajectory premised on attaining a state of wellbeing. A definition of occupational justice includes the notion of empowerment. As a process, *empowerment* is the devolution of power from the occupational therapist to the person served. This transfer of power supports the development of an occupational life trajectory based on what is meaningful for the person.[8] Enablement is based on point-in-time needs. In the case of occupational therapy practice it involves, for example, providing devices, retraining programs, or art mediums for self-reflection. Enablement requires that we see people as they appear before us. Empowerment, on the other hand, goes further into the future and moves beyond mundane daily life. It is premised on building an occupational life trajectory that is based on the construction and experience of meaning in everyday life.[9] *Meaning* is defined as the interpretation of experience and actions according to a value system that has been internalized by the person and/or imposed by the social context in which that person is imbedded.[1,10] Empowerment helps people build meaningful lives within the context of their situation. *Spirituality* pertains to the experience of meaning in life in everyday occupations.[1,11] It is through experience that meaning is constructed.

Abrupt changes in everyday life may be imposed either by design or circumstance.[1,3] In these instances, the transformation of spirituality (as experienced meaning) is often substantial and pervasive. This transformation involves a worldview as well as goal orientations.[2] What people do, how they do it, and why they do it may become affected. What makes the change profound is the spiritual transformation that accompanies these abrupt changes in occupational lives. There are also changes in the worldview. To understand spiritual transformation, as the gestalt of meaning and occupational transformations, it is necessary to move beyond a conventional point-in-time and point-in-place perspective called the here and now. Therapists must also move toward what will be, what could be, and what should be in the everyday life of the person concerned.[1]

PERSONAL ACCOUNTS

This section offers personal accounts provided by people who have been marginalized or who are at risk of being marginalized, and by occupational therapy students and occupational therapists. They represent personal transformations that occur when client and therapist interact.

Homelessness

Hank Brewer, who describes his situation below, was successful for many years in his employment and had a good social support network. Through a variety of misfortunes he ended up homeless. Two occupational therapy students, who met Hank through a fieldwork placement under the author's supervision, provide a joint personal account of the impact that Hank had on them. Both accounts offer personal perspectives of worldview and meaning schemes.

Hank's account: survival and homelessness

When we hear the word survivor, what do we think of? Someone shipwrecked on a deserted island, a person lost in the wilderness, or a castaway in a lifeboat. All these people have one thing in common, they will do anything they can in order to survive. And if or when they are rescued, we admire their strength and courage.

However, each day in all large cities in this country, we pass survivors of equal courage who fight hard to find food and shelter. But, is the will to survive any stronger in a person who kills a rodent in the wild in order to eat than in a person who shakes the ants and flies off a half eaten donut in a dumpster so he can eat? If you have not tried it, you do not know the courage it takes to ask a total stranger for spare change. In the next few paragraphs I will attempt to tell you my story of survival.

Over the space of just a few days, I had my truck and my tools taken. I was then unable to continue working and in only a few days my life was completely turned upside down. Unable to attain another truck and tools, I was forced out of work and had no income. It was then that my struggle to survive truly started. And I found courage to do what needed to be done to exist. For 2 months, I slept outside in good or bad weather and lived on handouts from friends and strangers.

Yes, there were social safety nets available to me. But, unlike the person lost in the wilderness who will rush to meet his rescuers, people on the streets will often for matters of pride, or whatever, run away from help. However, in my case, I finally realized that pride did not put food in my mouth, nor clothes on my back. And, I allowed people who became my friends and cared about me to help me, and with this continuing help I will turn my life around and walk again with purpose.

The stories of the people who survive the streets and those who work to help them would fill many pages. But I hope that this will give people some idea of what homeless people go through. And, the next time you pass one on the streets, realize that he or she is using every ounce of courage that he or she has – just to survive.

The Lonely Streets

You may think that I'm an old man
As I walk with shoulders bent
But I once had a young man's dreams
Now I wonder where they went

I once had a home and family
But choices forced them away
Now lonely days and tear filled nights
Is the way I have to pay

The city it is crowded
But we walk the streets alone
It seems that you're invisible
If you don't have a home

Now thanks to people out there
Who have shared my despair
I have a beautiful place to live
And friends who really care

I've been down and out
Despair staked its claim
But like phoenix from the ashes
I shall rise again.

– by Hank Brewer

Students' account   Heather Ivany and Kerry Hicks, occupational therapy students at Dalhousie University, saw the tremendous importance of learning to practice without borders when they learned to 'be' with Hank. That experience provided the seed for learning: 'Learning nourishes the seed but gives it no seed of its own.' [12]

Part of their fieldwork experience included meeting people at a drop-in coffee shop operated by a local not-for-profit housing agency. There they met Hank and began to work with him. This meant helping him to secure resources for himself and advocating on his behalf to other health and social service agencies. Here is their account of their work with Hank.

> A man who was once homeless wrote a poem today which talks about how his new friends helped him to see more hope in his life; he was referring to us. The occupation of writing is extremely meaningful to our client and it provides him with the opportunity and means to express his feelings and emotions. When we work with individuals such as this man it makes us proud to be in the field we are in. We really feel we are enabling change in his life and he has clearly communicated that back to us. When considering one of our favorite enabling principles, instilling hope, we strongly believe that we have done this effectively in this man's life. The poem's words are from a man who was without hope and someone rekindled that hope for him. He feels it was us. We helped him to believe in himself and also believe that he has a meaningful future ahead of him. We can learn so much from people that have struggled and fought for their basic needs – their mere survival. For us we can only imagine what that must be like. It is like taking empathy to a new level.

Reflections   It is important to move away from the tendency to see Hank as a 'case', and instead to see his account and poem as providing a brief glimpse of his worldview and the meaning perspective in his everyday life on the street. We can also see the students' account as providing a transformed perspective of meaning wherein they moved from seeing Hank as marginalized to seeing him as a person who could empower himself. The meaning of that experience can be captured in the following words from Tennyson:[13]

> *A still small voice spoke unto me,*
> *'thou art so full of misery,*
> *were it not better not to be?'*
> *Then to the still small voice I said:*
> *'let me not cast in endless shade*
> *what is so wonderfully made.'*

Hank taught the students about hope, and woven into the notion of hope is the desire to lead a life that is built on meaning that can be constructed.

Meaning that can be experienced is the essence of spirituality.[1,11] He taught the notion of survival, defined by him as the meeting of basic biological and spiritual needs. The words of both his account and his poem suggest that survival is more than food, clothing, and shelter. He taught the students about the systemic barriers, such as access requirements to social assistance policies and affordable housing programs, that keep people from constructing and/or experiencing a meaningful life trajectory. Perhaps most important of all he taught the 'meaning' of survival. Simply, this means engaging in the day-to-day occupations that permit one to survive biologically. At a deeper level, it means engaging in occupations (such as writing) that serve to provide meaning that can be experienced. In other words, the students saw and touched the spirit of a survivor. They learned that holding onto the possibility of an occupational life trajectory (i.e. hoping) was pivotal to survival. Survival is not merely biological; it is spiritual. In seeing 'what is so wonderfully made',[13] in Tennyson's words, they were also able to see and experience those forces, including policies in the social service system, stigmatization of homeless people, and policies in the healthcare system, that kept their teacher from realizing his occupational life trajectory and hindered Hank from being who he wanted to be. In other words, they learned about occupational apartheid and some of the barriers that society erects to keep people in place at the margins of society. When the students talked about Hank's ability to transcend his homelessness with the help of friends and colleagues, they learned about occupational justice and discovered that there are forces which they could engage to combat those systemic barriers. Even more important than providing support and believing in him was helping their teacher to break down the barriers. It was about activism and advocacy, which included working with Hank to attain appropriate financial assistance, and helping him to find affordable housing, and access appropriate health services.

All were involved in a mutual transformation of meaning. Hank began to believe that it was possible to transcend the barriers that society had erected. The students believed that they could make a difference, and that in order to do so they had to engage with their teacher in a way that made it possible to dismantle barriers and recreate a meaningful life. After their engagement, all those involved had transformed their understanding of what it meant to be a homeless person and what it meant to be an occupational therapy student.

Living with Alzheimer's disease

In the accounts below Sandra Groves, whose husband has Alzheimer's disease, discusses the initial service that was provided for her by the healthcare team, which included occupational therapists, and her daughter Brittney, aged 12 years, discusses her own experience of 'being' with her dad. Their accounts should be read not as 'cases', but with the notion of uncovering how Sandra's and Brittney's worldviews and meaning perspectives changed not only because of Alzheimer's disease in the family, but also because of the services provided and the everyday occupations in which they now engage.

Sandra's story

The healthcare providers were caring in their dealings with us but at that time the thought was on what was best for my husband alone, not realizing the impact on Brittney and myself. Brittney was told she had to move out of her room so that her Dad could have it because it was in a straight line from the hallway. They decided she should take our old room and that the room down the hall would be a good spot for me because I would be able to keep a better watch if he got up at night; it was between his bedroom and the front entrance. There are enough changes to the family dynamics when a person develops Alzheimer's without the home being turned into an institution-like setting. Things like handicap bars, shower seats, mates taking on the responsibilities that their partners can no longer handle on top of their own responsibilities are one thing; but being separated from each other in your own home, not by choice, is really hard to get used to when you've slept in the same room together for all the years of your marriage through the good and bad times. Alzheimer's takes away a lot from a family but Brittney and I work very hard to make our lives as normal as possible under the circumstances for all of us. Unrealistic? Not really. Reality is that we are a family first and Alzheimer's is an intruder that has to be dealt with as best as we can without losing that closeness any sooner than we have to.

Brittney's story

My Dad is in later stages of mid-stage Alzheimer's. I have watched him go from the guy who taught me to ride my bike, fish, took me to car, recreation vehicle (RV), and boat shows, to someone who can't drive anymore, who has to use a wheelchair to go fishing, or attend car, RV or boat shows. He spends his days doing kiddy puzzles and telling the same stories many times over. He's my Daddy, even though the Alzheimer's is slowly taking him away from me, I'll love him no matter what.

They say miracles come in small packages but they can come in big ones too. My Dad is big and if he hadn't developed Alzheimer's I wouldn't have met so many nice people, or learned that I can do things that people don't think I can do, like using power tools when my Mom and I built a fence for our side yard and a wheelchair turn-around addition to our front deck this summer so we could still have BBQ's with Dad, which we like doing. This taught me that I can find a way to do things if I set my mind to it; I've learned to accept that my Dad isn't going to get any better and there's nothing that will help him and that what I used to do with him I now do with the other people in my life. Even though it is hard to live with Alzheimer's in the house there can be something good come from it also.

An occupational therapist sees occupational therapy as a marginalizing agent

Nancy Rushford, an occupational therapist, suggests that occupational therapists are people who have histories that impact on their practice. Nancy's Jungian connection to her past illustrates very clearly that occupational therapists have a horizon that stretches back into their early years. In reading her account the reader should perhaps take note that practice without borders may suggest that the borders therapists need to transcend stretch far back into their own historical horizons. Furthermore, until those borders are recognized and dealt with, the marginalizing influence that therapists have on people remains an invisible force acting against the client.

Nancy's account

Some dreams lie etched in the back of the mind as if awaiting opportunity to be realized. I was 11 years old when a vivid dream impressed upon me an injustice that I was too young to comprehend, but would later realize represented marginalization; its pattern of injustice would weave into the narratives of the people whom I would meet during my first role in rehabilitation. Their stories now guide me, orienting me early in my career as an occupational therapist toward the sociopolitical dimension of rehabilitation and the potential for the profession of occupational therapy to promote social justice.

The Dream

I am aware that I am part of a scene unfolding, yet I have no real form. I am floating within a magnificent park replete with flower gardens and enormous trees. A narrow river divides the park. In the center of the river lies a beautiful stone bridge that permits crossing. The bridge is cradled on either side by two bushes. I am mesmerized by this bridge and find myself unable to turn away.

As if out of nowhere, a young man appears on the scene. I watch as he slowly and deliberately makes his way across the bridge. His left leg drags behind him awkwardly and his foot scrapes painfully against the stone with each laborious step.

The man is too slow and is not welcomed on the other side of the bridge. Instinctively I know that something terrible is about to happen and I am helpless to stop it. Suddenly, a hand reaches out from behind the bush and snatches the man from his position on the bridge. He disappears. I am chilled by an eerie sense of stillness. It is as if the crime never took place but failed to erase from my memory. I can feel myself getting heavier beneath the weight of this apparent injustice. I awaken suddenly, and as if to purge myself of its burden, I record the dream, immediately allowing myself to forget it.

The memory of this dream was sparked years later when I acquired my first job in rehabilitation which involved providing support to parents who had sustained an acquired brain injury (ABI). It was one of the few programs in the province of Ontario that attempted to address the needs of parents with an ABI *and* their children. Having suddenly lost their 'position' in life following traumatic injury, these parents found themselves struggling to meet the challenges of everyday life with few and fragmented supports. Many felt as if they had been relegated to the margins of society with unfair consequences not only for themselves but for their spouses and their children. These Canadian families had an important story to tell and resilience to reveal. Their words unexpectedly formed the narrative to my dream and brought it sudden clarity and present meaning.

I now see the dream as a metaphor for the experience of too many people in Canada with too few supports to gain or regain meaningful occupation in all facets of Canadian life. As an occupational therapist I am in frequent contact with people facing illness, injury, and disability. It is my belief that with that role comes a unique responsibility not only to bear witness to acts of injustice inflicted by society, but to respond wholeheartedly with efforts to equalize opportunities to participate in Canadian life. Some dreams lie etched in the back of the mind awaiting opportunity to be realized. This is my dream and I believe it needs to be realized.

The author's perspective transformation

Next I have chosen to share something that was experienced early in my own career because I believe that it demonstrates the notion of an occupational life trajectory and that sometimes these trajectories are not oriented toward self-actualization, but toward survival. It also demonstrates the impact it had on me, my worldview, and my meaning perspective. In reading this account, the reader should focus on the transformation of the therapist rather than on the person who triggered it. That transformation, for me, can be summed up in the following quote: 'How small is the life of the person who places his hands between his face and the world, seeing naught but the narrow lines of his hands.' [12]

We are all transformed by meaningful life-changing events that occur in the course of our lives. One of the most profound experiences for me as a therapist began when I was in the first year of my occupational therapy training. I was volunteering at a children's hospital where I met a young boy who was in psychiatric care for a variety of behaviors. I finished my volunteer work and continued my studies. Toward the end of my training I had a fieldwork placement in a juvenile detention center for young offenders where much to my surprise, I encountered that same young boy, now older, now in trouble with the law. I remember the feeling of astonishment and dismay when I saw him there; not at his behavior, but the fact that the system had let him down. Later, I graduated and moved on to other parts of Canada to practice. About 12 years later I moved back to the city where I had attended university and was involved with an inner city agency for homeless people. One day I noticed a young man who seemed vaguely familiar in his appearance. He recognized me and I remember his words to me as he approached me: 'Bet you never thought you would see me here.' It was the young boy from the hospital – the adolescent in the delinquency center. He sat down and told me his life story from the point of his residency at the delinquency center to the point where he was that day – alone and homeless on the streets of the city. I don't know what has happened to him since then.

All these years later I remember him. He proved to be an invaluable teacher for me. He taught me that people live life on a path; that the path is not always built on moving toward self-actualization, as motivation theory would have it. Sometimes life is built on surviving, when the environment is hostile and the safety net that the social system provides actually keeps you in the margins of society.

He taught me how the world was from his vantage point. I learned from him that the system not only fails people, it marginalizes people. It pushes them to the edge and keeps them there. I also learned about myself as a therapist. Reliance on clinical knowledge had kept me from seeing people's realities. The notion of what it meant to be a professional, and what was appropriate professional behavior, kept me from experiencing the meaning of those realities. Furthermore, both of these together prevented me from sharing in someone's spirituality, i.e. experiencing the meaning of another person's occupational life. I learned that people do live their lives first to survive and then to thrive. I learned that I, as an occupational therapist, had perhaps used models, concepts, theories, procedures, and documentation to create distance between the spiritual needs of the people I worked with and myself. I learned to value the meaning of helping people to reorganize their lives on a trajectory rather than simply seeing them as point-in-time clients. In other words, I realized that the people I see in the clinic are much more than people I see at particular points in their lives.

CONCLUSION

And yet how simple it is: in one day, in one hour everything could be arranged at once! The chief thing is to love others like yourself, that's the chief thing, and that's everything; nothing else is wanted – you will find out at once how to arrange it all. And yet it's an old truth which has been told and retold a billion times – but it has not formed part of our lives! The consciousness of life is higher than life, the knowledge of the laws of happiness is higher than happiness – that is what one must contend against.[14]

Wisdom occurs when knowledge and experience are merged together. The ability to fuse the ethical and spiritual dimensions together with the models, concepts, and interventions of the occupational therapy profession is the basis for practical wisdom. Practical wisdom is the ability to select appropriate actions that take into account the widest possible range of factors and their consequences for the situated person the occupational therapist is serving.[15] It is through practical wisdom that occupational therapists can enlighten and enable clients so that they may empower themselves in the contexts of their own lives. It is through practical wisdom that occupational therapists can uphold the dignity of the individual.

When therapists abandon practical wisdom they amplify the marginalizing forces acting against their clients. Forces such as policies and professional roles are imbedded in the systems in which occupational therapists work. Other forces, such as stigma, and reasoning based solely on pathology, are situated in the experiences of therapists as they engage with clients and their contexts. It is in these latter cases that forces can be transcended when practice is without borders – borders imposed by therapists' historical horizons and their reliance on professional knowledge. When we rely solely on models, concepts, and intervention strategies we negate the dignity of the individual. According to Garrett, Baillie and Garrett:[15]

> … *dignity resides not merely in the capacity for pleasure nor in the ability to make free choices but in the capacity for human interaction, friendship, family relations, and for the most broadly based social life as well as for union with the whole of reality … the individual person is not an abstraction that can be labelled simply as 'an autonomous being' or 'bearer of rights', but is a concrete individual whose life involves shared life in a particular community and sharing in some specific set of habitual social roles in that community. Thus, the individual and society are not opposed concepts.*

To embrace practical wisdom as a necessary tool of practice puts the therapist beyond models of practice and forms of intervention. To embrace practical wisdom is to embrace the humanity of occupational therapy the way it was envisioned by the pioneers of the profession.[16] Practical wisdom allows us to transcend our personal and professional borders and understand the spirituality of survival that many of our clients and their loved ones strive to create and recreate every day. Occupational therapy premised on the application of practical wisdom can be summed up in the following words adapted by Thibeault[17] from Anne Lang-Etienne: 'Occupational therapy reveals not only reality in its concrete form, but also one's inner world and its many facets. And this world, if we know how to decipher it, touches the very core of being, the meaning [in] life, and all that is essential.'

References

1. Urbanowski R. Spirituality in changed occupational lives. In: McColl MA, ed. Spirituality and occupational therapy. Ottawa: Canadian Association of Occupational Therapists; 2003:95–114.
2. Taylor E. The theory and practice of transformative learning. (Information Series No. 374). Columbus, OH: ERIC Clearinghouse on Adult, Career, and Vocational Education; 1998.
3. Mezirow J. Perspective transformation. Adult Education 1978; 28(2):100–110.
4. Goethe J. Faust. Toronto: University of Toronto Press; 1970.
5. Allahar A. Sociology and the periphery: theories and issues. Toronto: Garamond Press; 1989.
6. Kronenberg F. Street children: being and becoming. Research report. Heerlen, The Netherlands: Hogeschool Limburg; 1999.
7. Townsend E, Wilcock A. Occupational justice. In: Christiansen C, Townsend E, eds. Introduction to occupation: the art and science of living. Upper Saddle River, NJ: Prentice Hall; 2003:243–273.
8. Freire P. Cultural action for freedom: part II. Harvard Educational Review 1970; 40(3):452–477.
9. Etting D, Hayes N. Learning to learn: women creating learning communities. Re-vision 1997; (20):28–30.
10. Canadian Association of Occupational Therapists. Enabling occupation: an occupational therapy perspective. Ottawa: CAOT Publications; 1997.
11. Urbanowski R, Vargo J. Spirituality, daily practice, and the occupational performance model. Can J Occup Ther 1994; 61(2):88–94.
12. Gibran K. The treasured writings of Kahlil Gibran. Edison, NJ: Castle Books; 1975.
13. Tennyson A. Two voices. Online. Available: http://tennysonpoetry.home.att.net/tva.htm 14 Jan 2004.
14. Dostoevsky F, transl Garnett C. The dream of a ridiculous man. Online. Available: http://perso.wanadoo.fr/chabrieres/texts/ridiculousman.html 14 Jan 2004.
15. Garrett T, Baillie H, Garrett R. Health care ethics: principles and problems. Englewood Cliffs, NJ: Prentice Hall; 1989.
16. Punwar A, Peloquin S. Occupational therapy: principles and practice. 3rd edn. Philadelphia: Lippincott, Williams & Wilkins; 2000.
17. Thibeault R. In praise of dissidence: Anne Lang-Etienne. Can J Occup Ther 2002; 4(69):197–203.

Chapter **23**

Unlocking spirituality
Play as a health-promoting occupation in the context of HIV/AIDS

Elelwani L. Ramugondo

OVERVIEW

The information in this chapter is intended to help the reader:

- begin to understand the psychosocial issues linked with mothering a child with HIV/AIDS and how mothering an HIV-positive child brings forth existential questions on the meaning of life and dealing with death and dying, paying particular attention to the role of the context;

- explore the role of play as part of occupational therapy intervention with children living with HIV/AIDS;

- begin to appreciate how much involvement with any marginalized community requires true engagement, which often means exploring how much the professional persona can either facilitate or hinder the use of self as a therapeutic tool; and

- appreciate the resilience and spirituality that can be demonstrated by children and mothers living with HIV/AIDS.

INTRODUCTION

The growing incidence of HIV/AIDS in children as a cause of morbidity in the pediatric population is a major health concern.[1-6] Since the first cases of HIV infection in children were reported in the late 1980s, the numbers have risen throughout the world.[7] In South Africa, in 2002, the prevalence rate was estimated at 40% among rural mothers, with 6% of their children infected.[8] Advances in anti-retroviral therapy, prophylaxis to prevent opportunistic infections and treatment of these, and aggressive nutritional intervention, allow for prolonged survival for infected children.[9] This has led to quality of life emerging as a crucial outcome of care.

Literature suggests that challenges confronting families with an HIV-infected member and their coping strategies, even though similar in some ways to those faced by families with other chronic diseases, are in many ways also different.[10-12] These families are particularly vulnerable because of the high probability of the infection coexisting in both the parent and the child. Looking after a number of sick family members, coping with multiple family deaths from AIDS, and managing stigma and its consequences have been identified as consistent stressors.[12,13] The families also often live amidst extreme poverty and poor social conditions.[12-15]

For the child, the physical challenges of carrying the illness are immense. Common complications include lymphadenopathy, failure to thrive, hepatomegaly, respiratory distress, bacterial pneumonias, cardiomyopathy, and neurodevelopmental abnormalities.[16] These inevitably lead to decreased mobility and lack of motivation in the child. There may be little inclination to interact with the environment. For the caregiver of a child with HIV/AIDS, the interaction with the child may be restrained or overprotective, impacting more on the child's major occupational engagement, play.

With their voices mostly absent on the experience of living with HIV/AIDS, children's needs have often been adult-identified. Food, shelter, freedom from pain and sometimes education, are often what caregivers and policy-makers deem paramount.[17,18] It would be interesting to see what children, if asked directly, would indicate to be their priority needs. A high employment status has been found to correlate with better quality of life for adults living with HIV/AIDS.[19] This may be due to inherent qualities in work that allow for continued exercising of competence, social status and possibility for social interactions. It may not be surprising if children, also living with the illness, were to prioritize play and having a playmate over what adults deem paramount for them. In 2001 the author of this chapter initiated a project that attempted to explore the role of play in children living with HIV/AIDS in a number of informal settlements in Cape Town.

The children came from very poor living circumstances. Their caregivers were mostly their biological parents and were themselves living with HIV/AIDS. The caregivers were all women and had mostly been abandoned by their partners. Most of them had not disclosed their HIV-positive status to their relatives. Even fewer had discussed their HIV status with their children. Consequently, the children were unaware of their own status. The reason given for this was that discussing death with a child was taboo. It was clear from this response that for these women, living with HIV/AIDS was equated to death or dying. Secrecy around serious illness and the dying of children is said to be common in African cultures.[17]

This chapter reflects the lessons learnt when play, as valued by occupational therapists, was explored with these caregivers, who mostly lived in Nyanga, Crossroads, and Gugulethu. These are areas historically designated for black people in Cape Town. Although some parts have formal housing, others are characterized by shacks. These are structures that are erected using corrugated iron, wood, hardboard or plastic. Most of these materials are waste materials from factories, construction sites, or even dumps. It is not unusual to find a structure built from a combination of these materials. The legacy of apartheid in South Africa left black people limited access to land[20-26] and proper housing.

The living conditions of these women and the discrimination they face due to the legacy of apartheid and the social stigma attached to HIV/AIDS link very closely with two concepts that have emerged recently in occupational therapy: occupational injustice[27] and occupational apartheid.[28] The very confined spaces[23,25,26,29,30] these families are often made to live in severely restrict occupational engagement in a way that signifies the extent to which policy makers during the apartheid era failed to think of them as occupational beings. Limited education and the resulting limited access to gainful employment continue to deny them resources within which they can exercise choice.

Social stigma often creates barriers that prevent the families from participating in occupations that hold cultural meaning, or are appropriate. There are still instances when the children are not welcomed in crèches and preschools. This is in spite of legislation in the country prohibiting this. Sometimes parental fears restrict a child from being allowed to play with his or her peers. There are instances where a mother would stop her child from attending preschool to avoid explaining the child's frequent absenteeism due to recurrent medical complications and regular visits to the clinic. This, compounded by her own bouts of illness, may also restrict a mother from seeking a job or staying employed. There have also been accounts of churches discouraging HIV-positive individuals from attending services by linking HIV infection to sin.

There are many levels at which these individuals experience occupational injustice. Their human right to engage in occupations that could bring meaning into their lives and determine their quality of life[27] is continually denied by their immediate communities as well as being a result of a historical legacy. The fact that the injustice is selective in that it is determined by whether one carries HIV or not, or with regard to the legacy of apartheid, according to racial differences, makes occupational apartheid[28] a more apt description of the experiences of this population. Access to resources or to meaningful occupational engagement is reserved for others, but denied to those who, through no choice of their own, are deemed different and therefore less deserving, by people who hold power and are able to exercise it through multiple levels within societal, economic, or political systems. As occupational therapists, it is crucial that we are aware of the political nature of occupations, and how our practice may perpetuate discriminatory policies.

PLAY: RESEARCH AND INTERVENTION IN CONTEXT

The need to embark on the project arose in 1999 after the author had been working in an outpatients' clinic attached to a pediatric ward at Groote Schuur Hospital, Cape Town. Her role in the clinic was initially to provide ongoing assessment of the children's developmental milestones and input for the mothers on developmental stimulation of the children. This role evolved with time to include the encouragement of caregiver–child interaction and playfulness as a means through which the child can be enabled to engage with the environment. Understanding the caregiver's context and needs, role-modeling on how to create opportunities for play, followed by brainstorming around how play can be made possible in the home environment, were central.

The project that emerged was based on an assumed relationship between health and play. The focus was on the primary caregivers who did not have access to the clinic due to the fact that they fell under different hospitals' service areas, or through lack of finances for transport. In many cases these caregivers had children who had never received occupational therapy services. The project explored ways to promote play, playfulness, and caregiver involvement in the interaction between the caregiver and the child.

Specific goals of the project were:

- To gather qualitative information on contextual determinants of play and how the caregivers understood play. Focus groups and individual interviews were used.

- To collect baseline quantitative data on playfulness using the test of playfulness (TOP) version 2 by Bundy,[31] and caregiver involvement using the parent/caregiver involvement scale by Farran et al.[32] Although both these measurements were developed outside South Africa, they were chosen because they focus on aspects of caregiving and play that the researchers deemed universal across cultures. Instead of focusing on what is done, they concentrate on how things happen. The TOP, for example, focuses on playful behaviour rather than how or what the child uses to play.

- To formulate and implement a training program on play and playful behavior in mother–child interaction, with the caregivers. The process of action–reflection was used where caregivers and researchers planned together and revised parts of the implementation according to emerging needs.

- To repeat data collection after the intervention. The same methods as above were used.

- To establish the impact of the training program on playfulness, caregiver involvement and how play was understood. Themes that emerged and quantitative data were shared and tested against what the women had to say in meetings held during the last phase of the project.

The intervention

Initial qualitative information indicated that even though there was a general appreciation of play among the women before intervention, there were still factors around play that would limit how much it was fostered. The younger mothers believed a child should not play when sick, and did not see themselves as enablers of play. All caregivers thought bought toys were necessary for play to happen. This was a disturbing observation in light of the women's economic deprivation, against knowledge by researchers of unlimited resources of traditional games and songs that required very few, if any, material possessions. However, in the context of the occupational apartheid engineered during the apartheid era in South Africa, it was not surprising.

Leaving rural areas to seek jobs in the cities,[20,23,25,26,30] often following being forced out of arable land,[21–23,25] black people were uprooted from familiar environments, where they could engage in culturally meaningful occupations[22,23,33] in the space and time that was collectively self-determined. The move to urban areas often meant a complete displacement.[23,26,33] This was accompanied by a systematic devaluing of their familiar way of life, through educational, political, religious, and cultural mechanisms.[33–35]

Education and the media played a role. For example, history was reconstructed to portray white people as brave and shrewd while black people were portrayed as cruel and barbaric.[36] Over time the internalization of black inferiority was almost inevitable.[33,35,36] Many black people aspired to that which represented whiteness.[34,35] This was worsened by the displacement of families,[23,25,26] with the elderly being left in rural areas. Many opportunities for indigenous games and songs to be handed on from generation to generation were probably lost this way. Living in confined spaces, with parents commuting over long distances to labor that was often hard,[26] families who moved together struggled in transposing their occupations from rural areas to the urban environment. This was yet another expression of occupational apartheid.

Quantitative data before intervention pointed to less than adequate caregiver involvement on the parent/caregiver involvement scale,[32] and low levels of playfulness in the children using the test of playfulness version 2.[31]

The training included 16 workshops. These were run in the same venue the women used for their support group meetings in the community. This was done to facilitate contextualization and relevance of the training and also allowed drawing from available resources, which was thought of as supportive for carry-over and sustainability.

The training approach was mostly experiential and involved reflection-in-action. The women were encouraged to reminisce and tell stories of their own experiences of play as children. This story-telling served as a departure point for appreciating how much the children also needed rich play experiences. Games mentioned by some women, that were unfamiliar to others, were described and all participants were invited to play. This allowed brainstorming around the benefits of play, and a celebration of play as a valuable human experience. Playfulness as an overall approach to interacting with a child, regardless of ability, was highlighted. Time was also allocated to the making of playthings, using available resources.

Overall findings after intervention

Data collected after intervention suggested that there was a positive impact made on caregiver involvement and the children's level of playfulness. The themes that emerged from qualitative data were: play is linked to health and development; play happens anytime, anyhow; play affects the caregiver too; and a caregiver enables play.

WHY PLAY?

What encouraged the author to seek funding that would allow for a service based on play to be extended beyond the hospital clinic was what one of the mothers, who visited regularly, said: 'Yes I get it! When my child plays she's happy, and when she is happy, she looks healthy, and I am happy.' She realized the link between play and health directly from her own observation. It appears that she saw a change from the point when the child was not readily playful or engaging in play to a period of engagement, leading to a child who looked healthier. What is also remarkable is the positive impact this had on the mother. On further reflection on whether this momentous turning point for the mother should be surprising or not, additional insights emerged that are dealt with later in this section.

The link between play and health has been made by many,[37,38] including occupational therapists.[39] The ability to influence one's world or environment may be central to the almost magical power that play seems to be endowed with.[40] It has been established that human beings have an inherent drive to explore, meet curiosity needs and have some effect on their environment.[41] According to White, humans also have a biological need to feel competent as they act on the environment.[42] The satisfaction derived motivates successive attempts at being an agent of change.[42] What emerges from this is a perception of the self as a competent being, a notion which Bandura[43] termed *self-efficacy*. This is accompanied by a sense of agency that is essentially a belief that one is capable of exercising control over events around oneself. Other than providing resilience and ability to resist disease,[44] a sense of control in one's life is an important aspect of the notion of health that is broader than an absence of illness.

The process through which play ultimately leads to courage in a child has also been articulated by Reilly[45] and McAdams.[46] Children who repeatedly experience failure in their attempt to have an effect on the environment develop a sense of helplessness in the face of events in their lives, and have low self-efficacy.[47] A life-tone, in terms of exuding either agency or mistrust and resignation, is set on in infancy,[46] and can be argued to be central to the resilience that can be demonstrated during a health challenge. It follows, therefore, that health-promoting occupational therapy interventions with a child can be through play, as a vehicle through which the child can be equipped to adapt so that person–environment interactions can be performed with competence and satisfaction.[42]

Another view is that promoting play for its own sake, not only because it prepares a child for future engagements or sets an agentic life-tone, is a legitimate notion to pursue because play is a vehicle of meaning,[45] through which true self-expression can be achieved. Prompted by the editors of this book, the author reflected further on the role of spirituality in the way play becomes the vehicle of meaning. Continued sharing of stories with the women in the aforementioned project, particularly one called Flora, strengthened these reflections.

Flora is someone from whom this author has learnt a great deal and continues to draw inspiration. She shared the knowledge of her HIV status with her son from the time he was 7 years old. She also told him he was HIV-positive. The first comment she made, which was incredible, was that the project called her and the other women from the grave. When asked to explain, Flora said that by being encouraged to be playful with their children, the women were asked to look at their children differently, in a way that allowed them to see who the children were meant to be.

She told a story of when her son was hospitalized. He was in the ward with another child. They both had diarrhea. She came into the ward and found the two boys laughing. Flora's son had apparently found the size of the nappies they were both made to wear hilarious. She said that for the first time she could see through to her child's spirit. Having learnt from the project about the need to give oneself as a mother, and the child, permission to be playful, she joined in the laughter. What also emerges from this is that elements of play – humor, the ability to experience sheer joy and suspend reality – can be either encouraged or discouraged by primary caregivers in childhood. There have indeed been instances where the author observed children who seemed incapable of demonstrating these elements of playfulness to the extent that they continually carried blank expressions. Often such children have caregivers who are somewhat non-demonstrative of these elements.

This links clearly with what Robbins and Winnicott[48] said about the role of the mother in creating a 'holding environment' wherein a child allows its healthy, genuine self to emerge. Considering the equating of living with HIV/AIDS with death by the women, commented on earlier, and Flora's assertion that the project called them 'from the grave', it may be inferred that in allowing the child this space for true self-expression, a caregiver enables the child to reconnect with his or her own spirit, and with life itself. This returns us to an earlier question on whether it is surprising that a playful child would impact positively on his or her mother. Given that play has a role in how the human spirit locates itself, it should not be surprising that in expression, the spirit of the child will connect with that of the mother.

Living with HIV/AIDS disenfranchises both the mother and child from essential roles in life, through the overwhelming proximity of death. A mother who, instead of seeing a child, sees a 'dying being', will struggle to connect with her mothering role. In reconnecting with the child through play, she probably reconnects with herself, her mothering role, and her own spirit, since indeed spirituality is related to one's understanding of one's role in life. Frankl[49] proposes that it is possible to survive anything once one has found a reason to live. It seems, therefore, that play and playfulness did indeed unlock the sense of humanity or spirituality within the children, and as Flora indicated, in the mothers. If quality of life is deemed a crucial outcome of care for a child living with HIV/AIDS, promoting play where it is restricted is imperative.

LESSONS LEARNT

Working with communities can be both exciting and challenging. Some of the challenges can be overwhelming, explaining why the turnover of professionals who work directly with communities is often high. A few professionals, however, persist in their efforts. Some therapists will not work anywhere else except where they are directly involved with communities. What drives these people? What spurs them on? A number of observations made throughout the project may explain why some occupational therapists are inspired by communities and will continue working in situations that from a distance appear almost dismal.

True engagement

As members of a profession, it is essential to realize that we are products of a culture that represents particular worldviews and values. Our individual professional identities are covertly related to how we are successfully acculturated into the profession, and inadvertently impress upon how we behave toward those we regard as our clients. Regardless of our past heritage, most of us trained in occupational therapy have adopted Western values and have learnt to view professional practice through Western-based standards. It is not often that we interrogate our professional practice beyond these standards, regardless of how our conduct is perceived and responded to by communities from other non-Western heritages.

As researchers in the project, we learnt very quickly that we could not do research with the women without really engaging. The women challenged us at length on what our genuine interest in them was. In particular, they wanted to know the research assistant's HIV status. It emerged later that her speaking the same language as them allowed for a higher level of identification that simultaneously threatened their sense of safety with regard to confidentiality. It seemed a different language would provide the 'necessary barrier'. In other words, 'If you do not speak my language you probably do not come from where I do, so you won't disclose my status to people who know me.'

Even though speaking the same language was initially a barrier, as the women's trust developed it became a vehicle for true engagement. The women became confident in voicing their concerns and dissatisfaction when these arose, getting to a point where they could say, 'You are one of us, so we can tell you these things.'

It is imperative for professionals in communities to strive for self-awareness, particularly in unravelling their own prejudices regarding particular beliefs and practices. By not exploring how heritage and adopted identities inform present professional relations, important lessons can be missed, and the entrenchment of marginalization of certain groups will continue.

Resilience and spirituality

In reflecting on the experience of the project, the author realized that human potential and hope do not thrive on passivity. Potential is noted once an attempt toward attaining a goal is made. Hope also requires a vision of how things could be, and the anticipation of achievement. The author believes that hope involves having some understanding of how as individuals we are connected to the universe, a core element of spiritual wellbeing.[49]

Returning to the settings from which the women came, the author observed many elements of community living that pointed to the hope and human potential that can exist in apparently destitute situations. At a community level, the one apparent contrast noted was between the dilapidated condition of a number of shacks, and the spotlessly clean clothing hanging on the lines next to them. This highlighted the pride of these people, and the way in which they are able to use very limited resources to strive for self-expression that speaks of dignity.

On an individual level, a mother's description of her unfolding story points to remarkable resilience and immense hopefulness: 'Now I feel like a flower. Initially I was exactly the same as a flower that is dying. … I am now refreshed physically and in my soul' and: 'I asked myself whose child deserved this pain. When the window is closed you can't see anything but once it is opened you can see outside.' Another mother's description was: 'When I heard [I was HIV-positive] I was like a pineapple with its rough peels and didn't want anyone to talk about it. [Now] I am like an aloe that helps sick people.'

The comparison of self to an aloe plant here may indicate this mother's realization of her own resilience, which also extends to being able to help others. Spirituality, in the form of connectedness to others, is also expressed.

The words quoted above demonstrate the remarkable ability of human beings to adapt even in the most challenging of life circumstances. This supports what Schultz and Schkade[42] proposed in saying that it is in extreme life transitions that the most profound adaptation can be witnessed. This was particularly demonstrated in the lives of Flora and her son. Having been open with him about their HIV status, she was able to move from feeling as if their lives were merely waiting at the graveyard, to celebrating an expression of spirituality within him. It may also be argued that it is through resilience that we can find our own spirituality, and that spirituality, in turn, strengthens our ability to be resilient.

The role of support groups

For most of the women in the project, 'family' in the conventional sense meant the woman and her child. An example is one woman who said: 'I am taking care of my child who is HIV-positive. We are happy to have each other like a sunflower plant having the sun.' Support comes mostly from support groups. Some of the women made the following comments: 'There is a difference since I got up and looked for support,' and, 'Now the support group is like a tree with my shade to rest.'

This often leads to 'doing'[50] differently in a manner that perpetuates good health and wellbeing, as in the following comment: 'Now I've met with others and I am feeling well and I am getting good advice. I had to learn to behave myself. I have met real friends because it feels like all your old friends have left you.'

Support groups are powerful because they can allow for one's world to become congruous, as personal experiences are validated. There is also construction of meaning through social and cultural influences. The emerging values take up an interpretive predisposition, influencing judgement, decision-making and behavior, and shaping the meaning of daily life.[47] Support groups also facilitate connection with oneself and with the others, two of the spheres of connectedness[51] related to spirituality.

Professionals working with communities need to value the role played by the sense of belonging. Collectivism and interdependence, rather than individualism and independence, are what often underlie the ideals communities strive for. This needs to be acknowledged and allowed to inform any involvement strategy. Being part of a group, without any tangible output, may sometimes be enough to fulfill the needs of an individual. Just 'being'[50] within a support group went a long way in helping these women to start exploring the phenomenology of living with the illness from a positive perspective.

Fostering meaning

In the face of a multifaceted, threatening, and burdensome HIV status or illness like AIDS, many individuals often choose denial as a coping mechanism. This escapism can sometimes be experienced as better than confronting the battles that sometimes include being ostracized. There is ongoing debate on how professionals can help individuals deal with this dilemma. Most therapists strongly encourage disclosure so that individuals can confront issues and move on.

Rhem and Franck[12] propose a normalization strategy for families that eventually leads to the family interacting with others, based on a view of the child and the whole family as normal. This is a cognitive process used by families to redefine their lives and adopt strategies for the management of the condition. Family routines are maintained, incorporating the care and support of children and other family members. Whilst this can be viewed as a desirable process for any family to go through, it has been regarded by some as a typical Western response that could render professionals unable to fully appreciate and explore the range of social responses and processes available for the diverse cultural contexts within which families find themselves.[12]

Given that the project outlined in this chapter involved a lot of 'doing',[50] in the form of engagement for the caregivers in reminiscent play, and making playthings, it may be said that the distraction offered by this could perpetuate denial or be heavily based on the notion of normalization. One has to consider whether this 'doing' encourages an escape from the very real issues accompanying HIV/AIDS, and whether this is beneficial in the long run.

An assertion by occupational therapy is that clients are better served when the goal is not to help them adjust, but to help them become competent in controlling their own world. This can only be achieved through insuring that what is meaningful to the client is central to guiding practice. Perhaps the answer lies in facilitating processes where a relative balance between 'being',[50] with all the pain it may bring, and 'doing' can be struck. 'Being' can be facilitated through insuring space for reflection on what people value, and is helpful in building consonance within the self in 'doing'. Support groups could be one way of taking space to 'be' in a way that facilitates relevant and appropriate 'becoming'.[50]

CONCLUSION

Life is meaningful to the extent that future life stories are perceived to be unfolding in a way that speaks of coherence throughout one's life plot. An illness like AIDS, like many others that are incurable, can pose a serious challenge to how an individual experiences this congruity. What makes HIV/AIDS particularly formidable are the psychosocial issues that accompany it and the magnitude to which they extend beyond an individual within a family.

In working with a child who is HIV-positive the issues are extremely complex. Challenges commence from identifying what needs should be addressed first, extending to how any involvement should be approached. It is clear that any involvement should strive toward making a positive impact on the child's quality of life. As this cannot be achieved without insuring meaningful human occupation, play should be central. There is a lot that could have been added to the intervention portrayed in this chapter. Spiritual expression, as pursued through play by Simo Algado et al[49] with children survivors of war in Kosovo, could have been strengthened. The challenge, however, would have been in bringing caregivers who had not discussed HIV/AIDS with their children to a point where they did, and in helping their children confront issues of dying. As has been seen with mothers like Flora, it is in knowing what one is confronting that one discovers one's immense potential to be a survivor.

Primary caregivers are crucial for insuring that a child is provided with opportunities for meaningful play. When caregivers are also infected with HIV, they often need to be supported and enabled to foster play in the children. Appropriate involvement with caregivers should consider them in context. A deep exploration of environmental determinants (i.e. occupational apartheid, historical context), the caregivers' own experience of play both in childhood and as an adult, cultural conceptions of play, and an appropriate response to illness and dying, are required.

Acknowledgements   Deep gratitude goes to all the women involved in the project, who have a lot to teach humanity, to Peliwe Mdlokolo, whose appreciation for community kept the project afloat, and to Secure the Future of the Bristol–Myers Squibb Foundation, who saw value in supporting us.

References

1. Pillay K, Colvin M, Williams R, et al. Impact of HIV-1 infection in South Africa. Arch Dis Child 2001; 85(1):50–51.
2. Meyers TM, Pettifor JM, Gray GE, et al. Pediatric admissions with human immunodeficiency virus infection at a regional hospital in Soweto, South Africa. J Trop Pediatr 2000; 46(4): 224–230.
3. Wilkinson D, Dore G. An unbridgeable gap? Comparing the HIV/AIDS epidemics in Australia and sub-Saharan Africa. Aust N Z J Public Health 2000; 24(3):276–280.
4. Grant HW. Patterns of presentation of human immunodeficiency virus type 1-infected children to the pediatric surgeon. J Pediatr Surg 1999; 34(2):251–254.

5. Zwi KJ, Pettifor JM, Soderlund N. Pediatric hospital admissions at a South African urban regional hospital: the impact of HIV, 1992–1997. Ann Trop Paediatr 1999; 19(2):135–142.

6. Hussey GD, Reijnhart RM, Sebens AM, et al. Survival of children in Cape Town known to be vertically infected with HIV-1. S Afr Med J 1998; 88(5): 554–558.

7. Laufer M, Scott GB. Medical management of HIV disease in children. Pediatr Clin North Am 2000; 47(1):127–153.

8. Rollins NC, Dedicoat M, Danaviah S, et al. Prevalence, incidence, and mother-to-child transmission of HIV-1 in rural South Africa. Lancet 2002; 360(9330):389–390.

9. Brady MT. Treatment of human immunodeficiency virus infection and its associated complications in children. J Clin Pharmacol 1994; 34(1):17–29.

10. Mok J, Cooper S. The needs of children whose mothers have HIV infection. Arch Dis Child 1997; 77(6):483–487.

11. Pereira ML, Chaves EC. Being a mother affected with AIDS: reliving the original sin [Abstract]. Revista da Escola Enfermagem da USP 1999; 33(4):404–410. Online. Available: MEDLINE 13 June 2002.

12. Rhem RS, Franck LS. Long-term goals and normalization strategies of children and families affected by HIV/AIDS. Adv Nurs Sci 2000; 23(1):69–82.

13. White RT. Editorial. The AIDS crisis in Africa. Africa Update 2002; 9(2):1–2.

14. Dutra R, Forehand R, Armistead L, et al. Child resiliency in inner-city families affected by HIV: the role of the family variables. Behav Res Ther 2000; 38(5):471–486. Online. Available: ScienceDirect 12 June 2002.

15. Luzuriaga K, Sullivan JL. Pediatric HIV-1 infection: advances and remaining challenges. AIDS Rev 2002; 4(1):21–26.

16. Friedland IR, McIntyre JA. AIDS – the Baragwanath experience. Part II. HIV infection in pregnancy and childhood. S Afr Med J 1992; 82(2):90–94.

17. Lusk D, Huffman SL, O'Gara C. Assessment and improvement of care for AIDS-affected children under age 5. World Wide Web 2000. Online. Available: http:www.eldis.org/static/Doc12979.htm 08 November 2003.

18. Report to congress: USAID efforts to address the needs of children affected by HIV/AIDS (the Synergy Project). Washington DC: Synergy project; 2001.

19. Douaihy A, Singh N. Factors affecting quality of life in patients with HIV infection. AIDS Read 2001; 11(9):450–461.

20. Beinart W. Twentieth-century South Africa. New York: Oxford University Press; 2001.

21. Bundy C. Land, law and power: forced removals in historical context. In: Murray C, O'Regan C, eds. No place to rest: forced removals and the law in South Africa. Cape Town: Oxford University Press; 1990:3–12.

22. Claassens A. Rural land struggles in the Transvaal in the 1980s. In: Murray C, O'Regan C, eds. No place to rest: forced removals and the law in South Africa. Cape Town: Oxford University Press; 1990:27–65.

23. James D. The road from Doornkop: a case study of removals and resistance. Johannesburg: South African Institute of Race Relations; 1983.

24. Murray C, O'Regan C. Preface. In: Murray C, O'Reagan C, eds. No place to rest: forced removals and the law in South Africa. Cape Town: Oxford University Press; 1990:vii.

25. Platzky L, Walker C. The surplus people: forced removals in South Africa. Johannesburg: Ravan Press; 1985.

26. Surplus People Project. Khayelitsha: new home – old story. Cape Town: Surplus People Project; 1984.

27. Townsend E, Wilcock A. Occupational justice. In: Christiansen CH, Townsend EA, eds. Introduction to occupation: the art and science of living. New Jersey: Prentice Hall; 2003:243–273.

28. Kronenberg F. Street children: being and becoming. Research study. Heerlen, The Netherlands: Hogeschool Limburg; 1999.

29. Budlender G. Urban land issues in the 1980s: the view from Weiler's farm. In: Murray C, O'Regan C, eds. No place to rest: forced removals and the law in South Africa. Cape Town: Oxford University Press; 1990:66–85.

30. Sutcliffe M, Todes A, Walker N. Managing the cities: an examination of state urbanization policies since 1986. In: Murray C, O'Regan C, eds. No place to rest: forced removals and the law in South Africa. Cape Town: Oxford University Press; 1990:86–106.

31. Bundy AC. Play and playfulness: what to look for. In: Parham LD, Fazio LS, eds. Play in occupational therapy for children. St. Louis: Mosby; 1997:52–66.

32. Farran DC, Kasari C, Comfort M, et al. Parent/caregiver involvement scale. Nashville: Vanderbilt University; 1986.

33. Biko S. I write what I like: a selection of his writings. London: The Bowerdean Press; 1978.

34. Kallaway P. An introduction to the study of education for blacks in South Africa. In: Kallaway P, ed. Apartheid and education: the education of Black South Africans. Johannesburg: Ravan Press; 1984:1–44.

35. Molteno F. The origins of black education: the historical foundations of the schooling of black South Africans. In: Kallaway P, ed. Apartheid and education: the education of black South Africans. Johannesburg: Ravan Press; 1984:45–107.

36. Lamont R, Lobban S. A study of bias in Bantu Education Department school history books. Johannesburg: Faculty of Education University of the Witwatersrand; 1976.

37. Lindquist I. Therapy through play. London: Arlington Books; 1977.

38. Royeen CB. Play as occupation and as an indicator of health. In: Chandler BC, ed. The essence of play: a child's occupation. Bethesda: The American Occupational Therapy Association; 1997:1–14.

39. Parham LD, Fazio LS. Play in occupational therapy for children. St Louis: Mosby; 1997.

40. Schaaf RC, Burke JP. What happens when we play? A neurodevelopmental explanation. In: Chandler BC, ed. The essence of play: a child's occupation. Bethesda: The American Occupational Therapy Association; 1997:79–105.

41. Yerxa EJ, Clark F, Jackson JJ, et al. An introduction to occupational science: a foundation for occupational therapy in the 21st century. Occupational Therapy in Health Care 1990; 6(4):1–17.

42. Schultz S, Schkade J. Adaptation. In: Christiansen C, Baum C, eds. Occupational therapy: enabling function and well-being. 2nd edn. New Jersey: Slack; 1997: 459–481.

43. Bandura A. Human agency in social theory. American Psychologist 1989; 44(9):1175–1183.

44. Wilcock AA. An occupational perspective of health. New Jersey: Slack; 1998.

45. Parham LD, Primeau LA. Play and occupational therapy. In: Parham LD, Fazio LS, eds. Play in occupational therapy for children. St Louis: Mosby; 1997:2–21.

46. Polkinghorne DE. Transformative narratives: from victimic to agentic life plots. Am J Occup Ther 1995; 50(4):299–305.

47. Christiansen C, Baum C. Person–environment occupational performance: a conceptual model for practice. In: Christiansen C, Baum C, eds. Occupational therapy: enabling function and well-being. 2nd edn. New Jersey: Slack; 1997:47–70.

48. Robbins BD, Winnicott DW. Online. Available:http://www.mythosandlogos.com/Winnicott.html 09 November 2003.

49. Simo Algado S, Mehta N, Kronenberg F, et al. Occupational therapy intervention with children survivors of war. Can J Occup Ther 2002; 69(4):205–217.

50. Wilcock AA. Reflections on doing, being and becoming. Can J Occup Ther 1998b; 65(5):248–256.

51. Bellingham R, Cohen B, Jones T, et al. Connectedness: some skills for spiritual health. American Journal of Health Promotion 1989; 4:18–24, 31.

Chapter **24**

Inclusive education in Pakistan
An occupational therapist's contribution to teacher education

Debbie Kramer-Roy

OVERVIEW

This chapter shares my story of moving across both physical and conceptual borders. It shows how and why an occupational therapist ended up in teacher education, and how my background in occupational therapy helps me to promote inclusive education effectively through my role as a teacher educator in Pakistan. The chapter also shows how these experiences are preparing me for returning to occupational therapy per se, as I prepare local colleagues to take over the work in inclusive education and plan for the setting up of an occupational therapy department in the university hospital.

To understand why I am doing what I am doing, it is necessary to look back at my history as an occupational therapist. This shows how personal and professional experiences gradually shaped my ideas and vision of the fundamental issues in enabling persons with disabilities to attain their potential levels of independence and inclusion, or interdependence.

MY PERSONAL JOURNEY

I moved beyond my native country's borders as soon as I qualified as an occupational therapist in 1989 and have worked alternately in England and Pakistan ever since. My move to England gave me the opportunity to work in a general hospital, which helped the development of my clinical skills; however, it did not provide a significantly different sociopolitical context from my own and therefore did not challenge my rather reductionist conception (as I now see it) of occupational therapy.

My first stay in Pakistan made me move across conceptual as well as geographical borders, as I engaged in community-based rehabilitation (CBR) activities, as part of a primary healthcare project (see Ch. 13 for a definition of CBR). Because the CBR activities were not seen as a priority by the host project, this was not very successful in terms of establishing sustainable CBR activities, but it taught me a lot about the social, political, economic, and cultural barriers preventing children and adults with disabilities from becoming equal and fully participating members of society. Reading about and experiencing the realities of CBR in a sociocultural context wholly different from my own made me realize that increasing a child's independence in play and self-help skills has very limited value unless it is part of a much broader approach. This approach would seek to facilitate the community to accept all its members as equal and valuable contributors, who have the right to receive all necessary support to attain the best possible quality of life and to develop the skills needed to take up their roles and responsibilities. Although I did not use the term at the time, this is when I started to understand the need for a focus on *inclusion*, i.e. the need for full social participation and equal access to services. In other words, I became more conscious of the rights perspective of my work as an occupational therapist, through which I had developed skills of facilitating people's understanding of their position in society and their ability to act to improve it.

Before returning to Pakistan the second and final time, I obtained a Master's degree in Education and International Development: Health Promotion from the Institute of Education in London, in order to broaden my options for engaging in development work in Pakistan. Choosing to write in my coursework about disability related issues, such as the influence of culture and religion on parents' attitudes toward their children, helped me to reflect on my previous experience in the light of new concepts in the field of development studies, and from a more academic perspective.

Being offered a faculty position at the Aga Khan University Institute for Educational Development (AKU–IED) presented an opportunity to work in the arena of development that would have been impossible without attaining my Master's degree. However, I was initially reluctant to take what I thought might be a side step away from occupational therapy, fearing that I would lose my professional skills. In addition, the Aga Khan University is rather an 'elite' institution and I felt there was a danger of being distanced from those children whose participation in daily life, school, and society I really hoped to help increase. However, the opportunity to raise the awareness and skill level of mainstream teachers to enable them to include children with special needs effectively in their classrooms has made an extremely important contribution to the perception by faculty, staff, and students at AKU–IED of the 'problem' of children with special needs. An increasing recognition of hidden special needs present in children already studying in mainstream schools, as well as an increasing openness to granting admission to children with disabilities, are evident in the teachers and head teachers attending courses at the institute.

DEFINING OCCUPATIONAL THERAPY AND INCLUSIVE EDUCATION

Before describing what my work at AKU–IED actually entails, I will compare the underlying concepts and assumptions of occupational therapy and inclusive education, to show the ways in which they are compatible.

Occupational therapy

The World Federation of Occupational Therapists describes occupational therapy as 'a healthcare profession based on the knowledge that purposeful activity can promote health and wellbeing in all aspects of daily life. The aims are to promote, develop, restore and maintain abilities needed to cope with daily activities to prevent dysfunction [and] ... to facilitate maximum use of function to meet demands of the ... environment.'[1] Occupational therapists seek people's active involvement, facilitating them to be participants and partners in improving their occupational performance.[2] *Occupation* indicates all purposeful activity that people carry out to maintain themselves in self-care, productivity, and leisure, and to find meaning in their lives.[3]

Another important aspect of the occupational therapy approach is the structured, logical reasoning used to assess and define the person's strengths, needs, and social circumstances, to plan and implement the intervention, and to evaluate the outcomes. In my view, the combination of the therapist–client partnership with strong reasoning skills provides the essential ingredients of a good occupational therapy intervention, in which the outcomes are perceived to be successful for both the therapist, the person the therapist is working with, and the people in that person's environment.

Because of this broad view and the central importance given to the role of occupation in the health and wellbeing of each person, occupational therapy has never sat comfortably with the medical model of disability that underpins the health and education services most commonly provided to children with disabilities.[3] Occupational therapy's focus on seeing the person as a partner capable of making autonomous decisions, and the importance it ascribes to influencing the social environment to facilitate people to become as independent as possible and fulfill their required or desired social roles, are much more in line with a social model of disability. The tension of balancing the 'medical' and 'social' needs of the client and of clarifying this to others (notably the referring physician or the health insurance company, for example) is an ongoing challenge for any conscientious occupational therapist.

During studies for my Master's degree, I discovered a name for this balancing act of models in the World Health Organization's *International Classification of Functioning, Disability and Health*[4] (ICF–2001). The ICF – 2001 captures the need to integrate the various perspectives of functioning in a 'biopsychosocial model'. Studying a model of disability outside the occupational therapy literature helped me not only to become less territorial about my profession, but also to be comfortable in accepting and using alternative terminology for the concepts central to occupational therapy. Both of these are essential for my role at AKU–IED, which I will describe later. I contend that all occupational therapists engaging in a field that overlaps only partly with occupational therapy need to spend time studying and reflecting on the concepts and terminologies used, so that the evolution of their role does not alienate them from their identity as an occupational therapist.

Inclusive education

Inclusive education can be defined as 'the processes of increasing the participation of students in, and reducing their exclusion from, the cultures, curricula and communities of local schools.'[5] This clearly defines inclusion as a school improvement process, focusing on all children who are excluded for whatever reason, special needs being only one of these reasons.

A very important document in promoting inclusive education world wide is *The Salamanca Statement and Framework for Action*,[6] issued as an outcome of the World Conference on Special Needs Education: Access and Quality, which was held in 1994 and attended by government and non-governmental representatives from 92 countries. The Salamanca Statement sets out important principles and guidelines for developing contextually relevant inclusive education practices. Before specific guidelines for governments, schools, and other stakeholders are given, the main principles of and reasons for inclusion are stated as follows:

We believe and proclaim that:

- *every child has a fundamental right to education, and must be given the opportunity to achieve and maintain an acceptable level of learning*

- *every child has unique characteristics, interests, abilities, and learning needs*

- *education systems should be designed and educational programmes implemented to take into account the wide diversity of these characteristics and needs*

- *those with special educational needs must have access to regular schools which should accommodate them within a child-centered pedagogy capable of meeting these needs*

- *regular schools with this inclusive orientation are the most effective means of combating discriminatory attitudes, creating welcoming communities, building an inclusive society and achieving education for all; moreover, they provide an effective education to the majority of children and improve the efficiency and ultimately the cost-effectiveness of the entire education system.*[6]

It may be evident from this that inclusive education is essentially a human rights issue, which seeks to put an end to the notion that services for children with disabilities are a 'privilege' and instead asserts the right to equal access to and participation in mainstream schools for all children, regardless of their abilities or characteristics. This implies the responsibility of society and its systems to provide an environment in which all citizens not only receive their rights, but are also able to fulfill their responsibilities. Although few countries have achieved a situation anywhere near the ideal set out in the Salamanca Statement, many governments and non-governmental organizations have made significant progress in developing inclusive practices at school, local, or national level[7]. In many countries, including Pakistan, inclusive education is a very new concept and much advocacy and hard work will need to be done before it is accepted as a valuable contribution to achieving high quality education for all children as a preparation for full inclusion into society.

OCCUPATIONAL THERAPY AND INCLUSIVE EDUCATION

Where the occupational therapist tends to start with the child and aims to influence the school situation to benefit this individual child, inclusive education starts by challenging the system, encouraging it to change so that it becomes more able to include children with disabilities or other disadvantages, such as poverty, gender, or social problems. What they share is the endeavor to help the individual and people in the environment to work toward changes that will create optimal conditions for the child to participate fully in school and for all students to be able to contribute to building a more inclusive society.

In addition to this, the analytical approach of the occupational therapist can be applied equally to systems or situations, as to the individual service user. Being able to assess and define which aspects of various levels of the system (for example school policies, classroom practices, teachers' and parents' attitudes) are creating barriers or opportunities for the inclusion of children with special needs is essential for planning how to influence key players in the inclusion process. Similarly, evaluating the extent of success in this process is very important for fine-tuning the approach taken.[8]

INCLUSIVE EDUCATION AT AKU–IED

The Pakistani population is relatively very poorly educated. The adult literacy rate is 52% for men and 26% for women, whilst the net primary school enrollment rate is 49% for boys and 38% for girls.[9] There are many reasons for children not enrolling in school or dropping out before finishing primary school, including poverty, child labor, and cultural restrictions among some groups, affecting girls in particular. In addition, the population growth rate is so phenomenal (2.8%, with the population doubling between 1975 and 2000)[10] and the amount of government spending on education so low (2.7% of GNP),[10] that there are not even enough schools to accommodate all school-aged children.

Although no official data are available, those working in this field estimate that only 1 or 2% of Pakistani children with disabilities attend any school at all, whether it is a special school or mainstream school. A larger percentage of children who do not have an identified disability but have hidden special needs, such as mild intellectual, visual, or hearing impairments, dyslexia, or psychosocial problems, may get enrolled in school, but they are at a very high risk of dropping out as schools do not tend to cater for their special needs.

The AKU–IED aims to improve the quality of education in developing countries through educational programs, research, academic partnerships, policy initiatives, and a commitment to wider social development. It offers programs at Certificate, Diploma, and Master of Education degree level. All programs are grounded in the realities of school life, challenge participants' assumptions, focus on quality improvements, and develop sound teaching skills. At this time participants are mainly recruited from a large number of partner schools covering the Aga Khan Development Network, private (not-for-profit) schools, and government schools in Pakistan, Central Asia, and East Africa. Therefore it has a rich mix of students in terms of culture, language, and even educational background, which both enriches and complicates their learning together.

AKU–IED is grant funded (the main funding being provided by the European Commission and the Canadian International Development Agency) and in the grant proposal for its second phase (2001–2006)[11] it commits to incorporating the area of 'special needs' into its existing programs. It states that:

> *Throughout most of the regions which AKU–IED serves, little attention has been directed towards the education of the substantial minority of children with special needs, for example, those with varying levels of physical and intellectual impairment. AKU–IED will develop modules which deal with the identification, assessment and referral of special needs, the options for addressing them, and the potential of integrated schooling approaches and community support.*

Despite the official commitment to this area, during my first year at AKU–IED I had to direct a lot of my efforts toward raising awareness of special needs issues in education among my colleagues. Without their support I could not gain access to any of the participants who attended the courses at AKU–IED. I then started to conduct awareness-raising sessions in the existing courses, always careful to link up with the focus of the course, to ensure that participants would take interest. Even now these sessions remain an important activity, as new groups of students pass through AKU–IED all the time. The focus of these sessions varies from handwriting, through behavior problems, to international guidelines for inclusion, depending on the audience. In the sessions that focus on the child with special needs in the classroom, I tend to use the performance components (sensory-motor, cognitive, and psychosocial) from the adaptation through occupation model[12] as a structure for the participants to analyze what the cause of a child's difficulty with learning in school might be. A very successful activity I have used repeatedly is when participants work in groups, each of which is given a different 'impairment' (wearing a blindfold, wearing an oven glove, standing on one leg, using the non-dominant hand or the mouth, looking in the mirror, or copying an unfamiliar language script, such as Hindi) to find out the prerequisite skills for handwriting. These teaching approaches clearly reflect my identity as an occupational therapist, as they seek to make the participants (i.e. classroom teachers) independent in identifying the nature of the child's special needs, encourage them to apply analytical skills, and engage the participants in purposeful activities to facilitate their professional development.

I have also gradually increased the number of Master of Education (M Ed) modules in which I contribute to the teaching. Initially, only the teaching team of the Primary Education module was open to my input, but gradually the English, Social Studies, Mathematics, School Improvement and Educational Issues modules have become interested too, as I have always ensured that my input enriches the participants' understanding of the module subject, rather than distracting from it. Involvement in a large number of modules is important, because it helps the participants to understand that 'special needs' is not a side issue, but potentially affects everything they do as a teacher.

Through my growing experience of teaching large numbers of participants from a varied developing world context, I started to develop a working definition of special needs to reflect the reality in their classrooms. The definition is as follows: 'By special needs we mean any characteristic – whether obvious or hidden, whether temporary or permanent – which interferes with the child's learning at school and requires special attention.'[13] The definition reflects that special needs do not relate exclusively to 'disability', and that many problems identified by teachers affect a large proportion of children in school: poor nutrition, poor parenting skills, the complexities of living in extended families, domestic problems including violence, and child labor.

In September 2001 I reached the significant milestone of conducting a 6-week elective module for the M Ed students. Although the first offering was taught in face-to-face (classroom) teaching mode, it is now offered in open learning mode for which I have developed a comprehensive study package,[13] consisting of a study guide, reading package, and video materials with which the students work independently. Most of the interaction with the students is through an email discussion forum and through short weekly workshops. This is now an accepted and well-respected part of the M Ed program. The feedback from the course participants on the written materials has been very positive, for example: 'I really like the way it is written, it is as if you are sitting next to me, explaining it all to me.'

I am convinced that my experience as an occupational therapist, always explaining to people I work with, carers, and other professionals about difficulties, needs, possibilities, and rights, has contributed greatly to my writing style in this study guide. Interaction with the participants was also shaped by my occupational therapy approach, always seeking to advance the person's development in a way that enhances rather than damages self-esteem, while not avoiding the identification of areas that need improvement. This was evidenced by the feedback from one of the participants who wrote: 'Thanks for providing us [timely] comprehensive feedback. It really pushed me to think about the critical aspects of academic writing and [in my] understanding of slow learners. After having this feedback my confidence is raised ... and I'm hoping to be ... [a] torchbearer of inclusive education and ... lead others effectively in my context.'

Owing to the success of the module, a similar course is now also being offered at certificate level in which the participants study for 6 months part-time in open learning. For the first offering of this course we only have Karachi-based participants, although the aim is to enrol students from more geographical areas once a local support system can be organized. Again, most communication is through email, and in addition workshops are held at the beginning of the course and then every 2 or 3 weeks. This is an even more effective format, as the participants continue their teaching work whilst they study, immediately applying in their classrooms what they learn. This continuous practice base is very evident in the responses they give to activities.

As the work has grown, two local junior colleagues have been appointed to work alongside me and eventually take over the special needs program at AKU–IED. Both have backgrounds – like my own, to an extent – that sit more readily with the medical, reductionist model of disability, and they have needed to redirect their thinking and approach to understand and be able to promote inclusive education. The appointment of additional staff is an indicator of AKU–IED's commitment to inclusive education. However, a lot more proactive work will be needed before special needs and inclusion issues become an integral part of all the teaching programs.

In order to broaden the reach of the special needs program, I have founded the Pakistan Association for Inclusive Education (PAIE), which organizes monthly workshops and a short summer course, and publishes a biannual newsletter. PAIE has enabled us to build up contacts with many more schools, including the handful of private schools in Karachi that have taken a positive decision to include children with obvious special needs. This is a very brave step to take in the local situation; most private schools set entrance tests for their new admissions in order to take the highest achievers. As the quality of education in the government system is so poor and there are not enough private schools to cater for those who can afford it, the private schools can pick and choose the students they want to admit. This is a serious issue of inequity for all children, but even more so for those who experience any kind of difficulty with their schoolwork, as they have severely reduced chances of passing the admission test.

The few schools that do include children with special needs have been happy to collaborate with us, and our students have been able to do their teaching practice and even their Master's degree thesis research there. In addition, staff from three of these schools have taken the certificate course. This collaboration has shown, however, that despite their genuine desire to be inclusive, these schools find it extremely difficult to make this a reality at the classroom level. Although children with special needs are physically integrated in the classroom, in many cases their social inclusion is still limited, and in some cases their academic inclusion is hardly achieved at all.

To explore the best way of helping such schools to move closer to their ideal of becoming inclusive and providing effective education in a good social environment to all their pupils, the intention is to start a pilot project in 2004 to support and study schools that take a school improvement approach to becoming more inclusive. *The Index for Inclusion*, developed in Britain by the Centre for Studies in Inclusive Education[8] will be used to structure the pilot project. The Index uses lists of indicators pertaining to the culture, policies, and practices in the school which can be used to determine how inclusive it is, to plan for positive change, and to evaluate the outcomes. The Index has been piloted successfully in a number of developing countries and one of the intended outcomes is to develop a Pakistani version of it, in both English and Urdu (one of the official languages of Pakistan), adapted according to contextual differences. The outcomes of the pilot project will be disseminated widely in order to influence stakeholders, ranging from government policy makers to teachers in schools, in their journey toward building a more inclusive education system.

CONCLUSION

The professional knowledge, skills, and attitudes gained in my training and career as an occupational therapist have been an excellent preparation for promoting inclusive education in a mainstream teacher education institute. Working with large numbers of school teachers and heads, as well as sensitizing my colleagues at AKU–IED, has enabled me potentially to affect the lives of thousands of children with special needs, both by increasing the likelihood that they will gain admission to a mainstream school and by preparing their teachers to include them in school life and effective learning. My identity at AKU–IED has been simply 'faculty' and people have often been surprised to find out that I am not a teacher by profession.

In addition, my work in teacher education is impacting my identity as an occupational therapist. Despite the positive developments in my work at AKU–IED, my aim is still to hand it over gradually to my local colleagues who will carry the torch of inclusive education for their country. I have started to work for the Department of Pediatrics at the university hospital for 2 days per week in order to explore avenues to set up occupational therapy services and, in the more distant future, a pre-service occupational therapy education program within the Aga Khan University and hospital. My experience at AKU–IED is preparing me for a leadership and pioneering role in occupational therapy. In addition, it has enhanced my skills in teaching at tertiary education level, and in engaging in qualitative research and academic writing, which will all be of great help when seeking not only to set up a department, but also to lead local occupational therapists in developing a model of occupational therapy that is more appropriate to the Pakistani context. Encouraging occupational therapists to be actively involved in further developments in CBR and inclusive education in Pakistan will be a crucial part of this process.

References

1. World Federation of Occupational Therapists. About occupational therapy (information leaflet). West Perth: World Federation of Occupational Therapists; 1996.
2. College of Occupational Therapists. Curriculum framework for occupational therapy. London: College of Occupational Therapists; 1993:6.
3. Wilcock AA. An occupational perspective of health. Thorofare, NJ: Slack; 1998:22,166.
4. World Health Organization. The international classification of functioning, disability and health. Geneva: WHO; 2001.
5. The Centre for Studies in Inclusive Education. Inclusion information guide. 2002.

Online. Available: http://inclusion.uwe.ac.uk/csie/studnts02.htm#DefiningInclusion

6. UNESCO. The Salamanca statement and framework for action. Salamanca: UNESCO; 1994.

7. UNESCO. Salamanca: five years on. Paris: UNESCO; 1999.

8. Booth T, Ainscow M. The index for inclusion. Bristol: Centre for Studies in Inclusive Education; 2002.

9. McCarthy R. The quest for literacy in Pakistan. Guardian unlimited. 8 September 2000. Online. Available: http://www.guardian.co.uk/international/story/0,3604,365735,00.html

10. United Nations Development Program. Human Development Report 2002 – Pakistan. United Nations Development Program; 2002. Online. Available: http:// www.undp.org/hdr2002/indicator/cty_f_PAK.html

11. The Aga Khan University, Institute for Educational Development. Phase 2 proposal 2001–2006. Karachi: Aga Khan University, Institute for Educational Development; 1999:33.

12. Reed KL, Sanderson SN. Concepts of occupational therapy. Baltimore: Williams and Wilkins; 1992.

13. Kramer-Roy D. Inclusive education., Study pack for M Ed Elective Module. Karachi: Aga Khan University, Institute for Educational Development; 2002.

Chapter **25**

The return of the corn men
An intervention project with a Mayan community of Guatemalan *retornos*

Salvador Simó Algado, Cesar Estuardo Cardona

OVERVIEW

In this chapter we describe a 6 month occupational therapy project undertaken in 1996 with Mayan Indian families returning to Guatemala after 14 years as refugees in Mexico. Indigenous populations such as this are at even greater risk than usual when they are refugees. Since occupational therapy intervention guided by peoples' spiritual beliefs can be a powerful force for change, Mayan cosmovision was used to guide the project.

Reconsidering the project 8 years later in the light of new understanding about the human and ecological genocide we are confronting, the chapter urges occupational therapists to be more aware of the need to develop transcultural, holistic, and community-centered interventions, and to work as social activists, fighting for occupational justice together with the populations we have the privilege to serve.

In this chapter special attention is devoted to spirituality and to the development of occupational ecology.

The biggest treasure I have in life is the ability to dream; in the hardest moments I have been able to dream a more beautiful future.[1]

INTRODUCTION TO THE PROJECT

In 1996 Jose Maria Rodriguez, a social worker, and Salvador Simó Algado,[2] an occupational therapist, contacted a refugee organization called Comisiones Permanentes and offered their services as volunteers. From this they developed a project working with Mayan refugees returning to Guatemala from Mexico. It was an amalgamation of both disciplines, with the social worker focusing on education through leisure.

History of conflict in Guatemala – an injured, land

Inhuman are their soldiers, cruel their fierce dogs.[3]

Guatemala declared its independence from Spain in 1821. Its political and economic systems had been based on the exploitation of the indigenous communities, and little changed until 1945 when Juan José Arévalo and Jacobo Arbenz, presidents of 'the October Revolution' were elected. Cardoza y Aragon describes this period as 'the beginning of ten years of spring in the country of eternal tyranny'.[4] It allowed the beginnings of a labor movement and land reform, with some land being redistributed among the poorest people of the country and returned to its authentic owners, the Mayan people. In 1954 a Conservative coup d'état supported by landowners, clergy elite, and the CIA put an end to such progress[5] and began almost 50 years of military-dominated rule.

In 1960 a Cuban-supported revolt failed. The guerrillas fled into the hills where they continued a civil war against the military. From 1962 onwards the military stepped up its campaign against the guerrillas. Between 1978 and 1983 the Guatemalan army began a 'scorched earth' campaign in the countryside inhabited by Mayan Indians. The result was the destruction of 440 villages,[6,7] with 45 000 women widowed and 150 000 children orphaned.[5,8] There were 626 massacres attributable to State forces.[9] 200 000 Guatemalans were murdered and between half a million and a million and half were displaced, depending on the definition of displacement.[9] Mayan Indians began to flee to Mexico. The United Nations High Commission for Refugees (UNHCR) officially recognized 46 000 refugees. It was believed that another 150 000 Guatemalans went into hiding in the forests surrounding Chiapas, in Mexico.[10]

Improving political conditions made it possible, but not completely safe, for Mayan refugees to return to their beloved land[8] when a firm and durable peace was signed December 1996, ending 36 years of war. Those who go back are known as *retornos*.

The corn man and Mayan cosmovision

Today the Mayan people constitute more than 55% of the Guatemalan population. Their history reflects a proud past mired by four centuries of domination by *ladinos*, individuals of European ancestry. Mayan people established the first known villages in the Americas in approximately 2000 BC. By 100 BC Mayan land was divided into a system of states, each with its own complex social, political, and economic systems. The Mayan people demonstrated advanced knowledge, particularly in painting, pottery, medicine, mathematics, architecture, and astronomy. Our calendar is derived from Mayan astronomy, and we owe the zero and the vigesimal and binary systems to Mayan mathematics. By 1500 AD, the Mayan civilization was in decline.[11] The superior war technology of the Europeans had facilitated its conquest. From the sixteenth to the nineteenth centuries, the Mayan people were co-opted to work the plantations of wealthy European landowners, in conditions extremely close to slavery.

Mayan cosmovision – a resource for healing

In the name of The Heaven's heart, in the name of the Earth's heart…

(Mayan prayer)[3]

Almost all indigenous cultures reflect the sacred reality of life. We can listen to their wisdom in sayings such as: 'I am all the forces and elements that I touch. I am the wind, the trees, the birds, and the darkness'[12] or 'The sun, the moon, and the trees are the symbols of my continuity.'[13] (p. 17) Our Western societies, based on economic values imposed by capitalism, have forgotten about this sacredness.

The Mayans generated a system of myths of a holistic and religious nature that registered their perception of the world, the scientific measure of time, the movement of the stars, and the path of the earth in the galaxy. The myths link and interweave, possessing a vital force that generates the roots of thought and behavior.[14]

A non-anthropocentric cosmovision was created, where the multiple interdependence of beings is recognized. The cosmos is a flow of cyclical and changing energy. The universe is chaotic, generating life and death, but within an order. Human beings and nature participate in the same cosmic essence: *ajaw*.[15]

Ancient manuscripts and oral tradition show the conception of interdependence. This parity, seen not only as the unity of contraries but as a movement of complements, was indispensable. Woman and man were conceived as two in one, as were day and night, Heaven and Earth, and birth and death. The interdependence and complementarity of men and women was expressed in daily life as the unity of the unequal. There was an imaginary woman–mother–earth–life–sacred concept.[16]

Mayan cosmovision[2] refers to an articulated system of ancient symbols and meanings that represent cognitive and existential aspects of the community and of the individual. Cosmovision describes the place and purpose of all things in the universe. It influences every human activity and involves convictions, beliefs, habits, roles, and feelings. As a Guatemalan friend said: 'We are one in nature, we are unity in diversity.'

Mayan beliefs regarding the origin of illness, the role of the individual within the universe, and the meaning of evil and suffering guided the work of the project. The first author of this chapter learned about cosmovision by spending several days with an Ajgij, or Mayan priest. Mayan people believe that their ancestor, lxmucané, made men using white and yellow corn, so they are known as the corn men.

The Ajgij's goal is to maintain the harmony between human beings, nature, and God. The loss of this harmony is the origin of illness. As the Ajgij said: 'The Earth is my mother; the Earth is a living being. She feeds me, I live for her. We live from water, wind, fire, rain … If a person turns his back on nature, he'll become hopelessly ill' (personal communication, 1996). We are seen as spiritual beings.

Mayan philosophy clearly outlines the role of the individual in the community: you must work for your community using your talents and knowledge, leading to a focus on cooperation and respect for life. Human beings must contribute to the universe through their skills.

The meaning of suffering and the reason for the existence of evil were ever present issues for the community, embodied in the violence experienced by the refugees. Mayan philosophy grapples with the problem of evil and the Ajgij explained that 'in the Universe, Good and Evil exist in a never-ending fight in which we participate, as did our predecessors and the rest of the holy forces' (personal communication, 1996).

As enablers of the community, using a community-centered approach, we tried to develop the role of the Ajgij in our new community in Guatemala. As Bugental[17] has remarked, 'Therapists are the descendants of the ancient shamans.'

Life in the refugee camps

To get to know the story of the refugees' community we spent some weeks living in the refugee camps in Chiapas and Campeche, in Mexico. There were high levels of malnourishment, infant mortality, alcoholism, disability, and domestic violence.[18] The role of women was crucial, as they were responsible for the survival, in the face of violence, of both their families and Mayan society.[19,20]

The corn men's return

We have always lived here; we have the right to go on living where we are happy and where we want to die. Only here can we feel whole; nowhere else would we ever feel complete and our pain would be eternal.[20]

The first author of this chapter participated in two *retornos* (the return of indigenous people to their land), organized by UNHCR. Our first role was as human shields, giving protection to the refugees through an international presence. We accompanied two groups from Mexico to Quetzal and Esmeralda, in Guatemala, which were not their original villages. They returned with a mixture of feelings, including insecurity and fear, to the country where massacres had occurred and kidnapping, torture, and murder were everyday occurrences.

The new community

Naked land, awaked land, corn land with dreams ... corn land covered by the rivers of green water in the sleeplessness of the scarified jungles by the corn made corn sower man.[21]

One group of approximately 210 families, around 1200 indigenous people of mixed ethnic background, mostly Mam, Quiche, Ka-chiquel, and some *ladinos*, went to Quetzal, a completely new village constructed in the middle of the jungle. Life there was extremely hard. During the rainy season the community was essentially isolated. Food was scarce; many of the children were malnourished and some died.

An NGO offered medical services, and the community was organized by a cooperative, Cooperativa Union Maya Itza. There was a women's organization, called Ixmucane, an adolescent's organization, called Maya Tikal, and health and education promoters. Our role was to empower the people's own organizations to enable them to be the main characters in their own narrative, thus avoiding the creation of dependency.

Setting the goals of the intervention

The goals of the project were set in the light of observations in Mexico and Guatemala, and a visit to El Colegio de la Frontera sur (ECOSUR), a research center related to mental health studies, based in Mexico. However, it was vitally important for these goals to be agreed by the community itself, through a series of meetings with the different representative groups. This was a slow process, but showed us how important it is at times to forget our Western mentality and adapt to the tempo of local communities. Box 25.1 lists the problems that were identified.

Box 25.1   Problems identified by the project

Children

Unlike the children, parents and other adult relatives had suffered directly from the violence in Guatemala. These adults, in turn, transmitted some of their pain to the children, who then demonstrated secondary trauma associated with indirect exposure to violence. This secondary trauma manifested itself in malnourishment and mental health problems. Farias and Billings[22] found malnourishment in children at the Chiapas refugee camps to be positively correlated with post traumatic stress disorder (PTSD) in mothers, while Miller[23] found a positive correlation between the mental health of mothers and daughters.

There was no therapeutic support for these children, and their education was formal and rigid. No attention was paid to creativity and emotional development. Additionally, the children's cultural identity had not been developed. One of the children had cerebral palsy.

Adolescents

Yes, I remember the trip. We went with our fathers carrying all our things. One man was shot in the back. The army followed us into the mountains killing all who couldn't run. My father was carrying me; we ran fast. Those who remained behind died. My father told me they killed many women; they also killed their babies.

(Adolescent testimony)[23]

The adolescents of the community were anxious and angry. As they said: 'For us teenagers refugee life starts now, when we return to Guatemala.' They had grown to identify with the North American influenced culture of the Mexican cities. Some were even ashamed of their indigenous cultural heritage. One teen exclaimed: 'I am not indigenous; I want to be a *ladino*.' However, while they rejected the Mayan culture, it was apparent that many were not knowledgeable of it.

The adolescents felt both sadness and fear. Many felt that their life plans were being disrupted.

One said: 'All I can do here is sow corn'. Others remembered the violence left behind in Guatemala.[8]

Adults

I feel desperate here. There is only mud, snakes and malaria; my children are hungry.

(Adult testimony)

The long term symptoms of PTSD were prevalent, linked to the difficult psychosocial conditions associated with life as refugees and *retornos*.[24] Prior to leaving Guatemala, most of the adults had suffered one or more traumatic events, including the witnessing of tortures and rapes.[25] The symptoms of PTSD are given new life on returning to the place where the violence occurred. As one adult commented, 'We have returned to where it all happened. The same soldiers who massacred us are still living in the village.'

The author's previous experiences in Bosnian and Mexican refugee camps suggested that many seek to dull this pain with alcohol, which is then linked to poverty and domestic violence. Continuing loss of the indigenous cultural identity further fuels the despair.

Elders

In life we are walking like this. My life is sadness; I am just waiting for death. People say that the elders have no value. Nothing is as it used to be. They do not respect you; they have forgotten what our ancestors taught us.

(Elder testimony)

Life in the jungle was physically hard for the elders. Above all, though, they experienced anger and pain at the loss of their traditional role within the community. Customarily, elders were viewed as guardians of knowledge, who played an important role in passing on their wisdom to the next generation. Deprivation of this role represents not only a lack of usefulness for them within the community, but also loss of ancient knowledge on the part of the community.

SURVIVORS

The people were survivors, who had survived both the massacres before leaving Guatemala, and the hard life in the refugee camps. Now they were determined to start again in the middle of the jungle. They possessed many strengths, such as having their own organization. They had been able to create their own educational system, and the elders had maintained their traditional wisdom. They were willing to learn, to work, and, as Rigoberta Menchú says,[1] to dream and to create a more beautiful future.

The ocupational therapy intervention

Occupational therapy is both an art and a science. Our philosophy of intervention was based on a client/community-centered approach,[2,26–31] (and see Ch. 18) and on the use of holistic and transcultural occupational therapy,[2,26–31] where meaningful occupation is at the heart of the intervention.

Empathy, authenticity, and congruency are vital qualities. Communities possess extraordinary potential, and the role of the occupational therapist is similar to a catalyst, facilitating change and working with the resources that are already in the community. We must promote an inner locus of control and an inner responsibility in the community.

Holism means understanding the human being as a physical, psychosocial, and sociopolitical being, whose essence is spiritual, and who is immersed in an ecological and cultural environment.

Transcultural[2,26–30] occupational therapy not only means recognizing the beauty of all cultures, but also including culturally meaningful occupations in our interventions. Meaningful occupation is a fragile balance where the needs, potential, and the spirit of the person meet. This definition includes the spirit of the person, because the spirit is our true self that we try to express in all our activities.[32]

The project was based mainly on the Model of Human Occupation (MOHO),[33] and Box 25.2 sets out its goals using a MOHO related framework.

Intervention with the children

We used the workshop outline 'Playing to grow'[34] (see Ch. 18), training both the community promoters and the teachers to carry out this workshop. The children made contact with their cultural heritage through the legends and stories of Mayan culture, as related by the elders.

There was one individual-specific intervention for a 2-year-old child with cerebral palsy. The child's parents and a man from the community were trained as rehabilitation promoters, using the methodology developed by David Werner,[35] one of the founders of community-based rehabilitation (see Ch. 13 and Ch. 17).

Intervention with the adolescents

The adolescents received training in carpentry and community promotion. Through carpentry they were able to obtain economic benefits and work for the community; their first projects were wooden toys for the children.

Box 25.2   Goals of the project

The volitional subsystem

The objective was to prevent the loss of goals, interests, and values. We assisted community members in analyzing their new life situation in Guatemala, looking at their strengths and problems, identifying new goals, and confronting their new reality. We encouraged the recovery of the values inherent in Mayan culture, and in their cosmovision. Finally, we attempted to promote an inner locus of control through this empowerment, thus ensuring that the villagers saw themselves as the main characters in their life stories, and as survivors. This is an especially important consideration in humanitarian interventions, since traditionally such work has adopted a paternalistic position.

The habituation subsystem

The goals were to encourage adolescents in the role of community promoters and to return the role of

'guardians of ancient wisdom' to the elders. Finally, we attempted to discourage damaging habits such as alcoholism and its consequences (such as domestic violence) by promoting healthier ways of life.

The performance subsystem

The goals were to develop new skills in emotional expression among the children, in community promotion and carpentry among the adolescents, and the recovery of the traditional weaving skills among the adult women.

The environment

The goal was to develop income generating projects in order to address poverty. One of the most meaningful goals was the recovery of the cultural cycle of the community.

Box 25.3   The training of community promoters

Training took place over 3 months, each month having a different focus: work with children, with adolescents and with adults. The training program started with 20 adolescents, and 12 completed it. They participated in the selection of the topics (shown below) that were studied:

Working with children

- Areas and phases of childhood development: physical, psychological, social, emotional
- Stimulating creativity
- How to develop a preventive mental health workshop with the children: 'Jugando para crecer' (Playing to Grow)[34]
- Child animation techniques and gestalt therapy techniques.

Working with adolescents

- Mayan culture: past – who were they? Philosophies and values
  present – the indigenous reality of Guatemala today

- Alcoholism and its prevention
- How to help adolescents arriving with the new *retornos*.

Adults

- The role of mental health promoter
- Main problems: PTSD, depression, alcoholism, domestic violence
- Observation, relaxation and listening techniques.

It was very important for the adolescents undergoing training to reflect on their own experiences before attempting to help others. They dealt with their feelings regarding the refugee experience and the return to Guatemala. After the training, they were ready to help new adolescents arriving in new *retornos*.

Training the adolescents in community promotion (outlined in Box 25.3) gave us the opportunity to work with the feelings that they had expressed. This was done in an indirect way, as they practiced dealing with feelings of anxiety, fear, and sadness. Our experience with Bosnian refugees had taught us that clinical labeling of problems sometimes serves only to bring further grief. Cultural workshops were developed, where we compared Western with Mayan values, and we arranged visits to Mayan sanctuaries, such as Yatxilan. By these means, the teenagers recovered their pride in being Mayan descendants, and were able to embrace the best of the two worlds.

We focused our intervention on the prevention of alcoholism, working through role-play that introduced discussions about alcoholism.

Intervention with the women

As tears of a nation crying, it is the way the indigenous people express their joy in nature, in life. It is the voice of the silenced Maya nation which talks through their work.

(Seen under a display of Mayan textiles at
San Cristobal de las Casas Museum, source unknown.)

It was very important for the women to realize that they could change their reality. A weaving project was developed, similar to the successful weaving projects developed by Simó Algado in the refugee camps in Bosnia. It provided a meaningful activity that helped the women to earn the money they needed to survive; it also helped them to occupy their time purposefully, rather than continually reflecting on all they had lost. The women who knew how to weave taught those who did not. In this way, and in keeping with the transcultural philosophy of occupational therapy, we helped them recover this very important aspect of their culture.

We developed our work through the women's organization, lxmucane. Psychological support was offered to the women via the adolescent girls of the community, who were trained in listening and relaxation techniques in order to work with the women's thinking habits and the relationship between thoughts, feelings, and occupations. One of the weaknesses of the project was that, despite our intention, it was not possible to train the women from the association too, as they had heavy family workloads, and needed to prioritize projects generating money, such as weaving.

We worked with teachers, training them to support the emotional wellbeing of the children. Another important weakness was that we were not able to work with the rest of the men, who spent the full day working in the fields, so we had no chance to develop a project with them related with alcoholism. However, we believe that rebuilding the cultural cycle and recovering the traditional spirituality of indigenous communities such as the Mayans has a positive impact in combating alcoholism and addiction, which can be reactions to the lack of meaning in life.[36]

Intervention with the elders

Sons, wherever you stay, do not forget what lxpiacoc taught you, because it comes from the tradition of your ancestors. If you forget you will betray your lineage.[21]

Our main goal with the elders was to assist them to recover their traditional role as guardians and transferrers of ancient wisdom. Every week after Mass the elders met with the adolescents to teach them Mayan traditions, legends, and languages. In return, the adolescents took care of the elders. The Council of Elders was created, where they could discuss their problems and how to resolve them, and how they could continue working to preserve Mayan culture.

EIGHT YEARS ON – RECONSIDERING THE PROJECT IN 2004

The new context: a deepening human and ecological crisis

The components of the natural world are myriad but they constitute a single living system. There is no escape from our interdependence with nature: we are woven into the closest relationship with the Earth, the sea, the air, the seasons, the animals and all the fruits of the Earth. What affects one, affects all – we are part of a greater whole – the body of the planet. We must respect, preserve, and love its manifold expression if we hope to survive. [37]

The anthropologist Wade Davis[38] explains that world wide, some 300 million people, roughly 5% of the global population, still maintain a strong identity as members of an indigenous culture, rooted in history and language, attached by myth and memory to a particular place on the planet. These cultures account for more than 60% of the world's languages and collectively represent over half of the intellectual legacy of humanity. Yet, increasingly, their voices are being silenced.

Today, of the roughly 6000 languages still spoken, only 600 are considered by the experts to be stable and secure. Davis[38] maintains that a language is a flash of the human spirit, the filter through which the soul of each particular culture reaches into the material world; a language is as divine and mysterious as a living creature.

In conclusion, he considers the price of this loss: 'What is the worth of family bonds that mitigate poverty and insulate individuals from loneliness? What is the value of diverse institutions about the cosmos, the realms of the spirit, the meaning and practice of faith? What is the economic measure of a ritual practice that results in the protection of a river or a forest?'[38] (p. 15)

Referring to indigenous populations, Vandana Shiva[39] asserts that because colonialism now goes under the name of development, the exploitation process is omnipresent, legitimized by international financial institutions. The most irreversible destruction is the destruction of the cultural mechanisms of indigenous populations, mechanisms that protect both the people themselves and their natural environment. When these disappear, where will we find somebody able to teach us how to walk with tenderness over the Earth?

The survival of indigenous cultures is linked with the survival of the natural environment. Wilson[40] says that the rate of extinction is more than 50 000 species a year – that is 137 a day, 6 an hour. He concludes that if exploitative human activities continue to expand at the current rates, at least 20% of the Earth's species will disappear within 30 years.

Most significant of all, perhaps, has been the unchallenged traditional assumption that the loss is inevitable in the context of the advancement of human progress.[41] We do not understand that 'you and I do not end at our fingertips or skin – we are connected through air, water and soil; we are animated by the same energy from the same source in the sky above. We are quite literally air, water, soil, energy and other livings creatures.'[42]

It is possible to conclude that we are immersed in an ecological and cultural genocide, legitimized in the name of progress and executed by the political order.

THE ROLE OF OCCUPATIONAL THERAPY

Occupational therapists who are engaged in confronting this genocide, and working with its survivors should be aware, in their practice, of emerging issues, as described below.

Culture and transcultural occupational therapy

Isabel Dyck[43] explains culture as a shared system of meanings that 'involves ideas, concepts and knowledge, and includes beliefs, values and norms that shape standards and rules of behavior as people go about their daily lives.'

Michael Iwama[44] (p. 582) asserts that 'Occupational Therapy in its current construction and the ideologies that support it may be counterproductive and even oppressive to people who perceive, construct and live their realities along different beliefs, value patterns and worldviews.' He adds: 'If Occupational Therapy is to be developed into a service to universally benefit all, more culturally relevant epistemologies, theories and practice methods may be required.'

In order to avoid repeating a colonialist approach, Western occupational therapists need to become more aware that in their practice the situated meaning of a culture is an essential core concept. Thibeault (see Ch. 17) and Fransen (see Ch. 13) assert that successful community-based rehabilitation intervention depends upon this.

Cultural relativism asserts that fundamental notions of what is considered true, or morally correct, and of what constitutes knowledge and even reality itself, are socially constructed and vary cross culturally.[45] Cultural relativism can be helpful, but must be balanced with a human rights approach, as suggested by Galheigo (see Ch. 7). A transcultural occupational therapy philosophy, which introduces culturally meaningful occupations, must be developed.

The political nature of human occupation

Cardona[19,20] pointed out that politics are concerned with people's capacity and power to construct their own destiny. Occupational therapists are concerned with enabling people to help themselves to live dignified and meaningful lives. It can be argued that indigenous people world wide are restricted in this, or denied the opportunity to do so, due to man-made disabling conditions, which Kronenberg coined occupational apartheid (see Ch. 6).[26,46–52] Engaging in processes of change that are aimed at overcoming these complex realities requires occupational therapists to become critically aware of the political nature of human occupation and to develop appropriate sociopolitical skills and roles (see Ch. 6).[51,53–58]

The social justice model of health, a participatory, community model, can be a useful tool. Wilcock[59] defines it as the promotion of social and economic change to increase individual, community, and political awareness, resources, and equitable opportunities for health.

Occupational ecology

Wilcock[59] argues that human occupation (in the sense of human activity) has been the primary force in ecological degradation, and therefore requires urgent consideration and change aimed at ecological rehabilitation.

Do Rozario[60] established an ecological vision of occupational therapy, arguing that 'occupational therapists should work towards the harmonious relationship of people with their environment by empowering individuals and communities toward health, wellbeing, and sustainability through the use of interaction, occupation, and sociopolitical action.' This statement is congruent with the Ottawa Charter for Health Promotion[61] guidelines, which recognize the inextricable links between people and their environments that constitute the basis for a socio-ecological approach to health.

The ecological sustainability model of health, defined by Wilcock[59] (p. 240) as 'the promotion of healthy relationships between humans, other living organisms, their environments, habits and modes of life' can be a useful tool for occupational therapists. Based on biological and natural sciences, it is a holistic model with much in common with social justice and community development.[62]

In establishing a new relationship with our fellow human beings, the natural environment, and the cosmos, we need to learn from indigenous peoples and from different cosmovisions, such as East Asian cosmovision. This is described by Iwama[44] as arranging deities, nature, and humans as inseparable parts of a singular entity, where one's existence is no more important or meaningful than the next entity – be it a tree, a stone, a bird, or another person.

The first author of this chapter argues the need to take this development of an occupational ecology vision further, and defines occupational ecology as awareness of the ecological genocide we are confronting, along with proactive measures, through human occupation, to restore the balance with the natural environment.

There is a need to recover this connection between ourselves, the rest of humanity, nature, and the cosmos. We can understand occupation as the dialogue between the human being and the environment. If we want to survive, this dialogue must be based on veneration and respect. An Indian prayer says that 'we humans are no better but no worse than a rock, but our mission is to sing, to sing the World, to sing the Beauty' (source unknown). Occupational therapy can be a powerful song to preserve and celebrate the beauty of the world.

The meaning of suffering, the meaning of hope

Working with populations such as the Mayan *retornos* means understanding the meaning of suffering. Suffering and trauma may be easy words to say, but they are very painful to experience. They describe personal and subjective realities for each of us. In my own (Simó Algado's) experience, suffering means the feeling of physical pain, the sadness of loss or parting from a loved one, long nights in the middle of a dark winter, my mind in a storm, feeling alone in the middle of a crowd, and asking myself why I must keep on going.

When we are confronted with suffering we need to empower the spirit with hope, for ourselves, and for the people we walk with. And it is not easy. I will always remember the time when Islam, an 18-year-old Muslim boy, explained to me how he had been tortured for 8 months in a concentration camp. I can still see clearly the tears rolling down his mother's face. How can we transmit hope in these moments?

Nature must be our guide, teaching us that sunrise comes after the long night, and a joyful spring follows the coldest winter. This is the promise of nature, the promise of life. One day, sadness is no longer beside you, and spring comes back to your heart; the storm ceases, the light is bright, and you have come back from the land of tears.

CONCLUSION

A human being is part of the whole called by us universe, a part limited in time and space. He experiences himself, his thoughts and feelings as something separated from the rest, a kind of optical delusion of his consciousness. This delusion is a kind of prison for us, restricting us to our personal desires and to affection for a few persons nearest to us. Our task must be to free ourselves from this prison by widening our circle of compassion to embrace all living creatures and the whole of nature in its beauty.[63]

The problems faced by indigenous refugees challenge the occupational therapist, demanding the use of holistic, community-centered, and transcultural methods. They also challenge us as human beings. We live in that prison of illusion that Einstein mentions; to fight for the survival of indigenous peoples and the natural environment is to fight for our own survival, for we too are under threat of extinction.

We must learn from the indigenous populations to be careful how we let our moccasins fall on Mother Earth, being careful not to step on the souls of the new generations who are waiting their turn to live. We have inherited a world pregnant with life and beauty, and we must give back to its owners, our children, a world based on ecological sustainability, justice, and love. As Thibeault[64] says, we must become social activists so that, together with the populations we have the privilege to serve, we can co-create a more beautiful future and walk toward an occupational dream (see Ch. 9) called occupational justice.

We are challenged to take responsibility for our lives, develop a new outlook on our situation, and cultivate peaceful minds and the power of the heart.[65] Demetrio Matias says: 'in life you must sing with happiness, to pay homage to the beauty of the World, like the flowers, like the breeze. Even in the middle of the polluted fog, we must shine like diamonds.'[66] (p. 17)

It was such a beautiful privilege to walk with the Mayan community: to learn that man is blue, because he is the Heaven's heart, and that woman is green, because she is the Earth's heart; and to walk alongside survivors, whose spirit is embodied in people from the community such as José and Claudín, an elder couple, or Francisca, whose son Vidal has cerebral palsy. The images of José building his house or appearing with his yellow tricycle, or of Claudin preparing the corn, are unforgettable. Their faith and thankfulness had no limits. Francisca had previously lost a child in Mexico, but she was fighting to take care of all her family in the midst of poverty, and was always willing to learn more about how to look after Vidal, or to help any other member of the community. I thank them for their beautiful gift to me, a testimony of courage and love.

This chapter is dedicated to all the people with whom we worked, and who taught us so much.

References

1. Menchú R, Burgos ER. *Me llamo Rigoberta Menchú y así me nació la conciencia.* Mexico City: Trillas; 1998.
2. Simo Algado S, Rodriguez G, Egan M. Spirituality in a refugee camp. Can J Occup Ther 1997; 64(3):138–145.
3. Anónimo. *El libro de los libros de Chilam Balam.* Mexico City: Fondo Cultura Económica; 1963.
4. Cardoza y Aragón L. *Guatemala Las Lineas de su mano.* 1st edn. Nicaragua: Nueva Nicaragua; 1985.
5. Woodward RL Jr. Guatemala. World Bibliographic Series. Oxford: Clio Press; 1992.
6. Barry T. Inside Guatemala. Albequerque, New Mexico: The Inter-Hemispheric Education Resource Center; 1992.
7. Falla R. Voices of the survivors: the massacre at finca San Francisco, Guatemala. Cambridge, MA: Cultural Survival; 1983.
8. Lovell WG. A beauty that hurts. Toronto: Between the Lines; 1995.
9. Oficina de derechos humanosdel arzobispado de Guatemala. Guatemala: nunca más. Guatemala City, Guatemala: Oficina de derechos humanosdel Arzobispado de Guatemala; 1998.
10. Aguacayo S. *Los refugiados guatemaltecos en Campeche y Quintana Roo.* Mexico City: El Colegio de Mexico; 1989.
11. Sharer RJ. The ancient Maya. 5th edn. Stanford, CA: Stanford University Press; 1994.
12. Curtis E. The North American Indians. Hong Kong: Aperture; 1972.
13. Pigem J, ed. *Nueva conciencia.* Barcelona: Integral; 1994.
14. Girard R. *Origen y desarrollo de las civilizaciones antiguas de América.* Mexico City: Editories Mexicanos Unidos; 1977.
15. Hagen V. *El mundo de los Mayas.* México City: Editorial Diana; 1986.
16. Garza Tarazona S. *La mujer mesoamericana.* México City: Editorial Planeta; 1977.
17. Bugental J. The person who is the psychotherapist. Journal of Consulting Psychology 1994; 28(3):272–277.
18. Farias P, Arana M. *Aspectos psicosociales de la desnutricion infantil entre los refugiados guatemaltecos en Chiapas.* Segundo congreso nacional de salud publica. Cuernavaca, Mexico: 1991.
19. Meléndez Cardona CE. *Análisis situaciónal de ciudadanos mexicanos y refugiados guatemaltecos en el sureste de México.* Documentos internos. Mexico City: Centro Mesoamericano para la Promoción y Educación Rural Asociación Civil (CEMPERAC); 1996.
20. Meléndez Cardona CE. *Planteamiento estratégico: refugio, retorno, reinserción de población guatemalteca.* Documentas internos. Guatemala City: Asociación de Refugiados Dispersos de Guatemala (ARDIGUA); 1999.
21. Anonymars. Popol Vuh: *el libro sagrado de los mayas.* Mexico City: Oasis; 1977.
22. Farias P, Billings D. The impact of refugee women's social status on psychological health, child mortality and malnutrition. Paper presented at the Congreso Internacional de Antropologia y Ciencias Etnologicas: Desplazamiento, La Mujer y la Crisis Global. Mexico City. 1993.
23. Miller KE. The effects of state terrorism on children. Child Development 1996; 67:89–106.
24. Saenz I. Listening to the refugees: Guatemalans in Mexico. Links 1992/1993; 9(5):24–25.
25. Melville M, Lykes B. Guatemalan Indian children and the sociocultural effects of government-sponsored terrorism. Social Science & Medicine 1992; 34:33–48.

26. Simó Algado S, Mehta N, Kronenberg F, et al. Occupational therapy intervention with children survivors of war. Can J Occup Ther 2002; 69(4):205–217.

27. Simó Algado S, Thibeault R, Urbanowsky R, Kronenberg F, Pollard N. *La terapia ocupacional en el mundo penitenciario.* Terapia Ocupacional 2003; 33:10–20.

28. Simó Algado S. *El retorno del hombre de maiz, intervención desde la terapia ocupacional con una comunidad indígena maya.* Terapia Ocupacional 2002; 28:30–35.

29. Simó Algado S, Mehta N, Kronenberg F. *Niños supervivientes de conflicto bélico.* Terapia Ocupacional 2003; 31 (April):26–40.

30. Simó Algado S, Kronenberg F. *Intervención con una comunidad indígena maya.* Materia Prima 2000; 16 (August):28–32.

31. Canadian Association of Occupational Therapists. Occupational therapy guidelines for client-centerd practice. Toronto, ON: CAOT Publications ACE; 1991.

32. Egan M, DeLaat D. Considering spirituality in occupational therapy practice. Can J Occup Ther 1994; 61(2):95–101.

33. Kielhofner G. A model of human occupation: theory and application. 2nd edn. Baltimore, MD: Williams & Wilkins; 1995.

34. Miller KE, Billings DL. Playing to grow: a primary mental health intervention with Guatemalan refugee children. American Journal of Orthopsychiatry 1994; 64:346.

35. Werner D. *El niño campesino discapacitado.* Palo Alto, CA: Fundacion Hesperian; 1990.

36. Frankl V. *El hombre en búsqueda de sentido.* Barcelona: Editorial Herder; 1964.

37. Campbell B. Human ecology – The story of our place in nature from prehistory to the present. New York: Aldine de Gruyter; 1983.

38. Davis W. Light at the edge of the world. Vancouver/Toronto: Douglas & McIntyre; 2001.

39. Shiva V. *El vínculo sagrado con la tierra.* In: Pigem J, ed. *Nueva conciencia.* Barcelona: Integral; 1994.

40. Wilson EO. The diversity of life. Cambridge, MA: Harvard University Press; 1992.

41. Livingston J. One cosmic instant. Toronto: McClelland & Steward; 1973.

42. Suzuki D. The sacred balance. Vancouver/Toronto: Greystone books; 2002.

43. Dyck I. Multicultural society. In: Jones D, Blair SE, Hartery [?] Jones TRK, eds. Sociology and occupational therapy. London: Harcourt Brace; 1998:67–80.

44. Iwama M. Toward culturally relevant epistemologies in occupational therapy. Am J Occup Ther 2003; 57(5):582–587.

45. Marshall RC. Review of the myth of Japanese uniqueness. Journal of Japan Studies 1989; (15): 266–272.

46. Kronenberg F. Street children: being and becoming. Research study. Heerlen, Netherlands: Hogeschool Limburg; 1999.

47. Kronenberg F, Simo Algado S. Overcoming occupational apartheid: working towards occupational justice. Paper presented at the sixth European Congress of Occupational Therapy. Paris. 2000.

48. Pettersen BH. *Dolphin: arbeider mot aktivitetsapartheid.* Ergoterapeuten 2000; 43(11):7–10.

49. Tilburg van O. *Dolphin en de strijd tegen occupational apartheid.* Nederlands Tijdschrift voor Ergotherapie 2001; 29(4):141–144.

50. Kronenberg F. Juggling with survivors of the street: occupational therapy and clowns in Guatemala City. Paper presented at the thirteenth WFOT congress. Stockholm. 2002.

51. Kronenberg F. In search for the political nature of occupational therapy. MSc OT paper (unpublished). Linkoping University, Sweden. 2003.

52. Kronenberg F. Occupational therapy without borders: occupational justice education. Paper presented at the ninth European Network of Occupational Therapy in Higher Education. Prague. October/November 2003.

53. Kronenberg F. Understanding and facing up to the political nature of occupational therapy. Paper presented at the seventh European Congress of Occupational Therapy. Athens. September 2004.

54. Kronenberg F. WFOT position paper on community based rehabilitation. Forrestfield, Australia: WFOT; April 2004.

55. Kronenberg F. WHO International Consultation on CBR Helsinki. Forrestfield, Australia: WFOT; August 2003.

56. Cockburn L, Trentham B. Participatory action research: integrating community occupational therapy practice and research. Can J Occup Ther 2002; 69:20–30.

57. Urbanowski R, Kronenberg F, Pollard N, Simo Algado S. The politics of occupation. Paper presented at the 2nd Canadian Occupational Science Symposium, Toronto, May 2004.

58. Goldstein J. International relations and everyday life. In: Zemke R, Clark F, eds. Occupational science: the evolving discipline. Philadelphia: FA Davis; 1996.

59. Wilcock A. An occupational perspective of health. Thorofare, NJ: Slack; 1998.

60. Do Rozario L. Keynote address. Purpose, place, pride and productivity: the unique personal and societal contribution of occupation and occupational therapy. Proceedings of the seventeenth conference of the Australian Association of Occupational Therapists Darwin. 1993.

61. World Health Organization. Health and welfare Canada. Ottawa charter for health promotion. Ottawa, Canada: Canadian Public Health Association; 1986.

62. Potter VR. Bioethics, the science of survival. Perspectives in Biology and Medicine 1980; 14:127–153.

63. Einstein A. Quotation in Walsh MD, Vaughan F. Paths beyond ego. Los Angeles: The Putnam Publishing Group; 1993:266.

64. Thibeault R. Experimental and philosophical considerations on occupation and the genesis of meaning and resilience. In: McColl MA, ed. Spirituality and occupational therapy. Ottawa: CAOT; 2003.

65. Kornfield C. *Périlles et promises de la vie spirituelle*. Paris: Editions de la Table Ronde; 1998.

66. Matias D. *Brillar como diamantes*. In: Pigem J, ed. *Nueva conciencia*. Barcelona: Integral; 1994.

Chapter 26

Muffled cries and occupational injustices in Japanese society

Hiroko Fujimoto, Michael Iwama

OVERVIEW

This chapter illuminates the social context around the experience of marginalization and occupational injustice in Japanese society by chronicling families' struggles to raise children with special needs. In particular, the plight of children who live with the help of mechanical ventilators, and their struggle to enjoy similar freedoms and meaningful occupations to those of their non-dependent counterparts, are described. These vignettes offer glimpses of the occupational injustices evident in a particular context, which readers may then use to reflect on similar injustices that occur in other locations in the world. In conclusion, occupational therapists and other professionals are encouraged to become more comprehensively involved in such cases, while at the same time being advocates for occupational justice.

INTRODUCTION: WHAT ARE OUR *COLORS*?

Each of us can be described as having a unique *color* of our own. Features like personal values, character traits, experiences, age, gender, and socio-cultural background can contribute to our color. In Japan's collectively oriented societies, where uniformity is praised, individuals strive to keep their collective color monochromatic. The group may tolerate shades of a tone, but an individual's prominence is poorly tolerated. Lighter colors are preferred for the younger and more neutral in thought, who can easily be persuaded to match the group's color. Because the group's color explains who you are, Japanese people seem mainly interested in where you belong (e.g. which university you graduated from, whom you work with, your company name and profession etc.). Having a unique color makes it very difficult to belong. And when identity and a sense of well-being are contingent on the collective, as they are in Japan, belonging is everything.

Having relationships with others and belonging to groups are arguably the most important occupations of living as a Japanese. When my daughter was born with a severe disability, I felt isolated. I felt that my family could no longer belong in the mainstream of society and that my daughter would not be able to belong with her peers because her color was very different.

Injustice becomes acutely evident in the Japanese social context when people are excluded to the margins because of their color. It can also be unjust to coerce people to change their color in order to belong to a group. As an occupational therapist, I see and work with many people living outside of mainstream society who are fighting to belong again; and their inability to belong takes an enormous toll on their collective wellbeing. One of my young clients was bullied in nursery school. The parents asked the teachers to stop the bullying. To our surprise, the parents were told that nothing would be done about it. *Their child* was the one with problems and if the parents were not satisfied with the school, they were welcome to leave. They were also told that children with disabilities should go to 'where they belong'. I believe that an important tenet of occupational therapy is to accept each person's color, and not to try to change it. Occupational therapists may also be able to help find another color that will blend well with the person's original color and illuminate it. When our clients cannot belong to groups because of their color, occupational therapists may be responsible for evaluating and working on the group (or social environment) so that they might be willing to include a new color. Too often, however, we mistakenly apply a new color that appears to work, but that actually does not match the person's original hue. Without knowing, we may have applied the color of *our* choice on our clients in order to meet *our* requirements.

In this chapter, we offer a glimpse into occupational injustices or occupational apartheid[1] (see Ch. 6) that may go on everyday in Japanese society. You may find similar injustices that happen in other locations in the world. Our focus will be around the stories of families and their children with severe disabilities. These stories can provide glimpses of the occupational injustices evident in society. All of the children described in these pages use mechanical ventilators to help them breathe. Many of their counterparts are confined to hospitals because of lack of support to help them live in the community, but the children described here have families who were pioneers in bringing their children to live outside the hospitals. Often striving with no support, they set out to prove that, despite their severe disabilities, their children belonged with their families and their communities. 'Where are the occupational therapists?' you may wonder, while reading these vignettes. It seems to us that Japanese occupational therapists are conspicuous by their absence or by their complicity in maintaining the attitudes of the status quo. In this chapter we attempt to illustrate the struggle of people with different colors to fit into the groups of their choice and participate in their everyday occupations, and we offer occupational therapists the opportunity to expand their scope of practice in order to bring down the structures that disable and marginalize their clients.

SETTING THE CONTEXT: A PERSONAL STORY
BY HIROKO FUJIMOTO

In a collective society characterized by interdependence and the need to belong, it can sometimes be difficult to know who you are and what you really want. When I got married, I became 'Fujimoto's *okusan*' (wife). Often people would not call me by my name, but called me *okusan*. When my daughter was born, I was called 'Satoko's *okaasan*' (mother). Many people also addressed me as *okaasan* (mother), including doctors, nurses, nursery teachers, physical therapists, and occupational therapists. It felt strange to be called *okaasan* by people who were as old as my own mother or people who were even younger than me. When I was addressed as *okaasan* and not by my own name, it seemed that nobody was interested in what Hiroko Fujimoto wanted or felt, but they were interested in what I as Satoko's mom wanted and felt.

Just before Satoko was born, I was told that she would be born with severe disabilities and would likely not live for long. After she was born, I had to bear the pain of my own surgery, and the pain of the prospect of losing my first daughter so soon, as well as the fact that she was severely disabled. I sat in my room in the hospital, doing my best not to cry, trying to stem the endless tide of tears yearning to flow from my eyes. During my 2 weeks in hospital after giving birth to Satoko, none of the healthcare professionals wanted to talk to me personally. They came in and out of my room to perform their regular check-ups and routines, but they did not want to talk to me about 'her'.

When my breasts started to fill with milk after giving birth, I had to use an electronic breast pump to empty them. This physical pain was no match for its emotional toll, given the knowledge that Satoko would not consume the product of my exertions. As painful as it was, I was directed by the nurses to go to a room where all the new mothers went to breast feed their babies, because this was the 'monochromatic' rule. The mothers would go to this room and wait for the nurses to bring their babies to them. I sat in the room milking my own breasts into the machine, watching all the other mothers carrying their babies in their arms in happiness. At that time, I did not know that I should be angry and protest such maltreatment. I believe I was confused, feeling vulnerable, and oblivious to such violations of justice. This is how my new life with a daughter with severe disabilities started off.

The visiting hours in the neonatal intensive care unit (NICU) were very short. I visited her three times a week, 2 hours each time, for one and a half years. Seeing her for 6 hours a week didn't qualify me to be a mother, and Satoko probably didn't realize that I was her mother. I bathed her, fed her, changed her diapers, suctioned her, and put her to sleep under the supervision of the nurses. I always felt that I had to ask for permission to do anything to my own child, and though the staff in the NICU tried hard to make me feel at home, I didn't feel like her mother for a long time. But I cared for her and acted like an ideal parent, doing the best I could, so that she would get the attention she needed from the hospital staff.

When she came home for the first time at the age of 18 months, we finally became a family and it didn't take long to adjust to it. It felt as though she had been there all the time and we could no longer imagine a life without her. The three times a week mothering suddenly became full-time mothering. I also had another role as a full-time nurse. There was practically no one who could substitute for me in taking care of Satoko because of the complex procedures and her strong demand for her mother. The longest time that I could leave Satoko was for about 30 minutes with her father, and when I came back I would find her soaked in tears and pale from lack of oxygen. I could only take a bath when she was asleep, checking and listening to the monitor sounds every now and then. I could not take a shower because it made too much noise, and I would not hear the alarms. Apart from her everyday care as a child, she needed regular suctioning, maintenance of her mechanical ventilator and oxygen machine, catheterization every 4 hours, and an enema every night. Sometimes she needed to be fed through a tube. Every night all of the equipment had to be boiled and sterilized, and every week all of the tubes for the ventilator, including her tracheostomy cannula, had to be changed and sterilized. Imagine doing all that, as well as reading her stories, singing, and playing with her, and insuring that Satoko experienced occupations suitable for children of her age. I had no time to think of what I wanted or needed, what to ask for, or the future. All I could do was to live each day, without making any mistakes.

I regret to this day that I did not ask to go into the room when Satoko lay dying. When there are problems in hospital, parents are told to go out of the room and wait outside. Major or minor medical procedures are often performed away from the parents. When Satoko's monitor showed that her condition was fatal, we were told to go outside and wait. We made her fight for her life alone. While she was receiving resuscitation, we were not there with her. When we were allowed to go into the room again, she was lying there, her chest placid, no longer in need of her mechanical ventilator. If I had had the choice, or if only I had *known* that I had the choice, I would have held her in my arms until her heart failed to beat another beat.

AYUMI'S STORY

Ayumi is a teenaged student attending her local senior high school. She is in grade 11 now and dreams of becoming a nurse. Believe it or not, all through her school years her father has always attended school with her. She uses a ventilator 24 hours a day to help her breathe, due to her neuromuscular disease. All the schools that she has attended have forbidden her from attending school independently because she needed 'medical care', and her father had to stand in readiness in a nearby classroom all day in case she needed to be suctioned. Her family, as well as volunteer groups, have been lobbying the school board all of these years to let Ayumi participate in school without a member of her family accompanying her. They have advised the school board that anyone can suction her safely, as long as health professionals train them properly, yet to this day no teachers or assistants are allowed to support Ayumi beyond the boundaries of conventional teaching.

In grade 10 Ayumi's struggle was greater than she had ever experienced. When her class went on a 3-day school trip, she was not able to bathe in their accommodation because the bathing facility was too small and not structured to meet her needs. It was decided that she would use another facility nearby and she had to be transferred to that place by car. During her trip to the bath, Ayumi was admonished for all the trouble she was causing her company and reminded of her duty to be 'thankful'. Of course it was not Ayumi's wish to be excluded from attending the night gathering with her friends, nor to travel 30 minutes each way just to be bathed.

Japanese children, especially those with disabilities, are taught not to bother or trouble other people in mainstream society, and to be thankful. Asserting their rights is discouraged. The unspoken message is that they are unwanted, that they are a burden to society. Our children, who happen to have disabilities, appear to be deemed worthless by a collective that makes them feel as if they owe a debt of gratitude to 'able-bodied' people for taking care of them.

On another occasion, one of Ayumi's teachers who had been hired to assist Ayumi with her studies in her regular classroom refused to take notes for her.

Ayumi can use a single button switch to operate her computer, but it is impossible for her to take her own notes during class. The teacher seemed to feel that because Ayumi had not got satisfactory grades in her tests, she had not been working hard enough and was not doing her homework. This showed a failure to appreciate how Ayumi actually lived her life.

Ayumi commutes to and from school with her father by train. It is around 5 p.m. when she gets home. It takes her at least 3 hours to take a bath, with all the procedures involved, and to get settled on her couch before getting ready to do her homework. This does not include any time to watch TV or have fun after school, as most other girls her age would. Her parents spend hours typing her notes into her computer so that she can use it to study, and it takes Ayumi at least twice as much time as her peers to do her homework with her single computer switch. Ayumi and her parents work way after midnight, every night, to support her studies. Her parents put aside all other housework and make Ayumi's studies a priority. Ayumi's teacher did not seem to understand what Ayumi's life outside the classroom was like. Similar predicaments can occur with occupational therapists, who might prescribe exorbitant home programs for their clients and families without really knowing and appreciating the context of their clients' occupational lives. Accusing the client of non-compliance invariably results in increasing the client's sense of guilt.

One day, Ayumi typed out the following paragraph for her father. It is not often that she talks about her life in school, but she seemed desperate to tell her father about this:

Is my suctioning machine making too much noise during class? My class-mates told me so. Actually, the classmates told the teacher and she told me that they said it was noisy. You know that you were called before the 6th period to suction me today? I didn't ask for it, but teacher said that I should

Figure 26.1 Ayumi enjoys skiing in her stretcher. She later commented that she wanted to go faster!

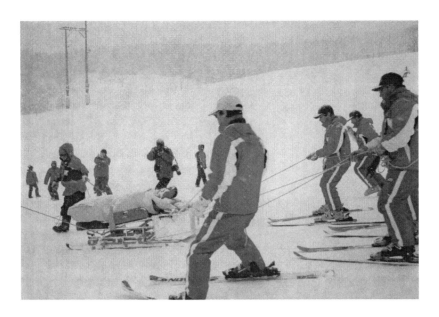

get suctioned during recess. I told her that I didn't need it, but she wouldn't listen to me. And you know that I always get suctioned in the hall (instead of in the classroom)? This is because the teacher told me to, because everyone might think it noisy.

No other student in her classroom is told to go out of their classroom to blow their nose, cough, or sneeze. Ayumi had to undergo suctioning for the sake of others' convenience, not for her own needs. Similar treatment can occur in healthcare settings. In hospitals or institutions, patients can be fed, medicated, treated, tested, or put to bed to meet the needs of healthcare professionals, rather than their own needs. Ayumi and her family have been striving against such injustice for a long time. Gradually she has been accepted as belonging in her school. Figure 26.1 shows her with her friends on a ski trip. The school has gradually become more understanding regarding Ayumi's participation in school activities. For Ayumi, it is important to be there and assert her need to participate and to be understood. Her father comments that her 'being there' makes a profound difference.

YUKIMI'S STORY

Yukimi had a progressive neuromuscular disease. She started using a mechanical ventilator when she was 2 months old. As she grew, her disease progressed and she was only able to move her eyes, eyebrows, and some of her fingertips. She communicated fully with these parts of her body. She was discharged to go home from hospital when she was 5 years old, with the help of many volunteers and supporters in her community. She attended a local nursery school and insisted on choosing and going to a local school with her peers. She loved school and her friends more than anything. Despite her parents' worries, nothing prevented Yukimi from

Figure 26.2 Yukimi in her favorite bathing suit after swimming in the river.

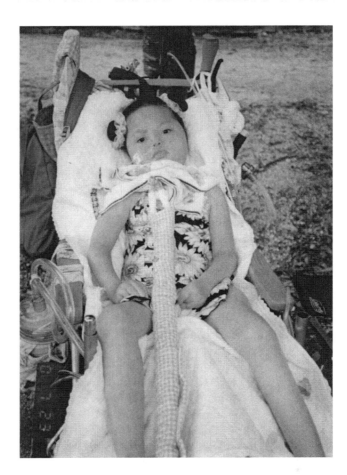

joining her friends. The children in her class soon learned voluntarily to read her 'language' and they invented many ways for Yukimi to participate in the class like everyone else. It was evident that going to school with her friends was a meaningful occupation for Yukimi and it kept her in good health. She would always get ill during her long school holidays because she could not go to school. Sadly, there were still some occasions and circumstances in which the school failed to prevent her from being marginalized from her mainstream peers.

Yukimi's school was on a hill. It was not easy for her mother to push her heavy wheelchair up the hill, so at first her brother and sister helped her to get to school. Soon, other children volunteered to help, pulling a rope that was tied to her wheelchair. Then other parents volunteered to help, too. However, teachers did not get involved in this and later it was suggested that the extra help required by students like Yukimi, with severe disabilities, prevented other students from being educated 'equally'. We can see that the 'equality' being referred to is one that excludes Yukimi.

It is very discouraging and difficult to have to explain to a child why they are being excluded when there are no tangible reasons. Yukimi loved to bathe and go to swimming pools (see Fig. 26.2). In the water, she was able to free herself and her limbs from the gravity that usually encumbered her.

It must have been a great feeling, once in a while, not to have the back of her head and back touching the sweaty seat of her wheelchair or a bed. Though she used a ventilator, her parents often took her to a local swimming pool and she often protested when it was time to come out of the water. In her school, swimming was a compulsory part of physical education, but the school decided that she could not participate in the class due to her health problems. Yukimi's home doctor, who had been seeing her since she was born, could find no reason to preclude Yukimi from participating in swimming classes, but the school insisted, reasoning that Yukimi had a high pulse rate, and that swimming could be dangerous for people with heart problems. So, she had to sit in the hot, humid Japanese summer for 2 hours each time watching her friends play happily in splashes of refreshing water. How could this 6-year-old child understand why she couldn't participate in occupations her friends enjoyed?

The image of a 6-year-old girl feeling the cruel realities of her limitations and disability is very sad. As an occupational therapist, I strive to empower our children by uncovering ways to maximize their occupational possibilities. Many children, however, are forced to learn to live within their limits in an unjust society. For Yukimi to ascend to the classrooms on the second floor of her school, it would take at least two and maybe as many as four people to carry her wheelchair and all of her equipment, including her ventilator, suctioning machine, and batteries. There are no elevators in the school. Though it would have been possible if a couple of adults had volunteered to carry her upstairs, the school wouldn't allow her to go upstairs because it seemed dangerous to them. Yukimi ended up staying alone with her assistant teacher in a separate room when her classmates went upstairs once a week during library hour. She was very much hurt by this decision, since joining in and spending time with her friends was a meaningful activity. She insisted that she would not stay confined in a room to wait for her friends, so she went to the bottom of the staircase. This way, she was able to 'walk' with her friends until they climbed the stairs without her and she would meet them as soon as the class finished upstairs. Later on, she told her mother, 'I wanted to go up with my friends,' but concluded, 'it is impossible.'

Occupational deprivation[2] and occupational coercion[3] into meaningless occupations can affect our health physically and mentally. When injustice is done, we try to adapt and cope with our life by becoming numb to our feelings and desires. As a consequence, we can become mentally unstable, lose self-confidence, feel incompetent, and even lose the ability to engage in meaningful occupations. It was of great concern to Yukimi when she found out that the second graders always used classrooms on the second floor. Her friends worried for her too. She was very scared that she would not be able to move up to second grade because of this. By the end of her first year, she still did not know how her concerns were going to be addressed. The night of her last day in school before the spring holidays (after which the new school year begins in Japan), she felt very ill. Two days later she passed away. She had symptoms of autointoxication, which she often had during her long holidays. This time, the symptoms were just too strong to overcome.

CONCLUSION

As occupational therapy continues its rapid expansion in Japan, making it perhaps the fastest growing occupational therapy enterprise in the world,[4] its practitioners and academics have largely yet to acknowledge and act upon commonplace occupational injustices that occur daily in Japanese society. Since the mid 1960s, when it was introduced to Japan's healthcare system, Japanese occupational therapy has maintained its strong skill-based scope of practice within the ideological framework of modern biomedicine.

Living and working in Japan as an occupational therapist and as a mother of a child with severe disabilities, I have become acutely aware of the many injustices that affect our own clients and other people in our society. Our challenge as occupational therapists who have been trained to enable our clients to live better lives, is to understand how to deal with injustices. People from all walks of life, from infants to elders, whose needs for fulfillment and wellbeing are social and occupational in nature, are overlooked for the sake of medically defined and prioritized needs. Occupational therapists, who naturally want to support their clients, come to realize that there is very little that they can do to meet their clients' needs. We too have our color, and might find the prospect of deviating from the monochrome too daunting.

Occupational therapists in Japan have yet to reconcile professional ideals that are moving increasingly toward occupation with a health system that persists in defining health according to disease and impairment. We need to recognize what occupational injustice is, refrain from participating in it, and garner the courage to fight it. There are so many injustices that we see and feel everyday, that occur right in front of us and not necessarily in some *other* location, and this is not just limited to Japan. We also need to employ a social perspective in our conventional approaches that seeks to understand how our own culture has developed affinity with and gives value to collectivism and social harmony. In Japan, social homogeneity and sameness are celebrated, and those who fall outside the boundaries of 'normal' are further stigmatized and subsequently marginalized.

Occupational justice[5] compels us to expand the content and meaning of occupational therapy philosophy and practice in a direction that society can understand and embrace, and thus helps to redefine occupational therapy's identity, which remains, at best, ambiguous in Japan. Most importantly, we wish to petition occupational therapists to distance themselves from societal forces that serve to stigmatize, oppress, and marginalize their clients, no matter what their color. May we truly bring tangible hope to those who await the emergence of occupational therapy's identity, which carries the promise of justice.

References

1. Kronenberg F. Street children: being and becoming. Research study. Heerlen, The Netherlands: Hogeschool Limburg; 1999.

2. Wilcock AA. An occupational perspective of health. NJ: Slack; 1998:145–149.

3. Fujimoto H, Takahashi R, Iwama M. Occupational justice – *sagyo joutai wo honrai arubeki sugatani*.

[Occupational justice – recognizing the state of occupational life of our clients.] Abstract. J Jpn Occu Ther 2003; 22(1):608.

4. Iwama MK. Toward culturally relevant epistemologies in occupational therapy. Am J Occup Ther 2003; 57(5):587.

5. Townsend EA, Wilcock AA. Occupational justice. In: Christiansen C, Townsend E, eds. Introduction to occupation: the art and science of living. Upper Saddle River, NJ: Prentice Hall; 2003:243–273.

Chapter **27**

The Occupational Therapy International Outreach Network
Supporting occupational therapists working without borders

Elise Newton, Beth Fuller

OVERVIEW

OTION, the Occupational Therapy International Outreach Network, is an internet-based network established in 2001 under the auspices of the World Federation of Occupational Therapists (WFOT). The OTION network currently consists of over 1600 occupational therapists and students, with connections in more than 120 countries throughout the world.

OTION's vision is an international network of occupational therapists working together to support and resource their colleagues in 'developing' countries and other challenging settings, for example working with people in marginalized situations in 'developed' countries. OTION aims to raise awareness about the needs and challenges in these settings; to facilitate the exchange of information and learning; and to enhance the contribution of occupational therapists in creating enabling and self-empowering environments. Ultimately, OTION should expand to include the many other professionals and organizations that work in this area.

The OTION story is an example of occupational therapists thinking globally and acting locally. It demonstrates how a simple idea can have a far-reaching impact. In this chapter we describe how and why OTION was developed, how it responds to the needs of occupational therapists working in developing countries, and how it can continue to evolve in the future. We hope the OTION story will encourage and inspire others around the world to share their visions and put their ideas into action. As Dom Hélder Câmara says so eloquently, 'when we dream alone, it remains a dream. But when we dream together, it is the beginning of a reality.'[1]

INTRODUCTION – WHY WAS OTION DEVELOPED?

The acronym OTION, pronounced 'ocean', captures the spirit and aims of the OTION network. The ocean is a connection between all occupational therapists around the world. Whether it is the Pacific Ocean, the Mediterranean Sea, the Amazon River, or simply the rain, we share the one body of water and it touches all of us. OTION symbolizes this connectedness and our shared responsibility to support our colleagues around the world and, through them, the individuals and communities they aspire to serve.

OTION is an international outreach network, a global forum for occupational therapists to 'reach out' to each other; to make contact and to become aware of the needs and challenges facing their colleagues; to share information and resources; to learn from each other; and, most importantly, to provide support and assistance when this is required.

OTION's concept of outreach is based on equality, respect, solidarity, and a commitment to mutual learning and development. Outreach is a two-way process. It is a conscious statement that OTION is not about the 'more established' or 'developed' parts of the profession helping or leading the 'less established' or 'developing' parts. OTION is about walking together for the mutual benefit of the profession as a whole and, ultimately, for the benefit of the individuals and communities occupational therapists work with around the world.

Recognition of the need for outreach was based on the first hand knowledge and experience of the founders of OTION of the realities of working in developing countries, realities that apply equally when working with marginalized or vulnerable groups in developed countries. These realities affect both locally trained occupational therapists and those trained elsewhere. They include professional isolation and lack of resources on the one hand, and the challenge of a complex social, cultural, economic, and political environment on the other.

At this point it is important to clarify our use of the terms 'developing' and 'developed' in relation to different countries. These terms are used because, in our view, they are the most commonly understood and relatively accepted terms for low-income and high-income countries. We acknowledge the inadequacies of the terms and point to the paradox that many people in 'developed' countries face circumstances akin to those in 'developing' countries, and vice versa.

PROFESSIONAL ISOLATION AND LACK OF RESOURCES

The problem of professional isolation is not confined to developing countries. In Australia, for example, many occupational therapists work alone in rural and remote areas.[2,3] This is increasingly recognized and action is being taken at various levels to facilitate the access of allied health and medical workers to resources, educational opportunities, professional support, and mentoring. Networking and technology are important elements of the response.[4,5] However, in many developing countries the occupational therapy profession is less established and has only very small numbers of therapists. In these countries, therapists often lack the organizational and structural resources to address the impacts of professional isolation.

In Bangladesh, a country of 138 million people, there are currently approximately 25 locally trained therapists and two therapists trained abroad. In Cambodia, a country of 13 million people, there are only four or five occupational therapists, all trained abroad, working with various non-government organizations. These therapists work in a situation where they have little access to clinical resources and few opportunities for continuing education. They are also largely without professional support and mentoring. Furthermore, the fledgeling nature of the profession and a limited understanding of the role of occupational therapy by governments and healthcare systems mean that day-to-day practice can seem like an insurmountable challenge. The experiences of Josne Ara Begum (a Bangladeshi occupational therapist), and Beth Fuller, one of the authors of this chapter, (an Australian occupational therapist), who both worked in Bangladesh highlight some of these issues in Case studies 27.1 and 27.2.

CASE STUDY 27.1   JOSNE ARA'S STORY

Josne Ara Begum trained as an occupational therapist in Bangladesh in the mid 1970s. Much of her early work involved the rehabilitation of Bangladeshi 'freedom fighters' who had survived the war with Pakistan in 1971. Of the small cohort of occupational therapists and physiotherapists trained at that time, all except Josne Ara and some of the physiotherapists left Bangladesh to work in countries like Canada and America.

Beth Fuller writes:

When I met Josne Ara Begum in January 1998 I encountered a quietly spoken, tired-looking woman, running a small clinic for children in a large room in desperate need of renovation, in the huge and chaotic public hospital in Dhaka. The furniture and therapy equipment, hidden under thick layers of dust, told of a once-thriving occupational therapy department. Josne Ara was only using a small corner of the room for her work. She was desperately keen for the occupational therapy students being taught at a local non-government organization, the Center for the Rehabilitation of the Paralyzed, to graduate. She would then have some colleagues again after having been the only occupational therapist in a country of 138 million people for the previous two decades. Sadly, Josne Ara died of cancer just 1 year after the first students graduated. The department has since been absorbed by the physiotherapists, as the government has not yet approved the establishment of occupational therapy positions in the hospital. This ongoing issue is now being managed by a new generation of Bangladeshi occupational therapists, with support and assistance from the foreign-trained volunteers who work with them.

(Used with permission of Josne Ara Begum's family)

Josne Ara is the perfect example of a locally-trained therapist who would have benefited enormously from contact and support from the international occupational therapy community. In 1998, as a volunteer at the Center for the Rehabilitation of the Paralyzed in Bangladesh, Beth Fuller learnt that the need for contact and support from the international occupational therapy community was also great for therapists trained abroad. She describes her experience in Case study 27.2.

CASE STUDY 27.2   BETH FULLER'S STORY

As a young therapist, and after having been in Bangladesh for only a few months, I found myself responsible for the coordination of the occupational therapy course; supervising interns and students in the hospital and on clinical placements in rural villages; supporting occupational therapy assistants in the hospital; and coordinating the team of foreign volunteer occupational therapists who stayed for approximately 6 months. My main objective for the year was upgrading the existing diploma level qualification to a degree level. This process involved 10 months of negotiations with Dhaka University regarding the rationale for this change, and then working with the WFOT Education Committee to have the curriculum recognized.

Working in Bangladesh as a therapist trained abroad meant working without clinical supervision and without the materials and resources I was accustomed to; being placed in a position where I was considered the 'expert' and expected to train and supervise others regardless of my own level of experience; undertaking tasks I had never imagined I would be doing; and facing hurdles and challenges that frequently seemed far beyond my capacity to address.

Josne Ara Begum and Beth Fuller made a significant contribution to their clients and to the profession in Bangladesh and they are by no means isolated examples. However, achieving the goals of pioneering occupational therapists around the world often requires the contributions of many people over a period of years or decades. In Bangladesh, the employment of paid occupational therapists in public hospitals is one such example. It is our conviction that many occupational therapists working in challenging settings around the world would benefit from the support of the international occupational therapy community, particularly through facilitating exchanges between therapists addressing the issue of professional isolation in different countries and settings.

THE CHALLENGE OF OCCUPATIONAL THERAPY PRACTICE IN A COMPLEX ENVIRONMENT

In addition to professional isolation and lack of resources, occupational therapists working in developing countries face a further challenge. The social, cultural, economic, and political environments they work in give rise to a multitude of complex and varied factors that impact directly and indirectly on individuals and communities. These factors range from the economic and social impact of globalization to national government health spending, and from cultural beliefs about health, illness, and disability to local practices such as cooking.

Providing effective intervention in this context is an ongoing challenge. The complex environment itself may adversely affect the impact of occupational therapy intervention. An occupational therapist may work with a girl with cerebral palsy to enable her to hold a pencil and form letters, but if she is not allowed to enrol in school due to legislation or policy, the therapy will have minimal impact. An occupational therapist may help a man with quadriplegia learn to use a sewing machine, but if he cannot access a loan to buy his own sewing machine because the bank thinks that disability is a curse, or if he cannot work in the tailoring factory because of poor accessibility, the therapy has not greatly improved his situation.

Addressing the practical and lived reality of an individual or a community in a developing country can take its toll on a therapist. Many who work in these settings were trained within educational models and frameworks based on circumstances found in developed countries. These may not always have prepared them adequately for working in a very different context. Clinical interventions such as teaching a girl with cerebral palsy to hold a pencil or teaching a man with quadriplegia to use a sewing machine simply do not go far enough. Occupational therapy intervention requires broader skills such as policy development, training, project management, and advocacy.

Kirsten Cresswick is an Australian occupational therapist who has worked in Cambodia for many years. Her previous role as 'advisor for children with disabilities' with the Disability Action Council (DAC) involved clinical intervention as well as consulting and training. The DAC plays a key role in coordinating, facilitating, and networking between individuals, organizations, government, and other institutions working for the wellbeing of people with disabilities in Cambodia. In Case study 27.3 Kirsten describes some of the factors that impacted on her work of establishing community accommodation for abandoned children with disabilities.

CASE STUDY 27.3

There are many factors that impact on the task of setting up community accommodation for children with disabilities in Cambodia. Attitudes about disability are founded on cultural beliefs but, in the case of Cambodia, they are also influenced by other factors such as war. There may be a higher level of empathy for people with disabilities because of the large number of people disabled by land mines. However, this is often associated with feelings of pity, which can also be a negative thing.

In Cambodia children in general, and children with disabilities in particular, are not always valued highly by society. There has been a reluctance to provide funding for issues relating to children's rights, such as access to education or improving quality of life. There has been a lack of understanding too about the need for community integration, given the fact that orphanage accommodation is seen to be more than adequate.

Another factor is attitudes of people, and in my experience particularly the older generation. During the war Cambodians were discouraged from making decisions, thinking for themselves, and because of the nature of war, had great difficulty thinking about the future. This can be seen today in people's inclination toward apathy, and reluctance to take risks, or to try something new and possibly to fail. Even Cambodia's closest neighbors, such

> *as Thailand, have very different experiences and, therefore, comparisons can be hard to make or learn from. Local funds are insufficient to sustain many programs, and people are reluctant to think of creative ways to sustain even relatively small programs.*
>
> *As a result of these and many other factors, progress toward these children making the transition from institutional to community living is very slow. There must be ownership, will, and commitment from within government and the community for this change to occur and be sustainable. In the meantime, non-government organizations, individuals, and international bodies continue to provide a large percentage of the support for people with disabilities in Cambodia, a situation that may in turn be a factor impeding change.*
>
> (K Cresswick, personal communication, 2004)

OTION emerged as a practical response to the needs of both local and foreign therapists in developing countries, which arise from the work in these complex and frequently isolated settings. The initiative was based on the assumption that if this isolation could be reduced, practice would be enhanced, therapists would feel more supported to remain in these challenging settings, and solidarity within the profession around the world would be strengthened.

FROM VISION TO REALITY – HOW DID OTION COME ABOUT?

OTION is a grass roots initiative of Australian occupational therapists and occupational therapy students. The April 1999 Occupational Therapy Australia National Conference in Canberra included among its themes the fostering of networking opportunities. A group of therapists and students who had worked in countries including Samoa, India, Bangladesh, and Cambodia, and others with an interest in this work, took advantage of the conference's goal of facilitating networking opportunities for delegates, and held a meeting to discuss 'occupational therapy in developing countries'.

The group quickly became aware of the many connections between Australian occupational therapists and occupational therapists around the world. They spoke of the great resources being developed; the wonderful work occurring under difficult conditions in developing countries; the insufficient number of therapists; and the lack of general awareness within the profession of the needs and challenges facing their colleagues.

Communication, networking, and access to information emerged as three significant areas of need. It became obvious that the most affordable and accessible means of contemporary communication, the internet, was the medium through which this support network would be possible. Thus the idea of OTION was born: a very pragmatic response to an identified need and one that is perhaps typical of the practical way that occupational therapists address problems. OTION simply aimed to show support and solidarity with occupational therapists working in very challenging settings; to encourage other occupational therapists to contribute to this work; to raise awareness about the inequities within the profession; and to work within existing professional structures to achieve this.

A small team of volunteers from the group took up the challenge of nurturing this vision into reality. One email to the international occupational therapy list server (http://www.otdirect.co.uk/images/occupther.txt) provoked a steady stream of emails from occupational therapists around the world interested in supporting the initiative. A list of contacts was started, and soon it became possible to respond to inquiries by putting people in touch with each other. The many hundreds of inquiries received confirmed the need for the proposed website.

In May 2000 a detailed project proposal and request for funding was submitted to the WFOT Council Meeting in Japan. The WFOT agreed to fund the development and maintenance of an OTION website and included OTION within its International Cooperation Program. In April 2001, 2 years after its conception, the OTION website was online. The interactive networking database and discussion forums were added a short time later. OTION was formally presented and launched internationally at the 2002 WFOT World Congress in Sweden.

OTION now operates through an internet site linked to the WFOT website (www.wfot.org). The OTION website creates a 'virtual global village', where occupational therapists from around the world can communicate, share information and resources, learn from each other and provide mutual support. To register with OTION, users simply complete and submit an online registration form. This enables access to the OTION website and its three main features: networking, discussion, and access to information.

A unique feature of OTION is the ability to make contact with other members. Information provided by members on the online registration form becomes part of the OTION networking database. This enables members to search under various categories, such as country or clinical area, generating a list of members who match the desired criteria. It is then possible to make direct contact with a person from this list by email. This feature has many practical benefits. For example, a therapist preparing to begin volunteer work in Nepal could make contact, even before leaving home, with others who are currently working in the country or the region or who had previously worked there. OTION also provides a valuable means of networking for occupational therapists in countries where there is no established professional association.

The OTION discussion forums have been very well used. Members are able to post a message online that can then be responded to by others. This area is regularly used to discuss a range of issues from the clinical to the ethical, the professional to the personal. Occupational therapists from around the world discuss issues ranging as broadly as mental health in India, jobs in Madagascar, occupational therapy in forensic settings, HIV/AIDS, student and volunteer placements, cerebral palsy home programs, asylum seekers, wheelchair distribution in Viet Nam, forthcoming conferences and events, and much more.

There is a wealth of information and resources available to support occupational therapists working in developing countries, and with marginalized populations. OTION makes this information more accessible by creating a central point of reference. The OTION resource directory provides links to relevant web-based resources, reference material, study options and more. This is directed specifically to occupational therapists who may have limited access to the internet, so resources can be found quickly. OTION also provides information to occupational therapists interested in working in developing countries, including links to organizations that publicize voluntary and paid positions.

Feedback about the OTION website from users and the WFOT has been very positive. Plans for a thorough evaluation of the website are under way, and will lead to further developments and improvements.

OTION IN THE NEW MILLENNIUM – AN EVOLVING MISSION AND VISION

OTION needs to evolve constantly in response to emerging needs, challenges, and opportunities. It has undergone many developments since its conception in 1999 but the possibilities for future enhancement are endless. It will take the contribution of many different people over many years to realize its full potential.

An immediate priority is ensuring OTION's ongoing sustainability. The voluntary commitment that brought OTION into being is not sustainable over the long-term. Strengthening the partnership with WFOT and sourcing appropriate sponsorship is vital. Broadening participation in OTION's management and direction by occupational therapists around the world is another important objective. A further goal is to develop partnerships with key stakeholders such as disability organizations, volunteer agencies, and government and non-government organizations.

The authors of this chapter have managed and steered OTION since its conception in 1999. Over this time we have identified a number of areas where, in our opinion, OTION and the profession could do better in supporting occupational therapists around the world. These include: contributing to the discourse around reconceptualizing the way occupational therapists work in developing countries; further developing OTION's potential to overcome professional isolation; and creating environments that promote occupational justice.[6] This list, discussed below, is by no means exhaustive, but represents the particular vision we have at this time for OTION's ongoing contribution to supporting occupational therapists working without borders.

Reconceptualizing the way occupational therapists work in developing countries

Occupational therapists need to develop an approach to working in developing countries that is appropriate to the unique circumstances found there. As discussed earlier, these include very low numbers of therapists and healthcare workers; populations that live predominantly in rural and remote areas and have little access to health care; inadequately funded health and social welfare sectors; governments that may not fully understand the contribution that can be made by health professionals; stigma about illness and disability; and widespread poverty. They also include the health and social impacts of forces beyond the control of individuals and communities, such as globalization, war and conflict, and international political and economic processes in the areas of trade, employment, and manufacturing.[7–12]

Occupational therapists need to expand their role beyond traditional clinical treatment to include broader capacity building and community development functions. This may involve adopting community-based rehabilitation (CBR) approaches and training people in the community to carry out therapy. It could include working to reduce stigma about disability, and lobbying, in collaboration with disabled people's organizations, for educational and workplace reforms and legislative change (see Ch. 24). Kirsten Cresswick, in her work with the DAC in Cambodia, provides a good example. Effectively fulfilling this role requires additional knowledge and skills in areas such as political, economic, and development processes, CBR, occupational apartheid and occupational justice, population health, health promotion, community development, capacity building techniques, and advocacy.[6,13–15]

These broader roles, in line with the CBR approach, also demand that occupational therapists work more collaboratively with other health and disability professionals, government and non-government organizations, and those outside the health and disability sectors. No single profession or service can deal with the multitude of issues at play in developing countries, and partnerships at all levels are vital. There is great potential for OTION to be broadened to include others working in this area, such as other allied health professionals, medical workers, teachers, primary healthcare workers, disabled people's organizations, non-government organizations, and government policy advisors. This expanded network would greatly increase the potential for collaboration, information exchange, and sustainable outcomes. Already, some Australian physiotherapists have expressed their interest in OTION and have presented this model to their profession internationally.

Overcoming professional isolation

Overcoming professional isolation requires a high level of awareness and interest within the profession of the particular needs and challenges in these settings, and encouraging the profession at individual, national, and international levels to become actively involved in alleviating this isolation in practical ways.

Individuals can become OTION members, and monitor the discussion forums on the OTION website to assist with inquiries from colleagues around the world. For example, an occupational therapist in a remote part of Africa requested ideas about expanding her role in a school for disabled children and a therapist working in a similar service in India responded to this. Offers to conduct tasks such as background research or locating resources could extend this contribution and practical assistance even further. Using contacts made through the OTION discussion forums or networking database, occupational therapists or students from different parts of the world could become 'email buddies', and share with and support each other.

Another function in which OTION could play a greater role is facilitating support of occupational therapists who are working in, or have returned from, particularly challenging settings. The risk of emotional trauma arising from such work is very real and the need for support and supervision is common.[16] Occupational therapists can use OTION to make contact with others who have worked, or are working, in similar settings and this may be a useful avenue for support. It should be noted, however, that this is not a substitute for more formal debriefing that may also be required.

There are also many opportunities for action at the national and international level. Professional publications can provide greater exposure to the work of occupational therapists around the world. Financial assistance to attend conferences and participate in continuing education would provide opportunities for therapists from developing countries to present and discuss their work. There is also great potential for further partnerships between universities, clinical services, and professional associations around the world.

Creating environments that promote occupational justice

The primary goal of occupational therapy is creating environments and conditions that enable people to participate in the occupations of daily life. Addressing the specific factors that prevent or hinder a person or community from engaging in the occupations of daily life, conceptualized in this book as 'occupational apartheid' (see Ch. 6), in our opinion should be 'core business' for an occupational therapist. Working alongside survivors of occupational apartheid to address and overcome the source of these factors is an area where occupational therapists should be much more proactive. Developing a working knowledge of the concepts of occupational apartheid and occupational justice is an important first step.

Creating occupational opportunities is integral to addressing occupational apartheid and achieving occupational justice. In many settings there is a long way to go to create environments that allow all people to become integrated into their local and broader communities and lead full occupational lives. In order to create occupational opportunities, occupational therapists need to identify, support, or establish initiatives that address the sources of occupational apartheid[17] (see Ch. 6). This could include projects such as working with microfinance schemes to ensure disabled people have access to small loans; ensuring that benefits of other development activities in the community are accessible to disabled people; and working with religious leaders to ensure places of worship are accessible and that superstitious myths which add to the stigma of disability are dispelled. Working to build capacity within the community for the full integration of disabled people is also important. Arole et al[18] argue that communities that are strong and self-determining are more empowered to support the needs of vulnerable members.

The scenarios presented earlier in the chapter can also illustrate this point. The occupational therapist working with the girl with cerebral palsy needs to consider working with governments or local communities, or advocating for changes to legislation to enable access to education for disabled children, in addition to direct clinical intervention. The therapist working with the man with quadriplegia may, in conjunction with the man and a local disabled people's group, lobby for access to microcredit loans for people with disabilities, or lobby for safer practices on building sites to reduce the incidence of this type of injury for others. Occupational therapists bring strength to this lobbying by offering a clinical evidence base to support the argument.

Setting up or working alongside disabled people's organizations is a powerful way to create occupational opportunities for individuals and communities. These organizations raise awareness about the issues that create barriers to occupational opportunities, and lobby for the implementation of appropriate responses. Disabled people's organizations are active at local, national, and international levels, so it should not be hard to find a group you can work with or support. Disabled Peoples' International (which can be accessed at http://www.dpi.org) is a good starting point.

Other international government and non-government organizations are also working actively to create occupational opportunities that empower people in marginalized situations around the world. These include the International Labor Organization, the World Health Organization, Oxfam International, and Amnesty International. Occupational therapists can find out about the policies and activities of these organizations, and contribute to their respective regional and country projects.

CONCLUSION

The strength of OTION's response to the task of supporting occupational therapists around the world is that it is a practical, grassroots, demand-driven tool that has enormous possibilities for networking and resource sharing. Ultimately, it is the hope of all those involved in establishing OTION that our direct support of occupational therapists will lead to the development of occupational justice for the individuals, groups, and communities with whom they work.

In this chapter we have outlined some of the realities facing occupational therapists working in developing countries and other challenging settings around the world. We focused on the issues of professional isolation, lack of resources, and the challenge of occupational therapy in a complex environment. Our conclusions lead us to propose three key issues for discussion and debate where, we believe, OTION and the occupational therapy profession can make a further contribution. These concern the need to reconceptualize the way occupational therapists work in developing countries; the need to further develop measures to alleviate professional isolation; and the need to create environments that promote occupational justice.

These issues in turn demand greater networking and collaboration with organizations and professionals outside occupational therapy. OTION is well placed to facilitate networking and collaboration among a much broader network, and a much broader range of issues. We look forward to the next stage in OTION's development, and hope that the OTION story has inspired others to join us. We can only repeat the statement of Dom Hélder Câmara quoted at the beginning of our chapter: 'when we dream alone, it remains a dream. But when we dream together, it is the beginning of a reality.'[1]

Dedication

We dedicate this chapter to two groups of occupational therapists. First, to those pioneers who are sharing their occupational therapy skills and their energy with people around the world. May your contribution and commitment inspire us all. Second, to the many occupational therapists whose support, encouragement, and participation has helped make the shared vision of OTION become a global reality.

References

1. Câmara DM. Undated. Online. Available: http://www.domhelder.com.br/ingles

2. Lannin N, Longland S. Critical shortage of occupational therapists in rural Australia: changing our long-held beliefs provides a solution. Austr Occup Ther J 2003; 50(3):184–187.

3. Hodgson L. Resourcing rural allied health: implications of the evaluation of the Allied Health Outreach Support Service. In: Gregory G, Murray D, eds. Rural and remote Australia: health for all by the year 2000. Fourth National Rural Health Conference. Canberra: National Rural Health Alliance; 1998:603–610.

4. McDonald J, Hannaford J, Cockfield G. The suitability of online technology to meet the professional development needs of rural and remote allied health professionals. In: Lennox D. Third biennial Australian rural and remote health scientific conference. Infront outback: evaluation and outcomes – making a difference in the bush. Toowoomba: Cunningham Center and Darling Downs Health Service Foundation; 1996:8.12–8.17.

5. Harvey D, Webb-Pullman J, Strasser R. Rural health support, education and training program (RHSET): where to now? Austr J Rural Health 1999; 7(4):240.

6. Townsend EA, Wilcock AA. Occupational justice. In: Christiansen C, Townsend E, eds. Introduction to occupation: the art and science of living. Upper Saddle River, NJ: Prentice Hall; 2003:243–273.

7. Turmusani M. Disabled people and economic needs in the developing world: a political perspective from Jordan. Aldershot: Ashgate; 2003.

8. Thomas M, Thomas MJ. Editorial. An overview of disability issues in South Asia. Asia Pacific Disability Rehabilitation Journal 2002; 13(2):62–82. Online. Available: http://213.203.162.14/old_sito/english/apdrj/July%202002-APDRJ.pdf

9. Abe-Nagata KK. Disability in East Timor and Cambodia. Asia Pacific Disability Rehabilitation Journal 2002; 13(1). Online. Available: http://www.aifo.it/old_sito/english/apdrj/Journal1-02/briefreports.htm#DISABILITY

10. Coleridge P. Community-based rehabilitation in a complex emergency: study of Afghanistan. In: Thomas M, Thomas MJ, eds. Selected readings in community-based rehabilitation. Series 2. Disability and rehabilitation issues in South Asia. Bangalore, India: National Printing Press; 2002:35–49 (Occasional publication of the Asia Pacific Disability Rehabilitation Journal). Online. Available: http://www.aifo.it/old_sito/english/apdrj/January%202002%20Selected%20Readings%20CBR%20II.pdf

11. Metts RL. Disability issues, trends and recommendations for the World Bank. 2000. Online. Available: http://wbln0018.worldbank.org/HDNet/HDdocs.nsf/65538a343139acab85256cb70055e6ed/33ed2bea9901edd6852568a20069e1c1/$FILE/Metts.pdf

12. Inclusion International. Disability, development and inclusion in international development cooperation: analysis of disability-related policies and research at selected multilateral and bilateral institutions.

Undated. Online. Available: http://www.inclusion-international.org/docs/pdfs/DandDanal.pdf

13. Wilcock A. An occupational perspective on health. Thorofare, NJ: Slack; 1998.

14. Thibeault R, Hebert MA. A congruent model for health promotion in occupational therapy. Occup Ther Int 1997; 4(4):271–293.

15. Twible R, Henley E. Preparing occupational therapists and physiotherapists for community-based rehabilitation. In: Thomas M, Thomas MJ, eds. Selected readings in CBR. Series 1. CBR in transition. Bangalore, India: National Printing Press;

2000:109–126 (Occasional publication of the Asia Pacific Disability Rehabilitation Journal).

16. Hewison C. Working in a war zone: the impact on humanitarian health workers. Aust Fam Physician 2003; 32(9):679–681.

17. Kronenberg F. Street children: being and becoming. Research study. Heerlen, The Netherlands: Hogeschool Limburg; May 1999.

18. Arole M, Arole R, Taylor CE. Jamkhed: a comprehensive rural health project. Oxford: Macmillan Education; 1994.

SECTION 4

Critical education and research

INTRODUCTION

In presenting discussion of research into and development of critical educational approaches to occupational apartheid, it is inevitable that we should turn to South Africa. Duncan, Buchanan, and Lorenzo (Ch. 29) describe how occupational therapists learning to work in the new context of a democratic society are prepared for political literacy. The link the University of Cape Town program makes between political literacy and the moral development of the student is of considerable significance for a profession whose antecedents include moral therapy. These issues are further underlined in Galvaan's chapter (Ch. 32), also from South Africa, an account of research into the lives of domestic workers whose needs are totally submerged in supporting their employers' daily living. And if there were any doubt about the centrality of politics to occupational therapy practice and education, it is made clear in Barros, Lopes, Galheigo, and Galvani's exposition (Ch. 30) of the Metuia project's social program of occupational therapy education, which engages with people whose most prioritized need is social inclusion, and finding the equipment to support themselves in advocating their rights.

These experiences are difficult and uncomfortable reading. Even for editors who have worked with human extremes consequent upon war and poverty, these examples of people asserting their basic rights in conditions of legitimated inhumanity are deeply shocking. Nonetheless, it might still be easy to dismiss them as something from another world, far removed from the comfortable and safe democracies many of this book's readers will come from. On the other hand, when one is immersed in the political activities of daily life which entail enabling people to maintain their integrity in the chaotic and dangerous environments to which they have been dismissed, it can be easy to assume that everyone in the wealthier societies lives a life free of real problems of social exclusion. The editors' own chapter (Ch. 31) draws together experiences narrated by several individual therapists working in both prosperous and impoverished societies, who have come to a realization and application of their awareness of occupational apartheid that enables them to address the needs of people who have hitherto been overlooked as partners for interventions.

The first principle we set out in Chapter 1, 'everyone is responsible for everything', has to be worked thoroughly through the educative practice underpinning an occupational therapy without borders. Thus, writing from the United States, Wood, Hooper, and Womack (Ch. 28) consider how an educational program centered on occupation addresses the principles and ethic of occupational justice and makes this explicit as a core of responsible practice. Also amongst the principles outlined earlier in this book are demands for recognition of the dependence of a public ethic on a personal value system, collective responsibility, the need for local actions to reflect global concerns, the recognition that change demands not only action, but a continuous process that goes beyond the immediate goals. Trentham and Cockburn (Ch. 33) set out a proposal for participatory action research to engage occupational therapists in person-centered practice with the needs of community groups and marginalized individuals.

This book was produced in order to provoke a discussion on the relationship between occupational therapy and the political, spiritual, and moral realities which contextualize the daily lives of the people we work with. Having advanced that discourse in collaboration with the authors here, we hope that occupational therapy, through reflection and research, will traverse the borders of philosophical confinement to engage with the fundamentals of occupational apartheid and injustice, which impact on the daily lives of so many people.

Chapter **28**

Reflections on occupational justice as a subtext of occupation-centered education

Wendy Wood, Barb Hooper, Jennifer Womack

OVERVIEW

This chapter explores occupational justice as an important, yet largely implicit, subplot of one educational program in occupational therapy. Excavation of this subplot was undertaken by evaluating materials from a curriculum revision process and culling findings from a recent qualitative case study of the program. Relevant educational outcomes were explored by inviting students and alumni to share their perspectives and experiences and then analyzing what they shared for evidence of awareness of, or effectiveness in promoting occupational justice, even when not named as such. Language, values, and beliefs congruent with occupational justice were found to exist, with varying levels of explicitness, in this program's vision and mission statements. Likewise, a variety of educational processes including curriculum themes, course design, teaching methods, and required assignments were found to embody an occupational justice perspective, as were ways in which faculty shared critical incidents from their professional biographies with students. It was concluded that students were afforded multiple opportunities for becoming infused with the ethic of occupational justice, and that some students and alumni were guided by this ethic in their practices. Nevertheless, how or the extent to which all students embodied and advanced occupational justice remained unclear. This identification and evaluation process, as applied to one curriculum, is used as a basis for reflecting on challenges that all educators in occupational therapy may face as they strive to infuse themselves, their programs, and their students, with the ethic of occupational justice.

INTRODUCTION

Various scholars have proposed that the practice of occupational therapy involves the telling of occupational stories as a means of creating future occupational stories that people and groups who receive therapy services, as well as the occupational therapists who provide them, regard as meaningful and important.[1,2] In this chapter, we propose that the education of occupational therapists likewise involves the telling and making of potentially invaluable occupational stories, ones which include main plots in addition to subplots that add intrigue, depth, and mystery. We tell an educational story here that has a main plot of an occupation-centered curriculum based on a foundation in occupational science. Yet our primary interest lies not so much in this prominent storyline as in an intriguing subplot: that of inviting occupational therapy students to become agents of occupational justice in partnership with the people they aspire to serve.

Our story is based on the occupational therapy program at the University of North Carolina at Chapel Hill (UNC–Chapel Hill) in the United States. It is important to stress that this program was not developed with the concept of occupational justice explicitly in mind, an omission that seems understandable given that occupational justice was only named as such in the mid 1990s.[3] Yet because many beliefs and principles inherent in the ethic of occupational justice arguably constituted the moral premises that first gave rise to occupational therapy in the United States in the early 1900s, similar beliefs and principles have presumably been implicit in the education of students at UNC–Chapel Hill since the program began. Accordingly, we searched for multiple examples of occupational justice as an explanatory subtext within the academic program and experiences of its faculty, students, and graduates – even when the words 'occupational justice' went unspoken. Our search began with materials produced through a comprehensive curriculum revisioning process initiated in 1995.[4] Additionally, findings of a qualitative case study of the program conducted in 2002 were re-examined for their relevance to occupational justice.[5] Other source materials were gathered from students and alumni who responded to our invitations to describe clinical incidents that clarified the relationship of education to practice for them. We made final decisions about what material to include predicated on the basis of clear relevance to occupational justice, as defined by Townsend and Wilcock.[3] Finally, all faculty members, as well as students and alumni who contributed to the chapter, reviewed an early draft of the chapter; with only minor exceptions, we incorporated suggested changes from this review process into the final writing.

Our purposes in this chapter are threefold. Most fundamentally, we seek to bring our subplot of interest – i.e. inviting students, through education, to become agents of occupational justice – into full light, revealing where this subplot is located, how it works, what ends it achieves, and what challenges and promises it holds for a future story about the education of occupational therapists. Secondly, by so doing we hope to provide other occupational therapy educators around the world with ways to locate and critically evaluate the presence and workings of the ethic of occupational justice in their curricula. Thirdly, we seek to reflect on our own search for the educational 'subplot' of occupational justice in order to help discern its implications for the future of occupational therapy education world wide.

Having established a goal of contributing to global discourse, we are obliged to offer a reflexive stance toward our position as authors. We are faculty members within a traditional research university in an economically privileged nation. Students enter our program having already earned baccalaureate degrees, and, after successful completion of 2 years of additional study and clinical fieldwork, graduate with a Master of Science in Occupational Therapy. For reasons due to privilege, access, and tradition, among other contextual factors, the examples of occupational justice and injustice we offer – both in the curriculum and in stories told by faculty, students, and graduates – may shrink in magnitude when compared with the experiences of some readers. Our examples largely depict challenges experienced in conventional social establishments and medical models of practice; they are thereby less focused on the broader sociopolitical implications evoked under the full scope of occupational justice. Yet within our cultural context and how we understand the practice of occupational therapy in the United States, we believe our examples illustrate how some UNC–Chapel Hill faculty, students, and graduates embrace their roles congruently with the principles of occupational justice.

Our chapter begins by addressing how occupational justice is implicit in the vision of occupational therapy and educational mission endorsed by faculty at UNC–Chapel Hill. We then explicate educational processes that may promote occupational justice. Stories of students and alumni are next examined for their value in illuminating educational outcomes of relevance to occupational justice. Lastly, we consider educational implications of imbuing occupational therapy curricula with the ethic of occupational justice.

EDUCATIONAL VISION AND MISSION

According to Townsend and Wilcock, the naming of occupational justice and the need to contemplate it as an important concept emerged from research on the occupational nature of human beings and from core principles of client-centered occupational therapy.[3] Occupational justice presumes that human beings are irrevocably occupational in nature; it values what is unique and indispensable in each person, no matter how marginalized; and it argues for the realization of the occupational potentials of all people toward the greater health of individuals, families, communities, nations, and, indeed, planet Earth. The converse of occupational justice, i.e. occupational injustice, results in three adverse situations, each of which can occur on individual and societal levels. *Occupational deprivation* refers to situations in which people's needs for meaningful and health promoting occupations go unmet or are systemically denied. *Occupational alienation* refers to situations in which people experience daily life as meaningless and purposeless. *Occupational imbalance* refers to situations in which sufficient variations in daily occupations needed to sustain wellbeing are rendered impossible due to personal or societal circumstances. The ethic of occupational justice calls forth a utopian vision of an occupationally just world: one in which these injustices are overcome and all persons are empowered in realizing their potentials through meaningful occupations such that they, and their interconnected worlds, flourish.

In 1995, the faculty at UNC–Chapel Hill created a vision of occupational therapy that now, in retrospect, clearly resonates with the principles of occupational justice.[4] Also utopian in nature, this vision imagined occupational therapists helping to sustain a world in which all people had opportunities to lead meaningful lives given their access to occupations that expressed their capacities and contributed to others. The vision was employed as a guiding beacon in redesigning not only the curriculum, but also admissions criteria that favored applicants who demonstrated sensitivity to issues of human diversity and experiences in community service. As importantly, the vision was employed to help students see, and deeply care about, how various occupational injustices can hurt countless people every day and almost anywhere – whether in first rate hospitals, typical nursing homes, poor communities, or materially rich lives that may nevertheless be experienced as empty or meaningless.[4,6,7]

The faculty's vision of occupational therapy also helped clarify their educational mission, the bare minimum of which was conceived of as insuring students' entry levels of professional competence. Yet the mission's highest calling was to endow students with resources such that, as their careers unfolded and built upon those resources, they became increasingly adept at providing occupational therapy services which they, simultaneously with the people and groups they served, experienced as deeply valuable and satisfying. Successfully launching graduates into such meaningfully contributory lifelong careers was thus held as the pinnacle of educational achievement, an aspiration inspired by a professional ethos akin to occupational justice.

EDUCATIONAL PROCESSES

Like its vision and mission, educational processes of the UNC–Chapel Hill program were designed to promote occupation-centered practices, not occupational justice. Yet on re-examination, various educational processes seem to inculcate in students the skills and values needed to enact an occupational justice perspective.

Curriculum themes   Curriculum themes manifest the core values and ideas inherent in the faculty's vision of occupational therapy. Seven themes, shown in Box 28.1, serve as conceptual building blocks upon which all courses, learning objectives, and academic content are constructed. Readers are also referred to Wood et al[4] for further descriptions of the content in each of these themes. Various beliefs presupposed within occupational justice are compatible with beliefs expressed through curriculum themes, including, among others, that humans need occupation to grow and thrive; that all people are entitled to health and a meaningful life, the realization of which requires access to occupation; that barriers to occupation are discriminatory and unjust; and that occupational therapists play important roles in insuring occupational access and promoting positive occupational experiences among those at society's margins.

> **Box 28.1 Guiding curriculum themes**
>
> - *Clinical reasoning* – Using and integrating multiple forms of reflection about clinical experiences to better understand therapeutic relationships, problems, situations, and possible solutions of direct relevance to recipients of occupational therapy services, at individual, family, group, and systems levels.
>
> - *Ethical reasoning* – Applying ethical standards of professional conduct and knowledge, analyzing problems and generating solutions based on a study of morality and responsibility to the greater good.
>
> - *Investigative reasoning* – Acquiring, communicating, and applying *knowledge* to provide evidence-based practice and help advance occupational therapy and occupational science.
>
> - *Occupation* – Employing occupation, or how people orchestrate time to fulfill needs and wants and create purpose and meaning in their lives, as a framework for professional activities.
>
> - *Humans as occupational beings* – Valuing and applying knowledge of the core relationship of occupation to human existence and multiple possible developmental trajectories across the lifespan.
>
> - *Occupation as a medium of change* – Providing, in collaboration with service recipients, meaningful occupations that enhance, sustain, or improve their development, quality of life, and health in context of traditional or new practice environments.
>
> - *Occupational therapists as scholars and change agents in systems* – Enacting the professional responsibilities to confront multilevel problems with occupation-centered solutions that reflect sound theory, research, and critical reasoning and to create progressive interventions that address occupational needs of marginalized people and groups.

Course design

Since curricular themes guide course design, it makes sense that various learning activities were also identified as having the potential to promote awareness of occupational justice and injustice, even without explicit use of the language. A course on the biomedical and phenomenological aspects of occupation weaves together study of medical diagnoses with study of illness narratives that highlight multiple levels of occupational deprivation experienced by some individuals due to illness or injury. A course on adult occupational development involves readings about members of minority groups who are deprived of access to important occupations, such as immigrant Hispanic women who provide in-home care for elders. Students also study a case example of older African American women who established child day care services in their rural community so that parents could sustain paid employment. A course on childhood occupational development explores how occupationally deprived environments detrimentally affect literacy development. A course on the history of occupational therapy and occupational science stresses the moral motivations of early twentieth century reformers who were dedicated to providing immigrants with access to meaningful work, healthy work conditions, culturally meaningful art, and play.

Teaching methods

Similarly, though in less obvious ways, teaching methods were identified as being germane to the promotion of occupational justice. For instance, the instructor in a course that addresses kinesiological bases of occupation was observed consistently to caution students against assuming that impaired body structures equaled impaired occupational engagement.[5] By highlighting the variability of movement across differing occupations and environments, this instructor battled the stigma that can develop when 'normal movement' is taught as the 'starting point' for intervention, thus discouraging students from assigning the status of disablement based on how people move.

Required assignments

We further identified required assignments that promoted beliefs and principles associated with occupational justice. For example, students complete literature-based research on questions they generate from illness narratives. Two recently researched questions of relevance to occupational justice are: how the context of psychiatric hospitals affects community reintegration,[8] based on *Girl Interrupted*;[9] and whether society promotes the devaluing of people's lives with the onset of disability,[10] based on *Moving Violations*.[11] For the history course, students construct their own intellectual and cultural histories of occupational therapy. Among other relevant topics, students have explored the roots of occupational justice in pragmatism, democracy, and the settlement house movement[12] and how humanistic ethics of caring historically promoted people's resilience through occupational therapy.[13] Building on a curriculum-wide commitment to community involvement, a course on community practices requires students to complete a major final project, conceived of as a culminating learning experience for the entire curriculum (see Bruner[14] for a discussion of integrating curricular 'works'). These projects involve creating innovative occupational therapy programs beyond the borders of traditional practices; students use a program planning model to document the unmet occupational needs of people and groups and then design, justify, and find funding for new programs that address those needs. One program used occupation to counteract the extreme occupational alienation experienced by loved ones of homicide victims in the year following the murder;[15] another sought to facilitate successful community reintegration of adolescents at risk for violent offences by ameliorating the occupational deprivation imposed by their institutional setting.[16]

Faculty professional biographies

Finally, findings in 2002 from the case study of the UNC–Chapel Hill program suggested that faculty professional biographies may advance the ethic of occupational justice.[5] Professional experiences of faculty were found to be key to the visions they held for graduates and conveyed through biographical stories. Oftentimes their stories promoted principles of occupational justice. We offer two examples. One faculty member told of significant experiences around racial segregation and desegregation which fueled her desire that students understand and respect the day-to-day experiences of African Americans, among other members of minority groups. Another faculty member shared her experience of two clients who were readmitted to rehabilitation wanting to live independently, a goal requiring their independence with transportation. This instructor stressed that practitioners had to partner with clients to gain access to needed community resources.

EDUCATIONAL OUTCOMES

Just as the curriculum at UNC–Chapel Hill has not been explicitly guided by the concept of occupational justice, neither have educational outcomes been evaluated with occupational justice in mind. What now seems clear, however, is that traditional and largely quantitative criteria for evaluating educational programs – such as how well students perform on fieldwork, their pass rates on certification examinations, their hiring rates, or a program's accreditation status – largely stop at the entrance into practice. Occupational justice requires a longer and more qualitative view, one that ascertains how graduates become agents of occupational justice over the course of their careers. We sought this longer view by inviting the perspectives of students and alumni. While respondents to our invitation comprised a self-selected group, their experiences suggest that students and alumni may undergo a developmental progression in understanding and becoming able to enact occupational justice.

Two students described required fieldwork experiences undertaken in the summers between their first and second years of study. Their vignettes represent, with varying degrees of explicitness, the curriculum themes of occupation, occupation as a medium of change, humans as occupational beings, clinical reasoning, and ethical reasoning. Both students also countered prevailing medical model practices with occupation-centered alternatives.

The first student told how, with her supervisor's support, she looked beyond traditional hospital practices to address the occupational needs of a woman who was severely depressed while awaiting bilateral leg amputations:

> We engaged her in an activity to give her insight, hope, and a vision of herself as an occupational being. By constructing a collage of what she wanted to do in the upcoming year, she saw beyond the immediate state of her health and envisioned the active person she wanted to be. We posted her collage on the wall in her room. Her family and nurses commented on how much she enjoyed the collage and how it seemed to boost her spirits. When working on her collage, she was more willing to participate in occupational therapy and benefited emotionally and physically from this therapeutic activity. I realized the power of occupation and the importance of creating an image of the client as an occupational being in the future.

The second student described her attempted advocacy for a resident of a retirement community who wanted to keep a treasured teapot in her room, a story with an occupational injustice subplot. Though unsuccessful in the experience described below, this student maintained an extensive involvement in political and other advocacy activities, on behalf of and in collaboration with people with mental illness.

> *June had been told that the cord to her electric teapot would cause her to injure herself and possibly trip and break a hip. Then there was the whole hot water thing and electrical situation. These concerns needed to be addressed since June made herself tea in the middle of the night. She told me the tea made her feel settled and ready to go back to sleep. Having her teapot allowed her to do this without causing a commotion with staff in the 'wee hours' of the morning. I tried explaining that maybe we could move the cord around and ask June to turn on the lights when she got up for her tea. I wasn't sure what would be the solution, but no alternatives were discussed. Nor was there discussion of her nightly ritual as being important. June described her tea as a necessity for sleeping well, but you could tell she just liked having this as her own private ritual. She enjoyed doing this. It was not only nice to have a cup of tea to relax, but it was something she did for herself that made her feel like herself. It was her routine.*
>
> *The teapot was taken away. This made me realize how much I had learned about what occupation really means to people and that many people without our education could just not see this many times. How powerful the seemingly ordinary can be.*

Two graduates of the program in 2000 submitted narratives evidencing multiple curriculum themes and an awareness of how their education helped them enact new practice models they found to be important and meaningful. A developmental progression in becoming able to promote occupational justice is also suggested. The first graduate noted:

> *Your request was well-timed with the contemplation of my journey thus far as an occupational therapist. If you had asked 6 months ago, I would have had little to say as I had had little occasion [in in-patient rehabilitation] to live and breathe my occupational science skills and know-how.*

Yet given a new position as a community-based occupational therapist specializing in helping older adults continue living in their own homes, this graduate was able to articulate what made her work possible:

> *It is a feeling, perhaps more than a skill set. A feeling of empowerment, in a challenging setting where occupational therapy is stepping outside of its frame. A feeling that I know how to talk about what I do (clinical reasoning skills, investigative reasoning skills) and know how to sell what I do (humans as occupational beings, occupation as a medium of change). A feeling that I know I can be successful at what I do (occupational therapist as change agent) because I have, in some capacity or another, wrapped my mind around the magnitude of a similar issue in the classroom.*
>
> *This applies to being able to identify needs within a population. It applies to being able to project where our program needs to be in 2 years to stay viable. It applies to being able to thread occupational stories with clients in real*

environments and real time. It applies to being able to stand my ground in a
community/workplace where no one has seen occupational therapy practiced
quite like this before.

The other recent graduate described how she is developing a position as a bilingual service coordinator for a county-wide infants and toddlers program:

My fieldwork directly influenced how I think and act as an occupational ther-
apist. The needs assessment process has proved to be an invaluable tool as I
draw upon it time and again while sitting on committees whose members con-
stantly overlook critical pieces, discuss issues, and offer solutions believing
their experiences alone constitute the real needs of the individuals we serve.
Thanks to our community practice class, I know what questions to ask. To cre-
ate a model program for the county, the manager and I discussed our vision in
meeting families' needs, which has led to these questions: What if we allow par-
ents to form their own 'support groups' that they coordinate and facilitate
while the 'professionals' sit back and provide support as necessary? What
opportunities can be created for parents to use their abilities since many are
craving to make contributions to society? How can parents organize their time
and routines to meet daily demands and support their children's development?

Since these vignettes are from individuals educated since the curriculum was revised in 1998, their use of current curriculum language is understandable. Yet because this language represented an evolution of the program's long-held beliefs, not a radical departure, many prior graduates presumably also embrace these same beliefs. A convened focus group of alumni supported this presumption by proposing that the program has historically been committed to instilling in students the critical thinking capacities, professional responsibility, and optimism about change required to enact progressive practices. Vignettes from individuals who graduated prior to the program's last major curriculum revision evidenced these values. For instance, a 1996 graduate described why she took a challenging new position as follows:

I realized taking this job would be like returning to school because of the
opportunities to learn. I felt destined to make this change because I had my
UNC–CH instructors' voices in my head telling me I would get out there and
do research, read publications, get published, attempt to change legislation,
and generally make a difference.

Finally, an alumnus who has directed two national programs supporting self-determination and self-advocacy of people with disabilities demonstrated determination in her pursuit of occupational justice (however unnamed) for a woman facing a steep uphill battle:

People who are not given choices of where to live, who to live with, where to
work, what supports they receive and by whom are not being allowed to live
as full occupational beings. Occupational beings need control over their own

> destinies and opportunities to make choices (and mistakes) in order to engage in the occupations/co-occupations important to them.
>
> An example is Mary, a 40-year-old mother of three children who has tetraplegia following an automobile accident 2 years ago and now lives in a nursing facility. Mary's dreams for her life are visions of herself as a true occupational being: being able to help raise her children, have her own house, be productive and self-sufficient, and choose who provides the assistance she needs. My understanding of the importance of engagement in occupations of one's choosing helps me continue to push for needed systems change so Mary can actualize her dreams.

CHALLENGES AND PROMISES

As suggested by the above vignettes, some students and alumni of UNC–Chapel Hill describe their work in language that resonates with the ethic of occupational justice. Those with more experience also evidence a growing confidence in their abilities to create and implement programs that reflect commitments to occupational justice and extend beyond the borders of traditional medical model practices within the United States. Through such venues as the program's vision statement, educational mission, and various educational processes, it thus seems reasonable to conclude that students at UNC–Chapel Hill are given multiple opportunities to become infused with the core principles and beliefs of occupational justice.

Yet that conclusion noted, it remains unclear how and to what degree occupational justice explicitly guides the professional practices and ideals of all students and alumni, let alone those whose vignettes we cited. We speculate that this vagueness is at least partly due to the fact that the language and clinical implications of occupational justice have yet to be systematically integrated into the entire educational program, even though students are exposed to occupational justice by multiple faculty members. If our speculation is correct, then educators around the world who desire to make occupational justice more prominent in their curricula, regardless of the particular educational systems or degree levels at which they teach, may face similar challenges to those involved in making occupation more prominent a few short years ago. Prominent professional language such as 'therapeutic occupation', 'evidence-based practice', or 'enabling occupation', and prominent practice models such as the Model of Human Occupation[17] or the Canadian Model of Occupational Performance[18] may need to be explicitly and repeatedly linked to the principles of occupational justice. Students may also need assistance in integrating the language of occupational justice within their professional practices, believing in the outcomes to which occupational justice points, and grasping how their expertise applies to attaining those outcomes.

The work of educational scholars concerned with transformational learning and with educating students to become deeply involved in their communities suggests several other factors that may influence the abilities of occupational therapy graduates to enact occupational justice.[19-21] Occupational justice may require an epistemological stance and self-perception beyond what some students can realistically achieve in entry-level professional programs. Graduates who see themselves as the recipients rather than crafters of knowledge, or as technicians of pre-scriptive practices rather than as creators of innovative practices, may not be epistemologically prepared to enact occupational justice. Such graduates may not yet grasp that vital knowledge and transformative practices can be generated within the particularities of each encounter of an occupational therapist with the people or groups that therapist wishes to help. Similarly, graduates whose identity does not include 'community member' may not be intra-personally prepared to enact occupational justice. Rhoads[21] proposes that critical community service entails a commitment to justice and democracy that is fundamentally 'tied to an individual's sense of self and vision for others.' This sense of self as connected to others is vital to enacting an ethic of care like that of occupational justice.

Currently, the occupational justice literature offers a vision and theoretical understanding for others as occupational beings; less explicated, however, is a vision and theoretical understanding of the epistemic, caring, and communal self-development of those who enact occupational justice. Systematically preparing graduates to become agents of occupational justice consequently presents challenges that occupational therapy educators have not yet explored in depth, as suggested by the paucity of relevant educational literature. To instill a level of consciousness necessary for transforming social worlds, educators may need to adopt a critical view of education, i.e. one which examines how education can propagate dominant cultural ideas and practices that may subvert occupational justice. In turn, such a critical stance could be instrumental in helping students, as expressed by Rhoads, 'recognize their own positionality and how various forces mitigate their ability to develop a critical consciousness'.[21]

The last decade has seen numerous calls from educators, scholars, and practitioners world wide to improve occupational therapy services; calls for change justified by various visions of 'best practice'. Yet whether 'best practice' is conceived of as being evidence-based, client-centered, occupation-centered, or something else, a larger question is begged: change for what end? More than a new content area or practice method to be mastered, occupational justice offers occupational therapists a meaning-making system that can inspire great occupational therapy: collaboratively created and occupation-focused interventions that are as valued by the people and groups they are intended to benefit as they are rewarding to the occupational therapists who provide them. The promise of occupational justice is exactly that it constitutes a system of beliefs through which therapists can interpret why they do occupational therapy, and thereby situate their clinical services, research, teaching, and other professional work in a broader system of meaning and caring. Without doubt, occupational justice is about action, but its action stems from a system of beliefs about people's occupational nature and what people thereby need, hence the damage that is wrought when those needs are not met. We believe that instilling the beliefs and principles of occupational justice through education can fuel a lifelong passion for occupational therapy. But as we have also discovered in this project, one challenge we face as educators is locating and critically evaluating the subplot of occupational justice in our educational programs, and then deciding how overtly and pervasively we are called to rewrite that storyline.

Acknowledgements

We thank the following students and alumni for their contributions on behalf of this chapter: Lauren Ashurst, Sally Bober, Shenyata Downing, Leila Ghassemian, Lori Goodnight, Shari Gorman, Shelly Harris, Liz Moe, Julie Pace, Michelle Patterson, Jodi Petry, Sue Porr, Julie Toporek, and Corinne Yenny.

References

1. Clark F. Occupation embedded in real life: interweaving occupational science and occupational therapy, 1993 Eleanor Clarke Slagle lecture. Am J Occ Ther 1993; 44:1067–1078.
2. Mattingly C, Fleming M. Clinical reasoning: forms of inquiry in a therapeutic practice. Philadelphia: Davis; 1994.
3. Townsend E, Wilcock A. Occupational justice. In: Christiansen C, Townsend E, eds. Introduction to occupation: the art and science of living. Upper Saddle River, NJ: Prentice Hall; 2004:243–273.
4. Wood W, Nielson C, Humphry R, et al. A curricular renaissance: graduate education centered on occupation. Am J Occ Ther 2000; 54:586–597.
5. Hooper B. Authoring lives in a subject-centered curriculum: an instrumental case study of graduate professional education in occupational therapy [unpublished doctoral dissertation]. East Lansing, MI: Michigan State University; 2002.
6. Palmer P. The active life: a spirituality of work, creativity and caring. San Francisco CA: Jossey-Bass; 1990.
7. Wilcock A. Reflections on doing, being and becoming. Can J Occ Ther 1998; 65:248–256.
8. Springer S. How does the context of a psychiatric hospital affect the ability to be integrated into the community? 2003 Apr 6; Presentation to the Division of Occupational Science, University of North Carolina at Chapel Hill.
9. Kaysen S. Girl interrupted. New York: Vintage Books; 1993.
10. Hildreth C. Do we as a society place a misguided mercy on the disability community by facilitating suicide through a perception that the value of life decreases with the onset of a disability? 2003 Apr 6; Presentation to the Division of Occupational Science, University of North Carolina at Chapel Hill.
11. Hockenberry J. Moving violations: war zones, wheelchairs, and declarations of independence. New York: Hyperion; 1995.
12. Wolcott N. Fighting for occupation: underpinnings of and opportunities for occupational justice in the United States. 2003 Apr 28; Unpublished paper completed as a graduation requirement of the Division of Occupational Science, University of North Carolina at Chapel Hill.
13. Malanga V. The role of philanthropic and humanistic ideals in caring: caring and doing influencing optimism, collaboration and reflective action. 2003 Apr 30; Unpublished paper completed as a graduation requirement of the Division of Occupational Science, University of North Carolina at Chapel Hill.
14. Bruner J. The culture of education. Cambridge, MA: Harvard University Press; 1996.
15. Stafford S. Survivor healing: a program to help homicide survivors regain the ability to live. 2003 May 2; Presentation to the Division of Occupational Science, University of North Carolina at Chapel Hill.
16. Zivica J. Life skills management from the inside out. 2003 May 2; Presentation to the Division of Occupational Science, University of North Carolina at Chapel Hill.
17. Kielhofner M. Model of human occupation. 3rd edn. Philadelphia, PA: Lippincott Williams & Wilkins; 2002.
18. Townsend E, Stanton S, Law M, et al. Enabling occupation: an occupational therapy perspective. Ottawa, ON: Canadian Association of Occupational Therapists; 1997.
19. Kegan R. In over our heads: the mental demands of modern life. Cambridge, MA: Harvard University Press; 1994.
20. Baxter Magolda MB. Creating contexts for learning and self-authorship. Nashville, TN: Vanderbilt University Press; 1999.
21. Rhoads RA. Community service and higher learning: explorations of the caring self. Albany, NY: State University of New York Press; 1997:212–227.

Chapter 29

Politics in occupational therapy education

A South African perspective

Madeleine Duncan, Helen Buchanan, Theresa Lorenzo

> **OVERVIEW**
>
> A strong sense of social justice and responsibility is critical for the practice of occupational therapy in a developing country such as South Africa. This calls for a transformational approach to undergraduate curriculum design in which no one culture, gender, or social class dominates the knowledge construction process. Attention to issues such as diversity, authority, governance, and power positions politics at the core of professional socialization. This chapter explores the relevance of politics in occupational therapy education in a democratizing society. It describes strategies for developing political literacy, for coping with the political dimensions of service learning, and for making politics explicit in assessment and evaluation. Deep learning methods to enhance attitudinal shifts are suggested and recommendations for addressing politics in the curriculum are offered.

FRAMING THE POLITICAL CONTEXT OF TRAINING

South Africa emerged from decades of apartheid after the first democratic elections in 1994. Speaking to the nation and the world at the installation of South Africa's first democratic, non-racial government, Nelson Mandela said,

> *We pledge ourselves to liberate all our people from the bondage of poverty, suffering, gender and other discrimination. Never, never and never again shall it be that this beautiful land will again experience oppression of one by another ... the sun shall never set on so glorious a human achievement.*[1]

Since this auspicious moment in our history, the process of nation building has resulted in one of the most progressive constitutions in the world. Based on the ideals of democracy, social justice, and human rights, it guides national governance and the rule of law as well as socio-economic redress for previously oppressed peoples.

The constitution also informs a range of progressive charters and policies that direct the development of all sectors of national governance and society as a whole. For example, the adoption of the primary health care (PHC) approach[2] as lead theme of the National Health Plan has led to substantial changes in the approach and structure of public health services, including occupational therapy. District-based services, encompassing the PHC philosophy, are guided by policies such as the White Paper on an *Integrated National Disability Strategy*[3] and the *National Rehabilitation Policy*.[4] Similar advances in other public sectors such as education, labor, industry, agriculture, and justice aim to provide a national infrastructure for the transformation of South Africa and its peoples. Inter-sectoral collaboration, an important PHC principle, positions health across all sectors of society, thereby opening up unprecedented opportunities for occupational therapy to become politically relevant. This means that the profession is poised to act upon and proceed from the motives of policy and good governance in meeting the health and development needs of the population.

BECOMING POLITICALLY RELEVANT

South Africa, called the 'rainbow nation' by Nobel laureate Archbishop Desmond Tutu, has a population of 47 million. Its distribution of wealth is considered to be the most unequal in the world with more than half the population living in poverty.[5] The country faces an HIV/AIDS pandemic as well as other diseases and mental health disorders related to poverty,[6] inequity, and structural violence. Addressing national health priorities within severe financial constraints has required the Department of National Health to take radical steps such as rapid de-hospitalization and downsizing of tertiary hospital services in order to create comprehensive health services at grass-roots level. Health professional posts, including those for occupational therapy, are completely inadequate to meet service and training needs at all levels of health care.

The Division of Occupational Therapy at the University of Cape Town (UCT) has therefore been proactive in engaging non-traditional service learning settings such as non-profit organizations and social development projects for the training of undergraduate students. Multi-sectoral learning exposes students to a range of sociopolitical realities that impact on the health of individuals, groups, and communities, and requires alternative interpretations of practice from those traditionally associated with the profession. Kleinman (in Swartz[7]) suggests that 'the trauma, pain and disorders to which atrocity gives rise are health conditions, yet they are also political and cultural matters. Similarly, to say that poverty is the major risk factor for ill health and death is only another way of saying that health is a social indicator and indeed a social process'. (p. 185) The shifts in service focus have required the alignment of the education program with the three proposed orientations to practice suggested by the World Federation of Occupational Therapists' (WFOT) *Revised Minimum Standards for the Education of Occupational Therapists*, namely *biomedical, occupational*, and *social*.[8]

The biomedical orientation deals with existing or at risk health conditions, the occupational with occupational risk, disruption, and deprivation, and the social with populations at occupational risk due to sociopolitical forces such as war and homelessness.

In order for occupational therapy to be relevant in a developing society, all three practice orientations are required. In other words, intraprofessional models and interdisciplinary frames of reference, particularly those informing an occupational view of public health,[9] poverty alleviation, and social development[10,11] need to take equal place with traditional individualistic, medical, and biopsychosocial models of practice. Working within a broad definition of health[2] enables occupational therapists to plan and monitor comprehensive occupational therapy services that promote social justice, equity, and community development through occupation.[9,12] A narrow definition of health such as that endorsed by the *International Classification of Functioning*,[13] *Disability and Health (ICF)* guides the provision of services that focus on the health concerns of individuals and their capacity to participate in society. Political literacy enables the occupational therapist to appreciate the motives of policy, power, and governance that inform these two approaches to health and to adjust practice paradigms accordingly.

DEVELOPING POLITICAL LITERACY

Political literacy provides the health professional with a frame of reference for understanding and responding to the organizational processes affecting authority, status, and organized forms of society. If students are to be well prepared for working in environments where poverty, structural violence, and overwhelming need are prevalent, they need to:

- understand how the politics of diversity, power and organizational development may influence the health of individuals, groups, and communities[10]
- be culturally sensitive and competent to meet the challenges of community entry[12]
- have a strong sense of agency, professional identity, and values in order to address change in their world of work[14]
- be emotionally resilient and morally mature in coping with the inevitable dissonance that arises in the face of inequity, injustice, and suffering[16]
- have good personal and practice management skills and the ability to administrate and deliver basic comprehensive (curative, rehabilitative, preventive, and promotive) occupational therapy.[12]

To achieve these outcomes an educationally transformative curriculum is indicated; one that shapes the ability for critical examination, interpretation, and understanding of available evidence as well as the ability to follow prescribed methods of practice or occupational therapy processes. The systematic exploration of personal and professional value systems throughout the undergraduate curriculum advances the conscientization of the developing practitioner as an agent of change in society. Freire[15] (p. 15) defines conscientization as 'learning to perceive social, political and economic contradictions and to take action against the oppressive elements of reality'. Emphasis needs to be placed on the transformation of beliefs, values, and feelings about power and the capacity of professionals to be self-determining through explicitly focusing on the affirmation of diversity and issues of power in curriculum design.

For example, at UCT attention is paid to the understanding and deconstruction of power by being alert to the following issues in the design of lecture content, tutorials, student writing requirements, and assessment forms:

- *Language*: What words are used, preferred, with whom, when, and why? Particular emphasis is placed on the deconstruction of languages that marginalize, oppress, or imply that power resides in the student or clinician rather than with the client, group, or community. For example, terminology that situates practice within the medical model refers to the person receiving occupational therapy as the 'patient'. This language may be appropriate in a hospital setting but is incongruent within community development projects where the therapist and community member are collaborators and partners in resolving health related problems.

- *Culture*: What assumptions and prejudices about people who are different from us have we internalized and how do these lead to the oppression of others?

- *Educational preparedness*: How do the personal educational history and prior life experiences of students influence the way they learn?

- *Stereotypes*: How do racism, ageism, sexism, as well as gender, class, disability, and religious bias, and other forms of discrimination influence the balance of power in relationships between people and lead to human rights abuses?

These sensitization strategies, which include a statement of intent, permeate the tacit and explicit structures of transformation imbedded in the undergraduate program.[14,16] The undergraduate occupational therapy curriculum is focused on occupation in a way that is similar to that described by Wood et al,[17] and is depicted in Table 29.1.

The content of the curriculum evolves cyclically and cumulatively over the 4 years, having horizontal and vertical connections within and between non-professional and professional subjects. Integration occurs through service learning from first through to fourth year across a range of sectors (for example education, industry, non-governmental organizations) and primary, secondary, and tertiary levels of the health service.

SERVICE LEARNING: PROMOTING POLITICAL AWARENESS

Students are valuable resources in contexts of overwhelming need and therefore render a supervised service from the first year of study. First year students are supervised by final years with guidance from faculty

Table 29.1 Focus for each year of occupational therapy training at UCT

Year	Focus
1	The wellbeing of the occupational human across the life-cycle. Occupation as means and end with reference to indigenous knowledge systems
2	Uncovering occupational performance and performance component needs. Health promotion through occupation
3	Preventative, curative, and rehabilitative occupational therapy approaches to health conditions in individuals and groups
4	Evidence-based and outcomes-based generalist practice within the South African context. Comprehensive occupational therapy program development and services across a range of sectors through an occupational perspective of public health.[9]

appointed staff. Fourth year students may have to work independently with indirect supervision from a university appointed occupational therapist/supervisor at sites that do not have full-time clinicians from any of the health related professions. The complexity of the professional demands of occupational therapy in a developing context is experienced when students grapple with cultural diversity, lack of resources, social disintegration, and poverty in the actual contexts of people's lives. Being 'thrown in the deep end' by having to work without the direct, one-on-one supervision of a qualified occupational therapist means students have to learn to be resourceful. They discover innovative answers to difficult questions through a gradual change of attitude and a willingness to let go of 'certainty'[18] and the need 'to make things better'.[19] Trust in prescribed protocols and processes such as those used in traditional, hospital-based practice is shifted to trust in solution generation through collaboration with a range of role players. Service learning initiatives are endorsed by the university's social responsibility agenda and supported by appropriate legal structures and safety policies.

Students report, in their service learning logs and tutorials, that they struggle to adjust to the slow pace of change. The apparent lack of motivation in communities and individuals to break the cycle of poverty or violence through hard work and commitment to development initiatives is demoralizing. They also find the apparent apathy or, alternatively, the expectation from consumers that they, the students, will bring money or tangible solutions, very difficult to process. Their anxiety is fueled by fear for personal safety while walking in unfamiliar neighborhoods, as well as by the lack of stable infrastructures, such as transport and central offices.

Dissonance leads to a range of defences such as projection and displacement of anger toward academic staff, regression to passivity and helplessness, splitting members of the health team, and acting out through unprofessional behavior. The containment and processing of these defences is paramount in maintaining the mental wellbeing of students and staff as well as their commitment to the ideals of the profession in a developing society. Service learning can be very demoralizing because students witness, and in some instances experience, the oppression of politics for themselves. They need to be empowered and contained through the praxis of engagement between educators, learners, and learning systems (i.e. contexts, people, texts) in a cyclical process of exploration, action, and reflection.[20] This praxis must be highly structured because it nurtures the development of self-directed practitioners who recognize that single answers to problems do not exist and that knowledge is relative, provisional, and socially constructed. An adult education approach ensures that students use deep learning methods that reinforce reflective rather than procedural practice competencies.[21,22] The following section describes some of the deep learning that has occurred for occupational therapy students at UCT as well as educational strategies to enhance this type of learning.

COPING WITH THE POLITICAL DIMENSIONS OF SERVICE LEARNING

Politics here refers to the particular sets of ideas, principles, and activities concerned with the acquisition and exercise of authority and governance that operate in a particular context, organization, community, or society. Enabling students to discern and 'read' political nuances is considered important for the development of the skills of citizenship.[23] Buchanan[24] and Lorenzo[25] researched the critical challenges faced and the strategies used by graduating students to cope during service learning in impoverished, under-resourced contexts where issues of politics regularly surface. Focus groups and textual analysis of service learning logs revealed that politics pervades the education process and that students are able, with support, to develop rudimentary adaptive, proactive actions in response to issues of power, authority, and status.

According to Lorenzo[25] students, whose comments are given below, became conscious of and developed actions in accordance with three dimensions of power similar to those mentioned by Nelson and Wright:[26]

- *Power to*: This approach to power comes from undoing the effects of internalized oppression by developing capacities and knowledge through collective action.

  There's a lot of interaction in the community between the OTs, social workers and coordinators – they are all working together. I found it quite different to a hospital setting where each one has their own little role because they need to be their profession. In the community a lot of the roles overlap and it's quite nice in that way because you do so much more than just to restrict yourself to being an OT only.

- *Power over*: Students recognized this form of power in situations where they had to gain access to 'political decision-making', often in public forums. By advocating for, and with, marginalized groups to be treated as equal partners, students learned to negotiate with community members, clients, and people in positions of authority.

  I decided I am not going to push them to come to the center. They are not mentally ill, they are fit and healthy and as an OT I am not there to heal them. I am just a resource. The issue I am dealing with is wellness not disease,

> *especially the work I do in the center … I must not be scared to let people learn about life and all its difficulties … coming from a caring profession you want to come and solve everybody's problems and you want to control the situation. You must not try to protect them … You are not there to control but to facilitate.*

- *Decentralized power*: In this approach power is seen not as a substance possessed and exercised by a person or institution but as an invisible, subject-less apparatus consisting of discourses, institutions, actors, and a flow of events beyond the control of individuals. It can only be understood through awareness of social dynamics. Students are encouraged to think at an organizational and discourse level about social issues and to journal their experiences of hidden power.

> *It's a journey that you go together, it's a life … the networks in the community are quite amazing. Everybody knows each other … you can't be up at the top looking down, you need to be on ground level … and amongst them … otherwise you don't see the small, little work inside.*

In her analysis of student service learning journals Buchanan[22] identified the following adaptive strategies that were being used by students during service learning:

- *Bracketing powerlessness*: Students who felt powerless in the face of overwhelming need found that, in order to progress, they needed to focus less on the need and more on identifying the small, observable steps they could take in making a difference in the lives of their clients.

- *Entering the lifeworld of the client(s)*: Students had to learn to appreciate the phenomenological experiences of clients in order to envisage what they could realistically do to bring about meaningful change. Cultural sensitivity and the willingness to enter the life world of the client or community paved the way for positive outcomes.

- *Negotiating transitions*: Students had to grapple with alternative ways of doing things by becoming resourceful, lateral thinkers. Transitions between the certainty of established treatment protocols and the uncertainty of inexperience and inadequate resources could only be resolved by critical, reflective thinking, and knowing how and where to access information and support.

- *Recognizing praxis*: A strong, theoretical grounding enabled students to make sense of emerging practice concerns. It was their ability to recognize the dialectic between theory and practice, rather than their technical, practical skills, that enabled them to arrive at reasonable solutions to complex problems.

- *Reciprocity of learning*: Students who were willing to equalize the relationship between themselves, their clients, and the community were more readily accepted into the various social systems that influenced service delivery. By letting go of their power as health professionals and being open to learning from their clients and the community they enabled the reciprocal flow of knowledge, skills, and attitudes. This is not an easy process, rather it requires substantial support and reflection.

MAXIMIZING THE LEARNING PROCESS

Educational strategies to support and equip students to grapple with contextual issues in creative, meaningful ways have been developed.[38] Table 29.2 captures some of the essential dimensions of containment

Table 29.2   Containment offered to students during service learning

What	How
Orientation	• Experiential learning is fostered through small group, problem oriented tasks in preparation for service learning, e.g. exploring safety and risk management strategies • Pre-placement information packages are provided[27,28] • Self-defence and personal safety classes are offered
Reasoning and Writing	• Reflection is imbedded in the curriculum in the form of journaling, logs, portfolios, and a range of other writing and debating requirements • Training in journaling, portfolio writing, and clinical reasoning[21,22] is offered
Peer learning and support	• Weekly tutorials with peers from similar placements are guided by input from an experienced clinician. These provide opportunities to teach and to learn from other students and especially their clients • Relying on the support of a friend is encouraged. Students are placed in pairs where possible. They find this support indispensable for learning
Supervision	• Students receive individual and small group supervision with regular written and verbal feedback from clinicians and university supervisors • A professional development program is offered to supervisors and clinicians to address service learning and educational issues
Access to Information	• Students are taught how to access information to guide their practice. They quickly embrace this approach and begin to collaborate in the knowledge construction process
Containment and support	• An open door policy enables easy access to academic staff • Designated academic staff monitor the progress of individual students • Referral to student counseling and academic development services is used when indicated
Discourse analysis	• Median groups facilitate values clarification and perspective transformation • Class constitutions allow students to process their learning in 'interdependence' with peers, thereby echoing the community development process about which they are learning • A systems approach to understanding organizational dynamics is used [16,29]
Feedback	• Information is received from other students who have been to the same placement. Hand over between students is built into the tutorial system • Records and resource files are kept to ensure sustainability of student-led services
Self awareness	• Students are encouraged to use their spirituality. Meaning and purpose are explored in a range of ways such as journaling and taking time to reflect or meditate. They are encouraged to substitute the urgency of 'doing something' with the ability to listen deeply to themselves and their clients • To develop their sense of agency, students are strongly encouraged to be independent thinkers, taking charge of their own learning and not following 'recipes' or expecting constant guidance. They find this liberating as well as daunting and develop confidence, over time, in their solution generating abilities
Formative curriculum	• The curriculum explicitly addresses human rights, ethics, transformation, professionalism, anti-bias training, and cultural competence to provide students with a theoretical frame of reference for practice[16,30]

offered to students prior to, during, and after service learning placements, containment being the diffusion of unease and distress by providing structure, support, and direction.

MAKING POLITICS EXPLICIT IN ASSESSMENT AND EVALUATION

Rapidly changing service platforms require flexible assessment methods to determine student competencies. Comprehensive primary health care and community-based rehabilitation does not involve taking the therapy that happens in hospitals or schools and transposing it to community centers or people's homes. It calls for a totally different practice paradigm and different methods of working, such as participatory action research, consultation with community health workers, or collaboration with consumers, traditional healers, and community leaders.[31,32]

Criteria for the assessment of students in traditional service settings, for example the individual, single case study treatment session, are well established and seldom include reference to the politics of practice, focusing rather on the technical performance of the student within the medical model. Expert clinicians know how to treat individuals or work with groups within established health or education contexts such as hospitals and special schools, using a range of therapeutic modalities. They are therefore familiar with the criteria for assessing performance skills and inferring therapeutic competence.

Inferring competence in primary health care practice requires assessments that elicit evidence about the ability to interpret, integrate, and address complex, multifaceted phenomena in intuitive, appropriate, and ethical ways.[33,34] Assessors have to listen and watch with expert ears and eyes for coherence in the students' approach to complex problems and their ability to make sense of political issues such as organizational dynamics, community unrest or culture-bound authority structures. They have to look beyond the student's technical skill in treating health conditions procedurally, for evidence of the student's ability to think critically and theoretically, understand deeply, and reason ethically about the health, occupational, and wellbeing needs of the public.

Against these requirements, we have found the development of criterion-referenced assessments for group and population focused practice to be particularly challenging. At present our assessment systems consist of multiple, complementary methods (e.g. portfolios, mind-maps, posters, video, practical demonstrations, workshops) that collect quantitative and qualitative evidence of a student's progress along the 4-year learning continuum.

The following assessment principles have proved helpful in ensuring the rigor of assessment:

- *Uniform marking criteria*: All assessments are based on a uniform set of marking criteria that spell out the structural indicators underpinning the various competencies being assessed.[35] These criteria are aligned with national higher education marking grades, levels of academic achievement, and quality assurance standards.

● *Holistic approach*: Use is made of the five unifying features of an integrated assessment suggested by Hager, Gonczi and Athanasou.[34] Each competency, for example professional behavior and interpersonal relationships, is evaluated with reference to knowledge, technical skills, problem solving skills, understanding, and ethics.

● *Alternative organizing frameworks*: Substantial deviation from the traditional occupational therapy process is introduced as an organizing framework for facilitating clinical reasoning. For example, the traditional medical model process of the 'referral, assessment, treatment, evaluation, discharge, follow up' cycle does not apply beyond the acute, curative context. By introducing neutral frameworks based on clinical reasoning and deep reflection, the student can depict competencies in using alternative, more appropriate processes such as Schön's reflective practitioner process[36] and Freire's action learning.[37]

● *Flexible writing guidelines*: Alternatives to the traditional case study format are used depending on service context. We make use of a flexible occupational therapy report form that allows students to mix and match between various sections according to the needs of the client, group, or community, the context, and models of practice. All three practice orientations (i.e. social, biomedical, and occupational)[8] are accommodated in the structure of the guidelines, as are opportunities to comment on the politics of the service.

TOWARD BUILDING THE FUTURE

This chapter has reviewed some of the critical issues for the training of occupational therapists in South Africa. Working toward social justice has called for the extension of occupational therapy into previously uncharted territories, such as communities that have been, or are being, subjected to violence, oppression, and pervasive poverty. By taking our social responsibility seriously we have had to align the training of occupational therapists with the political dimensions of a developing society.

We have suggested that a central theme in the professional, personal, and educational strategies used by students during service learning in contexts of overwhelming need and underdevelopment is power in all its forms; negative and positive as well as personal and social. Understanding power and how to work creatively with it has enjoyed particular attention in our curriculum as we believe this to be an essential competency for the challenges of practice in any society.

We have also proposed that at the heart of the education process should be an explicit commitment to addressing the 'being', i.e. the moral development of the student. Shaping attitudes that are radical in their commitment to political redress, nation building, and social change requires structures that enable students to contain and cope with the dissonance that arises in the face of oppression. Issues of power have to be recognized and creatively managed, reflexivity has to be inculcated, and cultural competency has to be explicitly reinforced during the process of professional socialization. These meta-cognitive and metaphysical competencies are considered essential for appropriate practice in any context.

References

1. Mandela N. Long walk to freedom. London: Abacus; 1995:747.
2. World Health Organization. Conference on primary health care: Alma Ata. Geneva: WHO; 1978.
3. Office of the Deputy President. Integrated national disability strategy. Pretoria: Government Press; 1997.
4. Department of Health. Rehabilitation for all: national rehabilitation policy. Pretoria: Government Press; 2000.
5. May J, ed. Poverty and inequality in South Africa: meeting the challenge. David Phillip: Cape Town; 2000.
6. United Nations Development Programme. UNDP poverty report 1998: overcoming human poverty. New York: UNDP; 1998.
7. Swartz L. Culture and mental health: a South African view. Cape Town: Oxford University Press; 1998.
8. World Federation of Occupational Therapists. Revised minimum standards for the education of occupational therapists. Forrestfield, Australia: WFOT; 2002.
9. Wilcock A. An occupational perspective on health. Thorofare, NJ: Slack; 1998.
10. Freire P. The politics of education: culture, power and liberation. Massachusetts: Bergin and Garvey; 1985.
11. Max-Neef MA. Human scale development. London: Apex Press; 1991.
12. Watson R, Swartz L, eds. Transformation through occupation. London: Whurr; 2004.
13. World Health Organization. International classification of functioning, disability and health. Geneva: WHO; 2001.
14. Watson RM. Competence: a transformative approach. World Federation of Occupational Therapists Bulletin 2002; 45:7–11.
15. Freire P. Pedagogy of the oppressed. New York: Herder and Herder; 1978.
16. Duncan M. Groups for perspective transformation. In: Becker L, ed. Groupwork in South Africa. Cape Town: Oxford University Press; In press.
17. Wood W, Nielsen C, Humphry R, et al. A curricular renaissance: graduate education centered on occupation. Am J Occup Ther 2000; 54(6):586–597.
18. Clarkson P. The achilles syndrome: overcoming the secret fear of failure. Dorset: Element Books; 1994.
19. Peck MS. The different drum. The creation of true community – the first step to world peace. London: Arrow Books; 1987.
20. Taylor J, Marais D, Heyns S. Community participation and financial sustainability. Action Learning Series – case studies and lessons from development practice. Cape Town: Juta; 1998.
21. Buchanan H, Moore R, Van Niekerk L. The fieldwork case study: writing for clinical reasoning. Am J Occup Ther 1998; 52(4):291–295.
22. Buchanan H, Van Niekerk L, Moore R. Assessing fieldwork journals: developmental portfolios. Br J Occup Ther 2001; 64(8):398–402.
23. Blackwell D. And everyone shall have a voice: the political vision of Pat de Maré. Group Analysis 2000; 33:151–162.
24. Buchanan H. South African contextual factors: impact on occupational therapy student learning, education and practice. Unpublished poster presented at the thirteenth World Congress of Occupational Therapists. Stockholm. June 23–28, 2002.
25. Lorenzo T. Developing competence for partnership: the voice of occupational therapy students in Cape Town. Unpublished poster presented at the thirteenth World Congress of Occupational Therapists. Stockholm. June 23–28, 2002.
26. Nelson N, Wright S. Power and participatory development: theory and practice. London: Intermediate Technology Publications; 1995.
27. Gilbert J, Strong J. Coping strategies employed by occupational therapy students anticipating fieldwork placement. Aust Occup Ther J 1997; 44(1):30–40.
28. Steele-Smith S, Armstrong M. 'I would take more students but …': student supervision strategies. Br J Occup Ther 2001; 64(11):549–551.

29. Lyndon P. The median group: an introduction. Group Analysis 1995; 28:251–260.

30. Occupational Therapy Division, University of Cape Town. What is occupation, how should OT be understood and what are the OT values at UCT? S Afr J Occup Ther 2001; 31(1):2.

31. Hermanus K, Lagerdien K, Watson R. A facilitator's manual for social action and development. Cape Town: Disabled Children's Action Group; 2003.

32. WFOT-CBR Project Team. Draft position paper on community based rehabilitation for the International Consultation on Reviewing CBR Feb–May 2003. Online. Available: http://www.wfot.org/Articles/CBRcomment.pdf 26 Nov 2003.

33. Gonczi A, Hager P, Athanasou J. National Office of Overseas Skills Recognition Research. The development of competency-based assessment strategies for professions. Paper no.8. DEET. Canberra: Australian Government Publishing Service; 1993.

34. Hager P, Gonczi A, Athanasou J. General issues about assessment of competence. Assessment and Evaluation in Higher Education 1994; 19(1):3–17.

35. Biggs J. Assessing learning quality: reconciling institutional, staff and educational demands. Assessment and Evaluation in Higher Education 1996; 21(1):5–15.

36. Schön D. The reflective practitioner: how professionals think in action. New York: Basic; 1983.

37. Hope A, Timmel S. Training for transformation: a handbook for community workers (Books 1–3). Gweru, Zimbabwe: Mambo Press; 1995.

Chapter **30**

The Metuia Project in Brazil
Ideas and actions that bind us together

Denise Dias Barros, Roseli Esquerdo Lopes, Sandra Maria Galheigo, Débora Galvani

OVERVIEW

This chapter aims to introduce the work being done by the Metuia Project, developed by occupational therapy teaching staff in three universities in the state of São Paulo, Brazil. Through the research, teaching, and development of an occupational therapy practice, the Metuia Project has worked on the theoretical basis for the setting up of occupational therapy programs in the social field. To familiarize us with the project, the chapter presents its principles and objectives and illustrates their practice with some story-telling and narratives from those involved, both students and users.

INTRODUCTION

The Metuia Project was created in 1998 in Brazil. *Metuia* means friend, companion in the native language of the *bororo*, a Brazilian indigenous people. The project, also known as Grupo Interinstitucional de Estudos, Formação e Ações pela Cidadania de Crianças, Adolescentes e Adultos em Processos de Ruptura das Redes Sociais de Suporte, is a research and development group formed by occupational therapy teaching staff and students from three different universities in the state of São Paulo: Pontifícia Universidade Católica de Campinas (PUC–Campinas), Universidade Federal de São Carlos (UFSCar) and Universidade de São Paulo (USP). The group also includes occupational therapists who work in the social field in the cities of Campinas, São Carlos, and São Paulo. The Metuia Project is organized in two branches, USP/UFSCar and PUC–Campinas, both of which have developed specific projects in each region.

The project sets out to develop studies, actions, and quality human resources in order to provide a better service for children, adolescents, and adults experiencing the breakdown of their networks of social support, a process described by Robert Castel[1-3] as 'disaffiliation' (see Chs 7 and 11.)

The Metuia Project has worked on the theoretical basis for the setting up of occupational therapy programs in the social field and on the development of an experimental practice. It seeks to achieve a deeper understanding of those who are disaffiliated because they are neither known nor recognized in the social field of occupational therapy.[4] In pursuit of this aim, one of the important interfaces of Metuia's activities is the fostering and development of occupational therapy practices in public places, community areas, and social institutions. The Metuia Project arises from a particular social and political context, within which occupational therapists in Brazil began to propose and develop community, territorial, (see Ch. 7) and open-setting initiatives. To achieve more inclusive actions, two axes were pursued:

1. The adoption of a critical standpoint in analyzing services and implementing actions, arguing in favor of an agenda through which social policies could make people's needs and demands their primary concern, disregarding the previous top-down approach.

2. The encouragement of an academic debate on the impact of the division of knowledge which gave precedence to specialized knowledge and resulted in reductionist strategies. This approach ended up reducing people to their symptoms, disabilities, and disadvantages, regardless of the complexity of the issues involved in their life conditions.[5]

ACTIONS AND OBJECTIVES OF THE METUIA PROJECT: CULTIVATING OCCUPATIONAL THERAPY IN THE SOCIAL FIELD

Occupational therapy is a field of knowledge and practice used in health, education, and social work. It combines procedures oriented toward the development of autonomy and the emancipation of people who, for different reasons, display temporary or permanent difficulty in being included and participating in social life.

The members of the Metuia Project share the belief that working in the social field requires an understanding of the reality and the living conditions of those in need. We also agree that the education of occupational therapists should take place through direct contact with the population who are taken care of by government and non-government organizations. Case study 30.1 gives a concrete example of this learning in context.

CASE STUDY 30.1   E AND L: LEARNING IN CONTEXT

As one of our teaching activities and as a strategy to get closer to street life we set out to get to know the territory (see Ch. 7), guided by the users of the My Street, My Home Association (AMRMC, see p. 423 below). E and L, who have no permanent or formal addresses, showed professionals and students around the city and neighborhood where they live.

E initially took us to the police station, which he told us was the first one established in the city. He told us that one of the strategies he used to make sure he got some lunch was to go to jail. He would hang around the police station looking for trouble until he was arrested. He would choose a day on which the duty officer was not, in his words, so 'harsh'. In front of the police station there is a tree, in which he sleeps. Taking shelter in a tree top is safer. 'During the day, street people are good, they don't get up to anything ... during the night it's all thieves who hang around.'

L, her partner, and a group of friends occupy the area underneath the overpass in front of AMRMC. There she transforms public space into private space by using pieces of cardboard and wood, mattresses, and chairs. She makes an effort to keep everything as clean and tidy as possible: we watch her sweeping the floor in front of the shack. She also attributes some rules to the space she has laid out; for instance, who can get in and when, who can touch her things. The exchanges in this group are extremely important, since some favors, such as washing her friends' clothes and cooking for them, guarantee her protection at night.

The Metuia Project aims to contribute, albeit in modest terms, to the improvement of social conditions in Brazil. According to the *Atlas of Social Exclusion in Brazil*,[6] 47% of 170 million inhabitants are living in what could be regarded as conditions of social exclusion. This map of exclusion shows that more than 25% of Brazilians live in precarious conditions, without income, job, or access to education, and 42% of the 5500 cities in Brazil have high levels of social exclusion. While the Social Development Index,[7] adopted by the United Nations, uses levels of education, longevity, and income as social indicators, the *Atlas of Social Exclusion* provides a broader picture of Brazilian social reality since it also uses other indicators: poverty, homicide levels, employment and unemployment rates, schooling, illiteracy, levels of inequality, and number of young people. Social exclusion has contributed to both social dissociation and social degradation in quality of life and has often led to the impoverishment of social and familial connections. This may be followed by a series of breakdowns in social participation and failures in the constitution of social ties, causing a sort of social and occupational emptiness in community life. Case study 30.2 illustrates that even children are aware of this social exclusion and inequality.

CASE STUDY 30.2   THE MAP OF SOCIAL EXCLUSION: INEQUALITY EXPRESSED IN A MODEL

Once during an occupational therapy session in Projeto Gente Nova (PROGEN, see p. 418 below), a group of children aged 8–10 years old were invited to build a model of their neighborhood out of cardboard and matchboxes. We, the teaching staff and students, expected that they would reproduce the area they used to live in (houses, school, church, PROGEN). We planned to use it to talk about their community, its organizations, life and friendship, cooperation and solidarity, conflict and daily violence, and the children's expectations.

However, the result was quite different. After the first two plain matchbox houses were ready, one girl requested more cardboard and asked if she could build a wall. Receiving the answer that this was their model and they could do whatever they wished, the group carried on building houses with higher fences. They asked for a light blue piece of paper for a swimming pool. When the model was complete, it was clearly divided into four areas, set on the four corners of the board. On one of the corners were two plain houses without fences, one very poor and damaged and another with a well tended garden: 'the houses of the poor' the children said. On the other corner was a two-storey house with a large swimming pool and high walls between it and the neighborhood: 'the house of the wealthy'. The other corner reproduced a smaller scale version of the previous one, which they named 'the house of the middle class'. There was only one collective area, located on the fourth corner: a supermarket and a branch of McDonald's.

The model did not show their neighborhood, the Vila Castelo Branco, as it really is but instead represented the ideas those children had about living in an unequal society, giving a subjective picture of social relations in a way the children were able to understand and express.

Vulnerability is produced by a combination of the precariousness of work and living conditions and the frailty of social bonds. The instability of working life has degraded one of the foundations of social integration. A secure means of survival performs an essentially integrating role in society and ensures the protection of individuals, families, and communities against major life risks.[2] Family and one's culture, described as 'close protection' by Castel,[1] are important to the weaving of sociability and solidarity networks. Lack of emotional support and economic relief causes people to feel a mixture of abandonment and helplessness. Culture, as a dimension where common values are shared, nourishes dialogue among people and constitutes in itself a system of interaction which creates and maintains social ties and social meanings. These two support networks hold a great integrative power. Thus disaffiliation is not only a state but a way of being (an ethos), lived in a time scale that can be either permanent or temporary. Case study 30.3 gives an example of the disintegration of a neighborhood.

CASE STUDY 30.3   VULNERABILITY AND DISAFFILIATION: ONCE A 'BEAUTIFUL NEIGHBORHOOD'

Projeto Gente Jovem (Young People's Project) in the city of Campinas is located in a working class community whose first name was Vila Bela (Beautiful Neighborhood). During the military government (1964–1985) its name was arbitrarily changed by those in power to Vila Castelo Branco, the name of the general who was the first military president. Vila Bela remained as a small area within this neighborhood, and came to be dominated by drug dealers. Today, 'Beautiful Neighbourhood', as it was once known, is just a reference to a specific place where drug trafficking runs free.

The Vila Castelo Branco, however, came to reflect the rapid urbanization fostered by the 'economic miracle', as the military proudly referred to their economic policies. In fact, social development did not follow economic growth and social inequality sharply increased under military rule. The Vila Castelo Branco, once a working-class region, is now home to people barely struggling for their lives. Campinas became an important technological center with universities and multinational companies, and this fostered the migration of people, even those with no qualifications, who were looking for jobs. Lacking consistent and adequate social policies, Vila Castelo Branco is an example of a poor neighborhood following the path to disaffiliation. In the absence of housing policies, three to four generations share the same houses. Despite further building in the courtyards, parents and their children, siblings and their cousins share the same rooms and beds. Conflict and domestic violence are silent facts of life. Emotional suffering is a daily routine. Men are in short supply: many are in jail, have been shot dead, or are simply gone. The remaining ones are largely unemployed or involved in drug dealing. Consequently, street violence is high and children have got used to it, although they constantly show signs of the impact of stress and loss. After all, they have seen friends, neighbors, brothers, fathers, and mothers being killed.

Despite all of this, they show an unquestionable resilience, facing both hard and quiet times as part of life. Those who have followed the history of this neighborhood can testify to its gradual descent into vulnerability and disaffiliation. However, by the city's standards, the neighborhood is considered fortunate in having a large network of social support, with schools, a health clinic, a social rehabilitation center (a daily facility for mental health patients), a community program for young people, and many local initiatives built up by popular participation,[8] such as a small free market on Sundays, working cooperatives, and community day centers. Collective action has historically been a characteristic and an asset of this community; keeping this alive is one of PROGEN's objectives (see below).

It is essential for occupational therapists to accept the new challenges posed in Brazilian society today regarding the process of disaffiliation its population is undergoing. It is within this perspective that the Metuia Project operates, as its objectives and actions demonstrate (see Box 30.1).

Actions taken by the Metuia Project follow the dynamics of the occupational therapy schools involved and confront the needs and realities of the cities where the programs take place. Therefore, the actions vary according to the context and this may be better comprehended by looking at Metuia's two divisions: the USP/UFSCar division and the PUC–Campinas division.

Both divisions have established partnerships with governmental and non-governmental organizations with the intention of promoting cooperation, consultancy, and the development of future projects. For details see: http://www.ufscar.br/portugues/projetos/metuia

---

Box 30.1   The Objectives of the Metuia Project

1. To develop and disseminate knowledge in the field of social occupational therapy.
2. To develop the debate among occupational therapists on the role of the profession in community action.
3. To develop a critical awareness of the social function of occupational therapists through the characterization of the population assisted by them, with emphasis on territorial or community attention.
4. To study the features and living contexts of the population undergoing a breakdown in social support networks, namely deprived children and adolescents, homeless and unemployed adults.
5. To develop theoretical and practical knowledge about the use of activities as a means of development of self-confidence and production of personal and social meanings.
6. To develop theoretical and practical knowledge about occupational therapy actions that promote personal and social emancipation for the improvement of quality of life.
7. To make occupational therapy students and professionals aware of the importance of work in the social field.
8. To contribute to the qualifications of the practice of professionals and students, providing elements for their action in territorial and community programs and in social institutions.
9. To enable professionals and students to develop a practice where the people's and communities' stories are heard, and the solutions for their own needs are fostered in an action that is jointly built and historically contextualized.

SHARING EXPERIENCES AND LIFE STORIES

Working with vulnerable young people: Projeto Gente Nova

The Projeto Gente Nova (Young People's Project), known as PROGEN, is a 20-year-old community-based non-governmental organization (NGO) in the city of Campinas that has a 12-year-old cooperation agreement with the PUC–Campinas. Programs designed for the young people and their families have been developed by a member of PUC–Campinas teaching staff, along with second, third and fourth year occupational therapy students. The foundation of the Metuia Project contributed to the debate on the programs developed by occupational therapists and provided a theoretical and methodological framework for work that has been carried out.

PROGEN caters for around 180 young people a day, divided in two shifts which correspond to non-school time (i.e. mornings or afternoons). When young people arrive at PROGEN they have some free time to warm up, play, chat, and have some lunch. They then take part in 'talking time' when they sit in a circle and share their experiences and problems, play games, discuss previously chosen themes, sing songs, define their own rules of engagement, and choose the activities they want to join. It is a good opportunity for them to learn better ways of resolving conflicts and developing tolerance, since the right to speak and the need to show respect for what others say are both assured. The talk is funny and serious, a sharing of good and bad moments. While the young people chat about ecology, community life, day-to-day violence, and human rights, solidarity with others and a critical attitude toward the reality they live in are cherished and motivated.

After this, they attend different workshops, such as cooking, craftsmanship, playing music, circus, theatre, or horticulture, run by *social educators*. This position was created at the beginning of the 1980s, when the number of street children started to increase in major Brazilian cities. The role of social educators was to approach street children, first making contact and then drawing them into a social support network. Since that time, the title of social educator has been attached to many of those who work in the social field, whether they be former street children, artists, craftspeople, volunteers, university students, or primary school teachers. The aims of these social educators are to provide occupational experience and satisfaction, to develop skills and creativity, and to foster a sense of belonging and respect.

Occupational therapy sessions are offered as an alternative activity. The only requirement to participate in these sessions is the willingness to do so. The difference between workshops and occupational therapy sessions is clear for all those involved (professionals, students, and users) and lies in the approach to activity. Workshops focus on the processes of learning, manufacturing, and participation in pre-selected activities in which participants are motivated to perform. The occupational therapy sessions, in contrast, start from a basis of free choice and problem-solving methodologies. They consequently run in a less structured and directed way and involve a higher level of problem solving. The whole process, from the initial choice to the final outcome, is seen as a means of developing self-knowledge, self-esteem, communication skills, and conflict resolution.

In 2003, besides offering weekly group sessions to children and pre-adolescents, occupational therapy took part in a different program, the Projeto Agente Jovem (Young Agent Project). This is a federal governmental program, providing guidelines and subsidies for developing different community programs in the country. Adolescents are invited to become protagonists in their own communities and receive a fairly small sponsorship. After some months of preparation, they become responsible for developing activities in schools, nursing care facilities, social centers, public areas, and so forth.

A member of the occupational therapy teaching staff is part of the professional team, and also participates in daily meetings with PROGEN's team to discuss particular needs and problems that children, adolescents, and families are facing. The team meets to discuss strategies to strengthen their social support networks and to think about suitable approaches for coping with difficulties in relationships. Planning of further actions is also carried out.

Occupational therapy intervention is expected to help bridge the gap brought about by inequality, but not by making young people conform themselves to the reality around them; rather, it should make them aware of their condition, help them to strengthen their cultural roots, and give them the opportunity to discover the potential of social organization.

Occupational therapists may also help to build up this bridge through engaging people in the expression of ideas and emotions, helping them to understand their expectations, and developing their reflexivity and communications skills. Occupational therapy sessions can help people to understand the world they live in, and to speak out against social injustice, but in a way that it is neither self-destructive nor violent. To do this, people need to develop a sense that life has something worthwhile to offer them, something they may be able to construct for themselves by themselves. This process starts to take place through the experimentation involved in activities such as graffiti, painting, newspaper writing, drama, varied craftwork, and games. Occupation enables people to get in touch with the human need to do and create, and to transcend the basic needs of survival. D's story in Case study 30.4 illustrates this.

CASE STUDY 30.4   IMAGES OF THE CITY, IMAGES OF DAILY LIFE

D, aged 11, had lived in Vila Castelo Branco since he was born. His family was considered fairly well-off by the standards of his local area. He lived with his grandparents and sister and had a room of his own. At first he had lived with his mother, but after some time his grandfather had decided to raise him and his sister because of their parents' drug abuse. When his grandmother died and the grandfather remarried, things started to get complicated. D got used to being told by the new wife, under the eyes of his silenced grandfather, that he would become exactly like his mother. This was when he joined Projeto Gente Jovem. He was a lively young man who enjoyed doing graffiti and was approached by other kids to do some sketches for them.

His drawings showed the pattern expressed by most graffitists: concrete buildings 'sprouting' from the ground, and his name imprinted amidst the concrete in an ambiguous image that suggested belonging somewhere and, at the same time, being squashed by it. On top of the buildings he would draw a huge moon or rising sun: light in the dark, the warmth of life, it wasn't clear what this signified. Below, in capital letters, he would inscribe the abbreviation of the name of the soccer club he supported fanatically. With small variations, he would repeat the same theme over and over, changing only a few details.

One day he came to the occupational therapy session sad and upset. Having ordered him to be home before 10 p.m., his grandfather's wife had made him sleep outside when he was late. With no other place to go, he had slept in the dog's kennel and arrived covered in dog hair. In silence, he sat down and worked on a picture he had sketched the week before – the same buildings and moon/sun. He used a pyrograph, a device much enjoyed in the occupational therapy sessions, to engrave his drawing in wood. He finished his work, laid it on the table, and walked around. After a while, he turned the device on and completed his work. He changed the moon/sun into an exploding bomb, artistically adding a graceful lit wick. At first he was afraid of being reprehended and said: 'I spoilt it'. Then, recognizing our expressions of admiration, he understood the force of what he had done. Quietly, he enjoyed one of those moments when so little means so much and we feel internally connected with our own self and with everybody around us.

Working with the homeless: Projeto Minha Rua, Minha Casa

Since 2003 the USP and UFSCar division has focused its work and teaching on the non-governmental organization (NGO) known as Associação Minha Rua, Minha Casa (AMRMC), the My Street, My Home Association. This NGO is located in a place lent by the city's administration, beneath an overpass in the center of São Paulo, a city of 10 million inhabitants. Above is the traffic, speeding people on their way to different places. Below are the street and a community day center which seeks to create life alternatives. This could be described as a place of tension, a borderline:[9] it demonstrates tension between private and public life, between collective memory and individual story, between exclusion and participation, between teaching and learning.

The AMRMC was created in 1994, through a partnership between a sector of the business community and a catholic organization. In July 2000 AMRMC and the USP/UFSCar division of the Metuia Project agreed to become partners to provide support to the community while allowing teaching and, more recently, research to take place.

AMRMC became a refuge for street people in São Paulo's town center, where an estimated 8600 people live on the streets. We consider as street people both those who use public places as the location for daily activities such as sleeping, feeding, and working, and those who stay overnight in shelters because they are homeless. Case study 30.5 gives the perspective of one of these homeless people.

CASE STUDY 30.5   EVERYBODY WANTS TO WORK: NARRATIVE FROM THE STREET

M, a user of AMRMC's services says:

The thing is ... we live here, many people arrive here, most of those who arrive here at the square come from other states, they come to São Paulo looking for a job ... like ... a better life, don't they? Then what happens is the Government doesn't give them the opportunity ... people who live here in São Paulo, many people do a lot of charity work for the street people, they give food, but others despise us, run from us ... we are hard-working people and when we ask for some work ... they get scared ... they say: 'Ah! ... we don't have any'. Many come to the streets to look for a job, but sometimes they don't find an opportunity and so they rob someone ... they end up in a police station or in a prison. People who have good sense think differently ... they do something ... they sell something .... But you can see that even for peddlers there is no opportunity ... everything is the Government's fault; because peddlers are not thieves, they want to work, peddlers want to work ... everybody wants to work, no matter what ... getting honest money, but the Government doesn't give the opportunity to anybody ... then what happens ... the violence comes from above ... it doesn't come from here.

Every day between 8 a.m. and 6 p.m. around 150 people come to AMRMC, where they engage in cultural, leisure, and daily living activities (e.g. self-care and getting meals). They are invited to take part in groups debating themes such as drug abuse or to join income generation projects. P, who uses this community day center, describes his experiences in Case study 30.6.

P, who uses the AMRMC center says:

I arrive at the association at 8 a.m. Here I have breakfast, lunch, and afternoon break. I wash my clothes, not all of them, but some, using the spare money I have to pay the laundry; my shirts continue to be washed at the laundry, for how much longer I don't know; this will probably be the last time. Then I continue to live as I used to before ... truthfully I think that the dream is over, there is no hope ... unless [there is] the prospect of a working collective ... I see no prospect for me to come back to the labor market ... while I'm here I'm responsible for reading the newspaper, I read the classified sections daily ... they don't help ... caretaker, gatekeeper, lift operator, cleaner, street sweeper, [in] everything they refer to age ... maximum 45 years old, you understand. The age limit is given, they ask you to have completed primary school to sweep the streets, they ask for documents, proof of residence, water and electricity bills ... these things ... and they inform you at the end ... age limit 45.

AMRMC have a multidisciplinary team composed of educators, social worker, occupational therapist, psychologist, and a coordinator. The work of nearly 40 volunteers makes possible the expansion of educational programs, leisure and cultural activities, or specialized services, such as psychotherapy and legal counseling. Short-term courses and weekly supervision are offered for the volunteers. In case study 30.7 a student gives his view of his work in the center.

G, an occupational therapy student in 2002, says:

I never imagined doing my supervised practice with the street population and my choice was not driven by an intense desire to do so, but by an inclination to get to know people I've never had any contact with and whose presence is a constant feature of daily life in São Paulo town center. This daily presence makes people ignore them, because they have busy lives, full of appointments, or they are afraid, due to the growing violence in the city, or they make judgements about people in the streets that are not always true. As I'm also part of this society, I believe there is some of this inside me, or rather there was, because my practice has contributed to the deconstruction of some of the labels I used (such as dangerous, vagrant, incompetent, ignorant).

The coordination and definition of guidelines and programs are carried out in weekly meetings. The practice of the AMRMC occupational therapy service is developed by a group composed of the NGO's occupational therapist, USP's occupational therapist, and students from USP and UFSCar. Together they have developed programs of collective action and programs of individual assistance. The first include groups involved in free experimentation with threads (tapestry, embroidery, etc.), jewellery making, and alternative income generation programs. The individual programs include the identification of specific demand, referral to other services, such as health services, training courses, and document provision services, and follow-up of users by the occupational therapist or the student. It is often essential to develop the role of facilitator of contacts between the users themselves and with the users of institutions, services, and other AMRMC programs. Where such bonds are formed, it is possible to initiate joint studies with the purpose of building dedicated projects (e.g. relating to housing, training, leisure, health, cultural activities, and personal relations). Hence, it is necessary to develop and use instruments for the interpretation of personal and social reality as part of a universe of complex interactions.

It is always essential that the role of occupational therapy is considered *after* the consideration of the features, problems, and concrete needs of the population in focus. It is vital to think about the social role that activities may embrace, inasmuch as they may serve as means of remaking narratives and social contexts and thus as resources for empowering people.

For us, the therapists who work in the field, it is essential to be able to uncover and interact with the needs expressed by the people we work with. To finish this chapter, we would like to tell the story of J from AMRMC (see Case study 30.8).

CASE STUDY 30.8 JOHN GUITAR: A FOLK ARTIST ON THE STREETS

J, generally known João da Viola (John Guitar – a viola is a folk guitar), is an artist going through difficult times, looking for support, an audience, and market recognition. He goes to AMRMC, which gives him support for basic daily activities such as getting meals, self-care, and doing his laundry, and provides a place to keep his belongings, a safe place to keep his documents, and a place to receive mail.

Through the workshops and cultural events developed by occupational therapists in the collective areas of the center, J is getting closer to achieving his ambition. His ways of dressing and relating to other people show a special style. He composes, sings, and plays folk songs.

J started to play guitar when he was 13 years old. Later, he found a musically experienced partner and started to do shows and recorded some albums. He used to travel around Brazil non-stop. He said the duo spent a long time on the road. On one of these trips, his partner died in a car accident. After that, J stopped playing for 9 years. He says he suffered in the country's economic recession, split up from his wife and arrived in São Paulo as a street person.

He came back to the guitar and to writing songs 3 years ago. He found a new partner with whom he shares most of his daily life, and they do shows at social institutions, record tapes in public parks, pass the hat round to get some cash, and seek sponsorship for their act.

The lyrics of his songs tell the story of his life, his thoughts, and his affinity with music. He says that the best way to interview him is through his lyrics; he likes to explain their meanings and the path of his inspiration.

The strategies of support that have helped J include accompanying him to shows, helping him to produce a video, looking for ways to widen his social networks, recognizing the important places of his life, producing a website to promote his work, and seeking places where he can perform beyond the support network of street people.

References

1. Castel R. *Da indigência à exclusão, à desfiliação. Precariedade do trabalho e vulnerabilidade relacional.* In: Lancetti A, ed. *Saúdeloucura* 4. São Paulo: Hucitec; 1994:21–48.

2. Castel R. *As transformações da questão social.* In: Belfiore-Wanderley M, Bógus L, Yazbek MC, eds. *Desigualdade e a questão social.* São Paulo: EDUC; 1997:161–190.

3. Castel R. *As metamorfoses da questão social.* Petrópolis: Vozes; 1998.

4. Barros D, Ghirardi MI, Lopes R. *Terapia ocupacional e sociedade.* Rev Ter Ocup USP 1999; 10(2–3):71–76.

5. Barros D. *Operadores de saúde na área social.* Rev Ter Ocup USP 1991; 1(1):11–16.

6. Pochmann M, Amorim R. *Atlas da exclusão social no Brasil.* São Paulo: Cortez Editora; 2003.

7. Human Development Report. Millennium development goals: a compact among nations to end human poverty. Online. Available: www.undp.org/hdr2003/

8. Midgley J, Hall A, Hardiman M, Narine D. Community participation, social development and the state. London: Methuen; 1986.

9. Bhabha H. *O local da cultura.* Belo Horizonte: UFMG, SAS/FIPE; 2001.

Chapter 31

Occupational therapy education without borders

Frank Kronenberg, Salvador Simó Algado, Nick Pollard

OVERVIEW

The opportunity to engage in occupational therapy education, to learn, experiment, and grow, is a tremendous privilege, giving its participants, whether students or teachers, scope to explore, develop, and achieve our personal potentials. SPIRIT of SURVIVORS–Occupational Therapists without Borders (SOS–OTwB) considers that an education which truly nurtures our abilities and commitment to respond to the diverse everyday occupational needs and rights of *all* should enable students and teachers to overcome obstacles to the profession's potential and promise. SOS–OTwB came about to enable students and teachers to reconnect with the spirit and challenge of the profession.

This chapter briefly describes the perspectives and objectives of SOS–OTwB education initiatives that have been carried out since 2000 in Sweden, Spain, Belgium, Canada, the United States, Guatemala, Portugal, Georgia, Denmark, England, Norway, Germany, the Netherlands, and South Africa. Participants in SOS–OTwB presentations, workshops, and courses, from Linköping University in Sweden (2000), the University of Vic in Barcelona/Catalonia (2002), and the European Network of Occupational Therapy in Higher Education in Tbilisi, Georgia (2003), share their views and experiences. In conclusion, we identify some educational challenges and offer recommendations to answer them.

INTRODUCTION

SPIRIT of SURVIVORS–Occupational Therapists without Borders (SOS–OTwB, see Preface) represents an innovative occupational therapy practice, education, and research network (formerly known as the Dolphin Association) started by the first two authors of this chapter in 1999. SOS–OTwB education initiatives are inspired by a vision of overcoming occupational apartheid (see Ch. 6),[1–10] and working toward occupational justice (see Ch. 9),[11–13] which implies a commitment to an occupational needs and rights approach to practice.[14–17] SOS–OTwB considers that practice, education, and research initiatives with marginalized people, especially those affected by occupational apartheid, should consist primarily of enabling them to explore and identify 'their own perceptions of what they are due in terms of fundamental freedoms and basic entitlements'[12] and supporting them 'to develop their capacity and power to construct their own destinies'.[18] This appears to correspond with the economist Amartya Sen's argument for 'a focus on the capabilities (substantive human freedoms) of people to do and be what they value', and offers occupational therapists a basis for evaluating justice.[19]

SOS–OTwB workshops and courses aim to enable the evaluation of these perspectives against the values and beliefs of occupational therapy. Who we are and what we do in the world is guided and informed by individual motives, aims, and considerations (the 'why' of our decision to become an occupational therapist), our professional philosophy, and our values and beliefs. This requires a deep reflection: we challenge participants to investigate their personal 'archaeology', to dig for and question their underlying assumptions, aiming to understand and experience more fully what drives us all, not just rationally but also at the heart and gut levels.

Pollard and Walsh[20] have argued that, as a feminine profession in thrall to a male-dominated medical model, occupational therapy has played down its base activities, such as domestic occupations or maternal skills, which are perceived as traditionally female, in favor of seeking professional status through an alliance with science. Occupational therapists need to reassert the core value of activities of daily living in practice, research, and professional development. People do not live in laboratories. We need to retain the personal aspect of daily activity, or we risk holing the ship of holism and disabling the essential personal component of owning the social change necessary to effect positive difference. Only then, we believe, can our principles inspire and give true guidance to the further development and maturation of our roles in the world as occupational therapists.

SOS–OTwB engages in conscientization or awareness raising,[21] exploring and questioning everyday local and global realities from different perspectives, such as the values and beliefs of occupational therapy,[22,23] the principles of Herbert de Souza (see Ch. 1), various human rights instruments,[24–27] and the way people who experience disabling conditions themselves look at and understand their realities. These exercises reveal how our professional actions can actually contribute to occupational apartheid or occupational absurdity (see Ch. 6) instead of enabling the people that we have the privilege to walk with and learn from to overcome their disabling conditions.

For example, the difficulty the profession has had in acknowledging its feminine origins and values in the male-dominated hierarchical world of medicine has served to hold back its development, and even to lead it into obscurity, while its female students have learned to repudiate 'women's work' in the pursuit of values which hold more scientific credibility.[20] At the same time, occupational therapists have been unable to gain postgraduate education in sufficient numbers to develop appropriate research skills to capitalize on the profession's strong narrative traditions of practice.[28] Learning to engage in dialectic discourse[29] about such issues also fosters a necessary critical awareness about the gendered and political nature of occupational therapy and its core construct, occupation.[1–4,20,30–33] The practice of examining our profession, daily living, and the world through many different glasses, and from different angles, enables engagement with the untapped potential of occupational therapy thinking and practicing 'without borders' (see Ch. 1).

SOS–OTwB educational initiatives aim to advance critical 'being, doing and becoming'[34] as 'a means of injecting a creative and transformatory element'[35] into the training of occupational therapists, enabling its participants:

- to become aware of their personal worth and potential group strength in order to help them gain confidence in themselves as thinking, active, capable human beings;
- to analyze and confront situations of occupational apartheid, occupational deprivation, and occupational absurdity;
- to identify and obtain the tools and skills they need in order to respond to occupational needs and rights at individual and community levels, enabling people to take charge of their health and their lives.[36]

These philosophical and theoretical arguments of occupational therapy become tangible when we share concrete SOS–OTwB practice and research initiatives with women in a prison in Zaragoza,[37] with Mayan *retornos* in Guatemala (see Ch. 25),[38–40] with survivors of conflict in Bosnia and Kosovo (see Ch. 18),[5,41] and with street children in Mexico[10] and Guatemala (see Ch. 19).[16] These accounts of the projects' origins, development, and evaluations provide inspiring and encouraging examples of occupational therapy without borders, i.e. occupational therapy outside traditional practice settings. The key role of networking is especially highlighted, in terms of collaborating with civil society organizations (CSOs), non-governmental organizations (NGOs), funding bodies, the World Federation of Occupational Therapists (WFOT), and the European Network of Occupational Therapy in Higher Education (ENOTHE), and presenting at national and international congresses. Although these practice experiences mostly took place in 'developing' countries, the aims of our workshops and courses are to explore *local* realities and identify situations of occupational apartheid, occupational deprivation, and occupational absurdity in the participants' own countries, home towns, neighborhoods, or workplaces (be it a healthcare institution or a university), and to consider possible strategies to confront these from an 'occupational therapy without borders' perspective.

The work of the third author of this chapter developed outside the formation of SOS–OTwB, through working with people with enduring mental health problems in the community and connecting them with adult education and survivor poetry organizations (see Ch. 21),[42–45] and with people with early onset of dementia.[46] There are many shared elements of working with local realities and with narratives with people whose mental illness and consequent marginalization had hitherto limited their access to educational opportunity, the means for self-expression, or their capacity for self-determination.[47]

ILLUSTRATIONS FROM WORKSHOPS AND COURSEWORK

This section of the chapter shares views and experiences of participants in SOS–OTwB education initiatives from Sweden, Spain, and Georgia.

Linköping University, Sweden

In February 2001 SOS–OTwB was invited to run workshops for groups of students and faculty members at the occupational therapy department of Linköping University in Sweden; this was the first occupational therapy program in Europe to express a special interest in our work. These encounters inspired the establishment of a local section of SOS–OTwB, which aims to encourage students to do practical fieldwork with marginalized groups in areas where occupational therapists have not traditionally worked in Sweden. Students have since worked at a probation center, a shelter for homeless people, and in a community project called *'Barn och ungdomars bästa: utgångspunkter för ett lokalt utvecklingsarbete i samverkan mellan Linköpings kommun och landstinget i Östergötland'* (For the benefit of children and adolescents: points of departure for local development work in collaboration between Linköping municipality and Östergötland county council).[48] This project is concerned with creating a basis for a continuous development work to promote the health of children and adolescents. These young people may be unwell, may have suffered bad treatment, may have a refugee background, and/or be youths with developmental problems, functional disorders, chronic illnesses, and/or handicaps. Degree projects about marginalized groups have been promoted,[49] and a poster presentation about the work done by the Swedish section of SOS–OTwB was presented at the WFOT conference in Stockholm 2002.[50]

Lena Haglund and Åsa Larsson, the occupational therapy program leaders of Linköping University, describe aspects of their program below.

We have students with both physical and mental disabilities, and we adapt our program through individual study plans so that they can pursue their studies. People with disabilities also use their experiences in teaching parts of the program. Sweden has strict laws on discrimination and a special ombudsman to support them. Linköping University has a person (who happens to be an occupational therapist) who supports students with special needs.

Students obviously need to develop an understanding of occupational apartheid and marginalized groups. The program has a responsibility to introduce both the faculty and students to concepts related to the Code of Ethics *of the Swedish Association of Occupational Therapists.[51] This states that occupational therapists shall respect human rights and the equal value of human beings. The program in Linköping emphasizes that occupational therapy is to be carried out in different areas, not only in the healthcare sector but also in the wider community. We already address community-based rehabilitation, and run a course called 'Occupational therapy in a changing society', where issues about marginalized groups and other topics are discussed.*

The current economical constraints in the Swedish healthcare sector will probably lead to the marginalization of more groups, as we can see in the community around us. We encourage students to undertake fieldwork in non-traditional occupational therapy areas and to meet new groups of clients. We also encourage them to raise public awareness that we can make a difference with people, for example those with a mental illness who live in the community, the elderly, people who are homeless, and those who are in prison.

The work initiated by the Swedish section of SOS–OTwB has made a difference; for example, the idea to visit the probation center came up in the group. We contacted them, went on a study visit, found a student who was interested, helped with the connection, and the student now works there. The work is not easy: it has to be taken one small step at a time, and relies heavily on the engagement of those who are involved. All the workshop participants, whether students, faculty members, or practitioners, agree that the SOS–OTwB mission is in line with occupational therapy philosophy. Many feel that advocating occupational justice is a professional responsibility. No one has left the workshops without new thoughts, ideas, and feelings about this issue.

The following reflections are from Lisa Wedin, a former student who was inspired by the SOS–OTwB workshop and carried out her final fieldwork placement at a shelter for homeless people in Stockholm.

In semester six you begin to understand what occupational therapy is really all about, what a powerful tool activity is, and how you can use it. This is a central focus of the Linköping occupational therapy program, consequently you have the opportunity to do fieldwork in non-traditional areas.

The subject of homeless people arose during a brainstorming session about the degree project. Why don't occupational therapists work with this population? To me it was obvious: homeless people had lost their ability to manage their everyday lives, and occupational therapy would be an appropriate intervention. Later, when I had a summer job at a shelter for homeless people, I saw the need for occupational therapy in reality. Doing nothing characterized the daily rhythm of the people at the shelter. They appeared to lack insight into their abilities and how to use these to make progress. My occupational therapy approach was very useful in looking at the whole person and thinking about appropriate activities as tools to facilitate their needs and wishes.

I decided to use my fieldwork practice to apply and test the value of occupational therapy with this population. My previous work there helped me to prepare and focus, but my plans were too ambitious. I could not even come close to accomplishing them during the 8 weeks of fieldwork. You do not know how much is realistically possible, but it is crucial to examine what you actually achieve for different individuals. I also learned that when you are going to practice in new territory it is essential to inform other personnel and the target group about what occupational therapy is, not once but ten times. Work is easier if everyone understands what you are trying to do.

I received a lot of positive reactions and I learned a great deal about occupational therapy. The occupational therapy role was often hard, demanding, and quite lonely. The most important advice I can give is to reflect on what you have learned yourself and what you have accomplished. Fieldwork is shorter in duration than you think, and you only have time to scratch the surface. Working in a non-traditional area is difficult but a lot of fun and rewarding. Think about how you can use your knowledge about occupational therapy and go and try it out. As a student you have the opportunities and conditions to do just that – to test and investigate what is possible!

King Juan Carlos University, Madrid and Vic University, Barcelona, Spain

At King Juan Carlos University in Madrid in 2001 and an extension of Vic University in Barcelona in 2002, SOS–OTwB presented a 2-week course covering a critical philosophical and theoretical examination of the rhetoric and the practice of the art and science of occupational therapy. This was informed and supported by concrete examples of occupational therapy practice without borders with people with a history of substance abuse, people in prisons, people who have suffered physical or sexual abuse, refugees, immigrants, street children, and young people and adolescents at risk. In the following narrative, Luis Fernández, an occupational therapist from Spain and participant in the Barcelona course, shares how this experience inspired and enabled him to conduct a research project with survivors of the street in El Salvador.[52]

My first contact with SOS–OTwB was as a student in the 'Psychosocial occupational therapy' course at the University of Vic in Barcelona in 2002. The 'Occupational therapy with marginalized populations' course has had a profound impact on my life, both at a professional level and especially at a personal level. During my training I was always wondering about the possibility of working as an occupational therapist in social contexts other than our traditional fields of intervention, and meeting today's global challenges. The course answered all my questions, and SOS–OTwB has been a motivating example for me.

Recently I have developed a research project about street children in El Salvador. The course has facilitated me in planning a major part of the intervention. I now wish to implement and promote occupational therapy programs which start from a common vision of health and occupational justice for all, with the aim of ensuring access to meaningful occupations for street children and addressing their situation of occupational apartheid.

I have learned so much with the children, especially at a human level. I have evaluated their occupational problems and needs, appreciating and considering their occupational narrative of moving from being victims to being survivors, understanding a holistic vision of the human being as a physical, psychological, social, and spiritual reality, with a life of meaning.

This people-centered approach has allowed me to visualize human beings with all their potentials and strengths, although sometimes they are immersed in extremely difficult conditions, such as the hostile environments in which street children live.

Guided and informed by the Canadian Model of Occupational Performance (CMOP)[22] (see Ch. 15), and the Model of Human Occupation (MOHO)[53] (see Ch. 14), I was able to identify the difficulties that these children are experiencing, taking into account the importance of the environment in which they are immersed. The street represents their place, their way of life, and surely their most immediate point of reference. In this environment, the children survive in a society that has rejected them, suffering repression from governmental institutions. The street is also the place where, among other activities, they engage in prostitution, delinquency, and drug trafficking, all of which can jeopardize their health, safety, morale, and dignity. Often they do not have a vision for the future, as for them 'there is no tomorrow or yesterday, life is an eternal now',[54] as life makes no sense, has no meaning.

As they live in an adult world they develop roles which are not age appropriate, and this makes it difficult to experience a sense of belonging, social identity, and consequently meaning. This conditions, among other things, low levels of self-motivation. Therefore, participation in meaningful occupations represents the medium in which they can reconnect with their being, and be aware of who they can become, thus redirecting their own narratives and experiences and re-establishing their place in society as survivors of the street and rightful citizens.

European Network of Occupational Therapy in Higher Education, (ENOTHE) Tbilisi, Georgia

In the following account, Hanneke van Bruggen, executive director of ENOTHE, describes that organization's collaboration with SOS–OTwB and how this led to the development of new approaches to occupational therapy education in Georgia.

In 2003 SOS–OTwB established a formal collaboration with the European Network of Occupational Therapy in Higher Education (ENOTHE). The general aim of this thematic network project is to enable educational institutes and professional associations to liaise, develop, and harmonize standards of professional practice and education, as well as to advance the body of knowledge of occupational therapy throughout Europe. One objective is to facilitate interaction and integration with occupational therapy education institutes in Eastern and Central Europe. ENOTHE is supporting and developing new projects and curriculum development in new occupational therapy institutes.

Over the last 7 years ENOTHE has developed three major projects, in the Czech Republic, in Georgia and Armenia, and in Bulgaria, Hungary and Romania. These are aimed at contributing to social change as well as reforming the higher education sector through the introduction and implementation of occupational therapy education and services. They include a general principle of training occupational therapy students to enable marginalized people, persons with disabilities, and their carers and families in both physical and social participation in the environment through occupation. ENOTHE members collaborate with local staff and students, with the direct involvement of client groups and their carers or families, to develop education modules, after each of which a small project is implemented.

Some of the most vulnerable groups, exposed to many health and social risks across East and Central European countries, are street children, refugees, or internally displaced people. This reality prompted ENOTHE to search for occupational therapists who had worked with these populations. In collaboration with SOS–OTwB, a module was developed in 2003 for the Georgian occupational therapy curriculum, focusing on street children and internally displaced people. To enable the implementation of their projects, one of the course assignments was to found a legally recognized occupational therapy association that could promote the profession in all fields and advance equal rights, equal opportunities, and social participation for all citizens. This led to the formation of the Georgian Occupational Therapy Association (GE-OTA).

The following section, illustrating the experiences and views of those involved in that Association, has been contributed jointly by the authors mentioned, who have also offered individual narratives within this section.

Georgian Occupational Therapy Association

Occupational therapy was first introduced to Georgia in 2001. The history of its development in Georgia is similar to that of other countries where conventional, traditional methods of medicine influence the process of adaptation of every new field comprising innovative ideas, concepts, and methods. Even in such mainstream fields as psychiatry and neurology, the introduction of occupational therapy has triggered complex social and system changes in our country.

In these circumstances, the implementation of occupational therapy ideas concerning marginalized populations proved to be especially interesting and challenging in Georgia. It contributed to the development of new forms of proactive thinking and new approaches in the field of occupational therapy as well as in the community.

Ana Arganashvili says:

> *Probably, due to my lack of experience and information before getting acquainted with this module, I found it extremely difficult to find a relationship between the street children and the concept of empowerment. I believe that one of the positive aspects of this module is the focus on supporting future occupational therapists in pursuing their professional identity. Consequently, although I had difficulty connecting certain concepts on a personal level, I managed to do this at a professional level and so developed a stable professional–personal attitude that served as a background for my further work and studies.*

Working with marginalized populations was especially interesting and meaningful for us, enabling us to understand the meaning of 'occupational therapy', 'function', and 'role' in society and to consider how the complex interrelationship of micro, meso, and macro aspects of key social factors

- going beyond cultural competence, and fostering cultural safety[67–69] (see Chs 10 and 13)
- developing and promoting community-based rehabilitation (CBR) entrepreneurship,[2,70] which includes knowledge of and skills in networking, forming creative partnerships, and fundraising[15,71–73] (see Ch. 27)
- understanding and learning to make use of humor[74,75] and 'clown-clusions'[76] in personal and social processes of transformation.

While this chapter has, we feel, been a just celebration of the work of students of SOS–OTwB education initiatives, with positive outcomes, we would like to conclude with a challenge. We have been concerned that whenever and wherever we have invited occupational therapy students and lecturers to stand up and express clearly and convincingly what occupational therapy is and why they have chosen it as a career, confident responses have been rare. Often this was laughed off as a typical professional trait; but how can such self-deprecation foster the development and realization of untapped potential that occupational therapy has itself proclaimed?

To us, occupational therapy goes way beyond merely solving technical problems. At its best, occupational therapy transcends the borders of being a profession. Occupational therapy can be viewed as a grand piano, a metaphor capturing the richness of both the art and science components that guide and inform occupational therapy practice. The keys of the piano are attached to strings which represent our principles, approaches, and the many different fields of knowledge that occupational therapy has the freedom to draw from, e.g. medical and social sciences, the arts. There are also strings we may not even have discovered or considered, yet, that might become useful and meaningful in responding to the needs and interests of the people we engage with.

Looking at it another way, the variety of keys of the grand piano of occupational therapy allows us to enable people and communities who experience disabling conditions to play anew the music of their lives. We should take to heart the words that the late violinist Isaac Stern expressed in the great film *From Mao to Mozart*:[77]

> *Every time you take up the instrument you are making a statement, your statement. And it must be the statement of faith, that you believe this is the way you want to speak. Unless you feel that you must live with music, that music can say more than words, that music can mean more, that without music we are not alive, if you don't feel all that, don't be a musician!*

Though of course occupational therapy's priorities are always and essentially a matter of debate, as long as there are people who are restricted in or denied meaningful and dignified participation in daily life, SOS–OTwB will aim, through stinging questions and advancing principles, to inspire occupational therapy education without borders. Together we can make use of *all* the keys that can enable the people we work with to play and experience again the music of their lives. We look forward to working with you.

Acknowledgements

We thank the following colleagues, and workshop and course participants for their contributions to this chapter: from Sweden, Lena Haglund, Åsa Larsson, Lisa Wedin; from Spain, Luis Fernández; from the Netherlands, Hanneke van Bruggen; and from Georgia, Ana Arganashvili, Tina Kavtaradze, Nino Rukhadze, Maia Bagrationi, Tako Tavartkiladze, Marina Gelovani, Rusudan Lortkipanidze, Nino Javakhadze, and Nino Okrosashvili.

References

1. Kronenberg F. Occupational therapy without borders. Paper presented at the thirtieth National Congress of the Occupational Therapy Association of South Africa. Cape Town. May 2004.

2. Kronenberg F. Position paper on community based rehabilitation. Forrestfield, Western Australia: World Federation of Occupational Therapists; April 2004. Online. Available: www.wfot.org

3. Kronenberg F. Occupational therapy without borders: occupational justice education. Paper presented at the ninth European Network of Occupational Therapy in Higher Education conference. Prague. October/November 2003.

4. Kronenberg F. In search for the political nature of occupational therapy. MSc OT paper, Linköping University, January 2003.

5. Simó Algado S, Mehta N, Kronenberg F, et al. Occupational therapy intervention with children survivors of war. Can J Occup Ther 2002; 69(4):205–217.

6. Kronenberg F. Juggling with survivors of the street: occupational therapy and clowns in Guatemala City. Paper presented at the thirteenth WFOT congress in Stockholm, 2002.

7. van Tilburg O. *Dolphin en de strijd tegen occupational apartheid*. Nederlands Tijdschrift voor Ergotherapie 2001; 29(4):141–144.

8. Pettersen BH. *Dolphin: arbeider mot aktivitetsapartheid*. Ergoterapeuten 2000; 43(11):7–10.

9. Kronenberg F, Simó Algado S. Overcoming occupational apartheid: working towards occupational justice. Paper presented at the sixth European Congress of Occupational Therapy. Paris. 2000.

10. Kronenberg F. Street children: being and becoming. Research study. Heerlen, Netherlands: Hogeschool Limburg; 1999.

11. Townsend E. Occupational justice: everyday ethical, moral and civic issues for an inclusive world. Keynote address presented at the ninth European Network of Occupational Therapy in Higher Education conference. Prague. October/November 2003.

12. Townsend E. Power and justice in enabling occupation. Can J Occup Ther 2003; 70(2):74–87.

13. Townsend E, Wilcock A. Occupational justice. In: Christiansen C, Townsend E. Introduction to occupation: the art and science of living. Thorofare, NJ: Prentice Hall; 2003.

14. de Gaay Fortman B. Persistent poverty and inequality in an era of globalization: opportunities and limitations of a rights approach. Paper presented at the Economic, Social and Cultural Rights Workshop. Nairobi. 14–16 April 2003.

15. Thomas de Benitez S. Green light for street children's rights. Brussels: European Network on Street Children Worldwide; 2002. Online. Available: www.enscw.org

16. Kronenberg F. WFOT discussion paper on CBR. World Federation of Occupational Therapists. April 2003. Online. Available: www.wfot.org

17. World Health Organization. International classification of functioning, disability and health. (ICF) Geneva, Switzerland: WHO; 2001.

18. Meléndez Cardona CE. *¿Qué es y para qué sirve la política? Educación para la Paz. Documento interno.* Guatemala: Oficina Pastoral Social Arzobispado de Guatemala OPSAG; 2001.

19. Sen A. Development as freedom. Oxford: Oxford University Press; 1999.

20. Pollard N, Walsh S. Occupational therapy, gender and mental health, an inclusive perspective? Br J Occup Ther 2000; 63(9):425–431.

21. Freire P. The politics of education: culture, power and liberation. South Hadley, MA: Bergin & Garvin; 1985.

22. Canadian Association of Occupational Therapists. Enabling occupation: an occupational therapy perspective. *Revised Edn.* Ottawa, ON: CAOT Publications ACE; 2002.

23. World Federation of Occupational Therapists. Code of ethics. Online. Available: www.wfot.org.

24. Human Rights Web. Online. Available: www.hrweb.org

25. Sinclair K. Disability rights as human rights. Australia: World Federation of Occupational Therapists; 2002. Online. Available: www.wfot.org

26. United Nations High Commission on Human Rights (UNHCHR). United Nations standard rules on the equalization of opportunities for persons with disabilities. Resolution 48/96. New York: United Nations; 1993.

27. UNHCHR. Human rights and disability: the current use and future potential of United Nations human rights instruments in the context of disability. New York: United Nations; 2003. Online. Available: http://www.unhchr.ch/html/menu6/2/disability_en.doc

28. Pollard N. Doncaster–Dumfries Part 1. Federation 2002; 24:13–15.

29. Habermas J, transl Lenhart C, Weber Nicholson S. Moral consciousness and communicative action. Cambridge, MA: Belknap Press of Harvard University Press; 1995.

30. Kronenberg F. Understanding and facing up to the political nature of occupational therapy. Paper presented at the seventh European Congress of Occupational Therapy. Athens. September 2004.

31. Urbanowski R, Kronenberg F, Pollard N, Simó Algado S. The politics of occupation. Paper presented at the second Canadian Occupational Science Symposium. Toronto. May 2004.

32. Thibeault R. Experiential and philosophical considerations on occupation and the genesis of meaning and resilience. In: McColl M. Spirituality and occupational therapy. Ottawa: CAOT Publications ACE; 2003:83–94.

33. Goldstein J. International relations and everyday life. In: Zemke R, Clark F, eds. Occupational science: the evolving discipline. Philadelphia: F.A. Davis; 1996.

34. Wilcock AA. Reflections on doing, being and becoming. Can J Occup Ther 1998; 65(5):248–256.

35. Barnett R. Higher education: a critical business. Buckingham, UK: The Society for Research into Higher Education & Open University Press; 1997.

36. Werner D, Bower B. Helping health workers learn. Berkeley, CA: The Hesperian Foundation; 2001.

37. Simó Algado S, Thibeault R, Urbanowski R, Kronenberg F, Pollard N. *La terapia ocupacional en el mundo penitenciario*. Terapia Ocupacional. 2003; 33:10–20.

38. Simó Algado S, Rodriguez G, Egan M. Spirituality in a refugee camp. Can J Occup Ther 1994; 61:88–94.

39. Simó Algado S. *El retorno del hombre de maiz, intervención desde la terapia ocupacional con una comunidad indígena maya*. Terapia Ocupacional 2002; 28:30–35.

40. Simó Algado S, Kronenberg F. *Intervención con una comunidad indígena maya*. Materia Prima 2000; 16(August):28–32.

41. Simó Algado S, Mehta N, Kronenberg F. *Niños supervivientes de conflicto bélico*. Terapia Ocupacional 2003; 31:205–217.

42. Ryan H, Pollard N. Poetry on the agenda for Scottish weekend. Adults Learning 2002; January:10–11.

43. Pollard N, Bryer M. Community publishing and rehabilitation: stories of ordinary lives. RED Journal (Doncaster and South Humber Healthcare NHS Trust) 2002; Winter:6–10.

44. Pollard N, Steele A. From Doncaster to Dumfries. OT News 2002; 10(11):31.

45. Pollard N. Notes towards an approach for the therapeutic use of creative writing in occupational therapy. In: Sampson F, ed. Creative writing in health and social care. London, UK: Jessica Kingsley; 2004: 189–206.

46. Jubb D, Pollard N, Chaston D. Developing services for younger people with dementia. Nursing Times 2003; 99(22):34–35.

47. Pollard N, Kronenberg F, Simó Algado S. Community based rehabilitation – a role for worker writers and community publishers. Federation Magazine – The magazine of The Federation of Worker Writers and Community Publishers 2004; 27(Feb):12–14.

48. Linköping Municipality. *Utvecklingsprojekt inom ramen för barn och ungdomars bästa*. (Development projects in the context of and for the benefit of children and adolecents.) Linköping, Sweden: Linköping Municipality; 2002. Online. Available: www.linkoping.se/bub/

49. Axelsson AK, Wedin L. *Stödjande och hindrande faktorer till aktivitet för hemlösa personer*. Uppsats Linköping. (Supporting and hindering factors for activity for homeless people.) Linköping University degree project. Linköping, Sweden: 2003.

50. Alfredsson Ågren A, Lygnegård F Persson A. Is occupational justice existing in Sweden? DOLPHIN-S, a vision! WFOT congress Abstract Book. CD–ROM. Stockholm, Sweden: WFOT; 2002.

51. Förbundet Sveriges Arbetsterapeuter. Code of Ethics. Nacko, Sweden: Swedish Association of Occupational Therapists; 2002. Online. Available: www.fas.akademikerhuset.se/

52. Fernández Martínez L. *Héroes del Boulevard: investigación sobre el consumo de drogas en los niños en situación de calle en la ciudad de San Salvador*. Masters

thesis. Universidad Rey Juan Carlos. Madrid, España. September 2003.

53. Kielhofner G. Model of human occupation: theory and application, 3rd edn. Baltimore, MD: Lippincott Williams & Willkins; 2002.

54. Ortiz A. *Vidas callejeras; pasos sin rumbos. La dolorosa realidad de los niños de la Calle*, 1st edn. Mexico City: Editorial Patria (Promexa); 1999.

55. Bagrationi M, Agranashvili A, Tavarkiladez T. Working with marginalised population using occupational therapy intervention in Georgia. Today's children are tomorrow's parents. Street children and abuse and neglect prevention. Journal Of The Network For Prevention Of Child Maltreatment. 2003; 12(May):67–73.

56. Mattingly C. Hayes Fleming M. Clinical reasoning: forms of inquiry in a therapeutic practice. Philadelphia, FA Davis; 1994.

57. Mattingly C. What is clinical reasoning? Am J Occup Ther 1991a; 45:979–986.

58. Mattingly C. The narrative nature of clinical reasoning. Am J Occup Ther 1991b; 45:998–1005.

59. Cockburn L, Trentham B. Participatory action research: integrating community occupational therapy practice and research. Can J Occup Ther 2002; 69:20–30.

60. Nelson D. Occupation: form and performance. Am J Occup Ther October 1988; 42(10):633–641.

61. Nelson D. Therapeutic occupation: a definition. Am J Occup Ther November/December 1996; 50(10):775–782.

62. Tenberken S. My path leads to Tibet: the inspiring story of how one young blind woman brought hope to the blind children of Tibet. New York: Arcade; 2003.

63. Pirsig R. Zen and the art of motorcycle maintenance: an inquiry into values. New York: Bantam Books; 1974.

64. Cyrulnik B. *Los patitos feos*. Barcelona: Geisa Editorial; 2002.

65. Molina Berrizbeita JP. A case for the human right of access to justice. Coventry, UK: University of Warwick; 2002. (mimeograph)

66. Kronenberg F. WFOT Helsinki CBR review report. Forrestfield, Australia: World Federation of Occupational Therapists; August 2003. Online. Available: www.wfot.org

67. Jungersen K. Cultural safety: *kawa whakaruruhau* – an occupational therapy perspective. NZJOT 2002; 49(1):4–9.

68. Jungersen K. Culture, theory, and the practice of OT in New Zealand/Aotearoa. AJOT 1992; 46(8):745–750.

69. Coleridge P. Disability and culture-selected readings in CBR. Series I. Bangalore, India: National Printing Press; 2000. Occasional publication of the Asia Pacific Disability Rehabilitation Journal.

70. Kronenberg F. The WFOT–CBR project team – enabling global collaboration in community based rehabilitation (CBR). Paper presented at the seventh European Congress of Occupational Therapy. Athens. September 2004.

71. Pollard N, Kronenberg F, Simó Algado S. Community based rehabilitation. A role for worker writers and community publishers. Federation Magazine – The magazine of The Federation of Worker Writers and Community Publishers 2004; 27(Feb):12–14.

72. Bornstein D. How to change the world: social entrepreneurs and the power of new ideas. Oxford: Oxford University Press; 2004.

73. Gregory Dees J, Emerson J, Economy P. Strategic tools for social entrepreneurs: enhancing the performance of your enterprising nonprofit. Whiley E Book; 2002.

74. Vanistendael S. *La felicidad es possible*. Barcelona: Editorial Gedisa; 2002.

75. Fernandez JD. *Hocia una pedogogia del humor*. Revista Ñaque: teatro, exprésion, educación 1999; 3(9):1–8.

76. Jara J. *El clown, un navegante de las emociones. Temas de educación artística 2*. Seville: PROEXDRA; 2000.

77. From Mao to Mozart – Isaac Stern in China. Film, directed by Lerner M. USA: Rhapsody Films; 1990.

Useful websites

Braille without Borders,
    http://www.braillewithoutborders.org
Caritas, http://www.caritas-international.de/
Child and the Environment,
    http://www.childandenvironment.org/

European Network for Occupational Therapy in Higher Education, http://www.enothe.hva.nl
Federation of Worker Writers and Community Publishers, http://www.thefwwcp.org.uk

Georgian Occupational Therapy Association,
  http://www. enothe.hva.nl/tp/ece/
  east-central-tempus-fapadag.htm (contact:
  ge-ota@gol.ge)
Linköping Universitet, Sweden,
  http://www.linkopingunversity.org
Norwegian Refugee Council, http://www.nrc.no/
Politics of Health Knowledge Network,
  http://www.politicsofhealth.org
Sheffield Hallam University, England,
  http://www.shu.ac.uk

Social Innovation Entrepreneurs Impact,
  http://www. ashoka.org
Spirit of Survivors – Occupational Therapists
  without Borders, http://www.sos-otwb.org
Universidad Rey Juan Carols, Madrid, Spain,
  http://www.urjc.es/
Universitat de Vic, Catalunya, Spain,
  http://www.uvic.es
World Federation of Occupational Therapists,
  http://www.wfot.org

Chapter **32**

Domestic workers' narratives
Transforming occupational therapy practice

Roshan Galvaan

OVERVIEW

This chapter introduces a research study into South African live-in domestic workers' experiences of engaging in occupations. It explores the process of problem identification and the necessity of applying sensitivity in the research method. The four participants' occupational profiles elucidate the challenges and barriers that they experience. An occupational therapy interpretation suggests how occupational therapists can contribute to promoting equal opportunities and facilitating the domestic workers' wellbeing.

INTRODUCTION

The occupational therapist's decision to embark on research has traditionally emerged from an academic or clinical cue. However, the profession needs to extend its borders, so that occupational therapists respond to communities' and populations' sociopolitical demands and needs. This requires an appreciation of what the needs are and a sense of how policy can be used to guide the occupational therapist's contribution to change.

The following chapter presents research into the occupational needs and rights of live-in domestic workers in Cape Town, South Africa.[1] It highlights the potential role of research in making the needs of marginalized groups explicit and suggests how this would contribute to social change and improving health.

PROBLEM IDENTIFICATION: SOCIETY AND CLINICAL PRACTICE

Clinical practice has traditionally been the source of many research topics in occupational therapy. This has led to research often focusing on occupational performance components and improving an individual's function. The author's research focus began in a similar way, while working with clients who had performance component deficits and presented at a psychiatric hospital. These beginnings prompted her to adopt a narrative style to identifying her influence on the evolution of the research.[2] This narrative, reflective stance is mirrored in this chapter.

The author worked as an occupational therapist in a psychiatric unit for women at a tertiary (specialist) level hospital. During this time, she encountered young, live-in domestic workers who developed psychiatric diagnoses such as substance-induced psychosis, depression, and bipolar mood disorder. These domestic workers were all black women, of rural origin, and under the age of 35 years. During therapy sessions, they shared how stressful it was for them to be away from home and how they struggled to adapt to the work environment. It appeared that their difficulty in adapting to their work contributed to them developing these diagnoses. Their descriptions alerted the author to the fact that much of what they did was work related. They had little access to alternative occupations that were more restful. The conceptualization of the research was guided by the need to understand the lack of diversity of opportunities and occupations experienced by this marginalized group in their daily occupational lives.

This knowledge was supported by the author's personal experiences as a 'colored' South African living in a home and a community where domestic workers were routinely employed. (The term colored here refers to the apartheid classification of groups of the South African population.) The author was conscious of the popular discrimination based on socio-economic inequalities and racial injustices and the class differences that often existed between the worker and employer (and employer's family).

The author needed to identify herself in relation to the status usually afforded to her in the community in order to be flexible in using different lenses with which to analyze the domestic workers' experiences. This resulted in the author dissociating herself from the stereotypical, paternalistic power position that existed between employers (and their families) and live-in domestic workers. As an occupational therapist committed to equality of citizenship and the transformation of South Africa, she considered the rights of these clients in terms of the South African constitution.[3] Discrimination against them was unconstitutional, a violation of human rights, and unethical. The author had to respect, protect, and advocate for clients' and communities' human rights. These human rights violations could lead to the development of occupational risk factors or dysfunction, or perhaps could be a product thereof.

The author's awareness of live-in domestic workers' needs led to further reflection on the South African domestic worker's situation. Domestic work was most common amongst black female South Africans and originated during apartheid.[4] This gender and race trend continues in post-apartheid South Africa. Black women were coerced by poverty in rural areas to undertake domestic work. However, they are regarded as easily replaceable, low skilled and of little economic value to their employers.[5] Employers undervalue their work so that it is viewed as unskilled, woman's work.[6] Devaluing domestic work is not unique to South Africa. Similar concerns have been raised for domestic workers in urban India[7] and in Canada.[8]

RESEARCH METHODOLOGY: SENSITIVITY IN APPROACH

Literature, particularly within the domain of human rights, has highlighted the plight of domestic workers, who are also often migrant workers,[9] and has outlined that domestic workers' poor work environments often endanger their health.[9] An occupational perspective raises questions such as: what are domestic workers' occupational profiles and how does this influence their health? The author viewed the right to health as a positive human right. This implied that if resources are limited or people's capacities to achieve this right are hindered, then human rights are potentially being violated. Consequently, the author decided to conduct a qualitative, ethnographic study into live-in domestic workers' experiences of occupational engagement.[1]

To avoid bias, the author was interviewed by an independent social worker with the purpose of bracketing her personal ideas regarding the study. It raised her consciousness of how her valuing of human rights and dignity positively influenced her approach to the live-in domestic workers. This process enhanced the researcher's ability to be receptive to the participants in the study.[10]

The majority of live-in domestic workers are marginalized, isolated, and are not affiliated to a trade union. Initially, gaining access to the small minority of 'organized' domestic workers was essential to ensuring the credibility of the research. Subscribing to the principles of ethnography[11] allowed the researcher to further insure credibility. These included becoming accustomed to domestic workers' circumstances and engaging in the research field for a prolonged period in order to establish trust with the participants.

The author became accustomed to the life situations and circumstances experienced by the participants.[11] Establishing contact with key informants, attending workers' forum meetings, and reading domestic workers' narratives achieved this. Sensitivity to the subjective elements allowed the author to be sensitive to the social class and economic difficulties that were peculiar to the live-in domestic workers' experiences of occupational engagement.

The author used snowball sampling, via a social scientist who had worked with domestic workers for many years, to access and contact three key informants (Hettie, Karen and Patsy – pseudonyms are used for confidentiality). This created the opportunity to explore personal accounts of what being a domestic worker was like and how this influenced what they did. Hettie was a proud domestic worker who was actively involved in the South African Domestic Workers' Union. Karen had experience as a domestic worker, but now worked at the Sea Point African National Congress constituency office. Patsy had recently left her job as a domestic worker and hoped to find an administrative job instead.

The author met with each key informant to discuss her research ideas and hear their opinions. They were skeptical of the researcher's concern, but affirmed the need for a study and highlighted some of the problems that they experienced as domestic workers. During discussions with them, they were convinced of the research's authenticity and agreed to contribute to accessing potential participants and to remain available for consultation. From discussions with the key informants, the author started to consider how the issues of gender and power related to the occupations that domestic workers engaged in. This broadened the author's views about domestic workers and their occupations.

The author also attended workers' forum meetings at the local parliament constituency advice office. These meetings offered domestic workers and those working in the hospitality industry an opportunity to voice their labor-related grievances and obtain advice or support from each other. This was a non-unionized forum where learners encouraged each other. Discussions at these forum meetings confirmed the need to explore domestic workers' occupational engagement. It became clear that these workers' work and living conditions had a profound impact on their choices of occupations. It also allowed the author to observe the unrestricted but respectful manner in which workers interacted and shared their stories, affirming that rich data could be collected through using either interviewing or a focus group.

THE PARTICIPANTS' OCCUPATIONAL PROFILE

Four participants were purposefully selected to participate in the study. These participants were able to communicate in English or Afrikaans; were between the ages of 22 and 35 years; of rural origin (including small towns close to urban areas, but poorly resourced); should have been in their place of employment for at least 3 months and have been working as domestic workers in Cape Town for a maximum of 2 years. The four participants were Emma (Case study 32.1), Victoria (Case study 32.2), Nomfundo (Case study 32.3), and Eliza (Case study 32.4), (pseudonyms are used for confidentiality). Their occupational profiles highlight some of the main challenges that domestic workers experience.

CASE STUDY 32.1 EMMA

Emma appeared as an energetic 25-year-old, Afrikaans speaking woman. The author met her at her employer's luxurious double-storied home. The house was empty as her employers had emigrated to America earlier that month.

Emma proudly related that she had completed high school and a secretarial diploma course. She described occupational experiences of triumph and joy that she had undergone during this time. One such experience detailed the creative manner in which she initiated and organized a netball tournament between different hostels whilst at college. Through these stories it became clear that Emma was a person who thrived on meeting challenges and had been a leader at school and college.

After completing her diploma, Emma was unable to find work in her rural home town. She thus resorted to working elsewhere as a domestic worker. After doing this for 1 year she returned home, hoping to find secretarial work. Unable to secure employment there, she went to work in Cape Town instead.

Emma had been working in her place of employment for 10 months at the time of the study. She had the responsibility of minding her employers' house until the weekend of the interview, when the house had been sold.

Emma was to start a new job on the day after the interview. Her employer had arranged that Emma could work for a friend. She made it very clear that she had to be interviewed before she started her new job, since she would no longer be allowed any outside contact or visitors. She vividly described the restrictions that she anticipated she would experience in this new job. This alerted the author to the reality of restricted choice when working as a domestic worker.

CASE STUDY 32.2 VICTORIA

Victoria was a pleasant, 26-year-old woman with a 4-month-old baby, Temba. She initially came to Cape Town to work as a pamphlet distributor and tea-girl for an Estate Agent. When the company closed down, she started work at a restaurant in Sea Point. Continuous conflict with the patrons and management of the restaurant about the multiple tasks she had simultaneously to complete made this job too stressful, leading to her decision to become a domestic worker.

Victoria sadly described how emotionally painful this time was for her. She missed home and had been especially concerned about the welfare of her mother, who passed away soon after Victoria started domestic work.

Victoria had worked for her employer for 2 years before Temba was born. Her employer would allow Temba to live with Victoria until he was 1 year old. Victoria felt unable to negotiate this condition and was very distressed because she wanted to be with her child. Also, since her mother had died, she did not have anyone at home who could care for her baby. Victoria illustrated the price that she had to pay for having Temba with her. She worked with her baby on her back or by her side. She had constantly to fulfill roles as a mother and a worker at the same time.

Victoria's work circumstances and her role as a mother impacted on the information gathering process. She did not arrive for the first meeting because her employer had given her extra tasks to do. She was late for the second meeting because she had to use her short time off to buy nappies for her baby as well as meet with the author. The third meeting lasted only half an hour because she had to fetch her employer's shoes. Victoria consistently apologized for being late and seemed genuinely embarrassed. Temba, who accompanied his mother, was cared for by Karen during the interviews. This led the author to reflect on the impact that dual roles and rigid working conditions could have on an individual.

CASE STUDY 32.3   NOMFUNDO

Nomfundo was a 27-year-old, smartly groomed woman from Khayelitsha. She was eager to participate in the interview, saying that domestic workers needed to speak out. However, she also needed much reassurance about the way in which the information would be presented. Her concern was about being exposed and that this could lead to her losing her job.

She explained that she had not completed her secondary education and had started to do a nursing certificate. She stopped when the college could not fund her any longer because of government retrenchments. Nomfundo had three young children who lived with her mother in Khayelitsha.

Nomfundo expressed distress about the nature and consequences of her job. She felt that her employers ill-treated her, but that she had no choice because she needed the job. She attributed her physical symptoms of illness, such as headaches and ulcers, to her experience of stress at work and her concern about her family's welfare. She also related how difficult it was to adapt to living and working in a new area.

CASE STUDY 32.4   ELIZA

Eliza was a 26-year-old woman from Bloemfontein with a 3-year-old daughter. She was recruited for domestic work by an agent who brought 'girls' (as she refers to domestic workers) from her hometown.

We met at a shop close to where she works and proceeded to her acquaintance's home for the interview. She was late for the interview because her employer had insisted that she performed some trivial tasks (in Eliza's opinion) before she left – doing a few arbitrary articles of laundry and waking the employer's husband in order to make his bed. She expressed immense irritation and resentment about these trivial tasks.

She had been at her current place of employment for 2 years. She expressed her frustrations regarding working long hours, not being given sufficient time off, and having to comply with her employer's whimsical demands. She also spoke of her sadness regarding not having had annual leave in the 2 years. This meant that she hadn't seen her 3-year-old daughter during this time. She hoped to go home for a week's holiday at the end of July. She worried that her daughter would not recognize her.

Managing and analyzing the research data

Each participant contributed to an audiotaped interview. Interviews were then transcribed by the author and participants were assigned pseudonyms. The data were managed using the QSR NUD*ST Vivo computer software package (available at http://www.qsr.com.au/). Content analysis was applied in order to identify, code, and categorize the primary patterns within the data.[12] Through content analysis the codes emerged from the data inductively. Each of these codes was then labeled. Similar codes were grouped together to form subcategories. These subcategories were then incorporated into the dynamic systems theory.[13]

The dynamic systems theory suggests that systems change with time and are complex, non-linear, and random. The complexity component was of most use to this study because it emphasizes that levels of variables exist within the passage of time.[13] It provided a way of analyzing how environmental factors interacted with other variables to form patterns of occupational engagement.

LIVE-IN DOMESTIC WORKERS' EXPERIENCES: OCCUPATIONAL THERAPY INTERPRETATION

Two of the themes that emerged from the analysis are described below.[1] The first theme, occupational restriction, describes how the domestic workers experienced being devalued because their occupations were controlled. The second theme, occupational reconciliation, describes the live-in domestic worker's occupational response to the stifling environment. The occupational therapist's potential contribution is then explored.

Occupational restriction

The domestic workers felt that they had no choice but to sacrifice their own education and undergo separation from their families in order to earn a living. Having accepted a job as a live-in domestic worker, the person is usually allocated a room on the employer's property. This room may be a little room inside the house, a shack outside, or any space that the employer chooses. Domestic workers have little say over exactly where or how they are accommodated, and living at the place of work then means being available to work whenever one's employer demands. They described the workload as unreasonably heavy, involving them in mainly purposeful work activities. The purpose behind these activities centered on earning a living and insuring both one's own and the family's survival. These activities dominated the domestic workers' repertoire and left little opportunity for choice and engagement in meaningful occupations. The long work hours also led to an overuse of work related capacities to the detriment of other dormant or potential capacities within the person.

The participants' work hours were ruled by the employer's schedule. This meant that they never knew and had little control over what time their work day would end. Living on the employer's property and relying on the employer for meals further restricted the domestic workers' freedom. The domestic workers concluded that they could never expect to rest in their rooms because their employers were inconsiderate. Being confined to their rooms resulted in them continuously ruminating over their dire circumstances. Victoria related how she was expected to return to work a week after giving birth. The domestic workers adapted their occupations to fit the employer-orchestrated environment, but were still treated in an inhumane manner.

Occupational challenges presented by the environment should match the individuals' repertoire of skills in order for them to experience mastery.[14] These domestic workers did not have the opportunity to apply or develop their repertoire of skills in order to achieve mastery within their overall occupational engagement. The environment was organized to match the employer's needs.

Occupational reconciliation

The findings illustrated that the different levels of the environment contributed to the characteristic occupational engagement experienced by the live-in domestic workers. Live-in domestic workers lack opportunities to develop or apply their full potential, are often lonely, and lack stimulation and resources within their rooms. Their opportunities to achieve their potential as occupational beings were limited. They were resilient in creating opportunities to nurture themselves despite these challenging circumstances; they reconciled their occupational engagement, rather than going through the process of and achieving occupational adaptation.[15] During occupational reconciliation domestic workers did not reshape their occupations to achieve a sustainable, desirable change. They gave way to their circumstances and engaged in limited occupations because of their restricted opportunities. They harmonized their occupational engagement without contesting the unreasonable occupational challenges. This allowed them to experience limited agency in their lives.

They networked with domestic workers by optimizing opportunities to contact others, such as being sent to the local café by their employers. They developed friendships that allowed them to feel cared for, valued, and emotionally comforted when they had problems. Through socializing with friends, they could exercise some degree of control. Domestic workers would negotiate to get a Saturday or Sunday afternoon off, sometimes one per month, which would be their opportunity to socialize. This helped them to compensate for the lack of control that they endured on a daily basis. It made their days off special, often because they could experience a sense of *ubuntu*, reminiscing about people at home or preparing traditional food. *Ubuntu* is an African concept that means 'I am because we are – I can only be a person through others'.[16] It describes a connection with others through a shared humanity and spirituality.

In response to their environmental limitations, the domestic workers harmonized their occupational engagement without contesting the unreasonable occupational challenge, reconciling their occupations within the constraints of their environment, coping instead of attempting to change their situation. The positive outcome of this occupational reconciliation is depicted in the sense of value and dignity that the participants described as they engaged in their occupations. The domestic workers do not experience occupational adaptation; they merely submit their occupational engagement to the restrictions of the environment.

Occupational therapy contribution

A supportive environment is required for health to be promoted;[17] domestic workers' work and living environments were quite the opposite. These workers were placed at risk of developing ill health because of the severe restrictions placed on their individual choices of occupations.

Considering the needs and rights of marginalized groups such as domestic workers can help us to explore occupational therapy's contribution to promoting the health of populations. Occupational therapists encountering domestic workers in clinical practice are ethically obliged to address the occupational risk factors and injustices that could lead to the development of impairments and disabilities. If we acknowledge this social responsibility, then how should we respond? Is this response limited to the clinical influence that occupational therapists have?

Consider the occupational therapist's contribution to assisting the domestic worker to negotiate with the employer regarding time off. The occupational therapist could use policy documents such as the Basic Conditions of Employment Act[18] in combination with skills training and could also advocate for change in employers' attitudes in order to reduce exploitation.

Occupational therapists could also use the techniques of occupational enrichment[19] to address the restrictions imposed by environments. The details of how occupational enrichment is applied need to be strengthened. Perhaps occupational therapists could collaborate with other stakeholders who are interested in promoting domestic workers' wellbeing. These stakeholders may include social activists and trade unions.

The author's research[1] was limited because she did not continue to work in the psychiatric or clinical setting and so discontinued her contact with domestic workers who accessed occupational therapy services. However, she had the opportunity to present her research findings at a research seminar organized by a social scientist who actively worked with the domestic workers' union. Attendants at the seminar included domestic workers, researchers working with the population, and representatives from the Western Cape Labor Department and the South African Domestic Workers and Allied Service Union. These attendants confirmed the authenticity of the research findings and expressed an appreciation for the unique lens of understanding that occupational therapy gave to the experiences of domestic workers. They saw this as further evidence for the need to promote an improvement in domestic workers' work conditions.

Raising awareness of live-in domestic workers' experiences creates access to information that would allow for increased sensitivity to the needs of marginalized groups. It also has the power to create instances where people advocate for change. The occupational therapy profession has the opportunity and social responsibility to contribute toward advocating with domestic workers so that they are enabled to optimize their occupational performance. Social activists and trade unions have illustrated that raising awareness and putting the needs of discriminated groups on the agenda can bring about policy changes. For domestic workers this has meant that they are included in the Basic Conditions of Employment Act[18] and have increased bargaining power with their employers. The position and capacities of domestic workers could be enhanced so that they become agents of change within their own lives. This would contribute to improving the quality of their lives.

CONCLUSION: TOWARD EQUAL OPPORTUNITIES AND WELLBEING

Occupational therapists appreciate the profound impact of human occupation on health and wellbeing at individual, group, and population levels. The role of the environment is a large mediating factor in this relationship. This research description has provided a glimpse of the insights that occupational therapists have into people's everyday occupational lives and the potential process of facilitating improved quality of life. It highlights the potential to use this knowledge to improve the quality of lives in marginalized groups. We are challenged to assume a political position in advocating with and for the rights of marginalized, disadvantaged groups of people in order to create shifts in the sociopolitical environment. An understanding of the impact of gender discrimination and geographic displacement on health urges occupational therapists to extend our scope of thinking beyond merely adapting the physical environment. The profession's occupational interpretation of health provides a powerful lens with which to contribute to the removal of occupational injustice[20] (see Ch. 9) and the overcoming of occupational apartheid (see Ch. 6).[21]

References

1. Galvaan R. The live-in domestic worker's experience of occupational engagement [Master's Dissertation]. Cape Town: University of Cape Town; 2000.

2. Munhall P. Ethical considerations in qualitative research. Western Journal of Nursing Research 1988; 10(2):150–162.

3. Constitution of the Republic of South Africa. Government Gazette. Pretoria: Government Printer; 1996:1–147.

4. Lessing M. South African women today. Cape Town: Maskew Miller Longman; 1994.

5. Grossman J. Summary of submission on basic conditions of employment. Cape Town: University of Cape Town; 1997.

6. Budlender D. The second women's budget. Cape Town: Idasa; 1997.

7. Dickey S. Permeable homes: domestic service, household space and the vulnerability of class boundaries in urban India. American Ethnologist 2000; 27(2):462–489.

8. Barber P. Agency in Philippine women's labor migration and provisional diaspora. Women's Studies International Forum 2000; 23(4):399–411.

9. Human Rights Watch. Treatment of migrant domestic workers with special visas in the United States 2001. Online. Available: http://www.hrw.org/reports/2001/usadom/usadom/0501-04.htm#p284 54979

10. Oskowitz B. Preparing researchers for a qualitative investigation of a particularly sensitive nature: reflections from the field. South African Journal of Psychology 1997; 27(2):83–88.

11. De Poy E, Gitlin, LN. Introduction to research: multiple strategies for health and human services. St Louis, MO; Mosby; 1994.

12. Patton M. Qualitative evaluation and research methods. London: Sage Press; 1990.

13. Gray J, Kennedy M, Zemke R. Dynamic systems theory: an overview. In: Zemke R, Clarke F, eds. Occupational science: the evolving discipline. Philadelphia: FA Davis; 1996.

14. Yerxa E. Health and the human spirit for occupation. Am J Occup Ther 1998; 52(6):412–418.

15. Schkade J, Schultz S. Occupational adaptation: towards a holistic approach for contemporary practice, part 1. Am J Occup Ther 1997; 46(9):829–837.

16. Mbigi L. In search of the African business renaissance: an African cultural perspective. Randburg, South Africa: Knowledge Resources; 2000.

17. World Health Organization. The Ottawa charter for health promotion. Ottawa, Canada: Canadian Public Health Organization; 1986.

18. Basic Conditions of Employment Act 1997. Government Gazette 75:1–179. Pretoria: Government Printer; 1997.

19. Molineux M, Whiteford G. Prisons from occupational deprivation to occupational enrichment. Journal of Occupational Science 1999; 6(3):124–130.

20. Townsend EA, Wilcock AA. Occupational justice. In: Christiansen C, Townsend E. Introduction to occupation. Thorofare, NJ: Prentice Hall; 2003:243–273.

21. Kronenberg F. Street children: being and becoming. Research study. Heerlen, The Netherlands: Hogeschool Limburg; 1999.

Chapter **33**

Participatory action research
Creating new knowledge and opportunities for occupational engagement

Barry Trentham, Lynn Cockburn

OVERVIEW

In this chapter, participatory action research (PAR) is proposed as a research methodology that responds to developments in the understanding of the occupational enablement process as well as societal shifts in health and social service provision, while emphasizing the need for the direct translation of knowledge creation into meaningful social change. We argue that PAR is an approach to knowledge development that is consistent with the values of occupational therapy and principles of occupational justice. From our experience on a variety of PAR projects, with injured workers, older adults, adult learners in a community literacy program, and mental health clients, this chapter outlines what we have learned about PAR. The assumptions and stages involved in the PAR process are described, using one PAR project as an example. Critical questions and lessons are raised, including ethical and political considerations necessary for work amongst community groups and individuals with inequitable power and resources and important points and contraindications to consider before choosing a PAR process. When carefully considered in light of its challenges and potential limitations, PAR can be a powerful tool to be used for the empowerment of citizens who are marginalized due to social, structural, or environmental barriers.

WHY PARTICIPATORY ACTION RESEARCH?

As occupational therapy educators and researchers, our understanding of the processes involved in the enablement of occupation is evolving. It is reasonable that there should also be growth in our understanding of approaches used to examine these processes. Practitioners and researchers in several fields have identified the need for an approach to knowledge creation and social change that acknowledges in its process and outcomes the impact of inequity, the determinants of health, client-centered practice, and cultural diversity.[1-3] Occupational therapists are also exploring ways to frame and understand the political nature of their work.[4-7]

The Ottawa Charter defines health promotion as the *process* of enabling people to increase control over their health.[8] Health promotion is equally and essentially concerned with creating the conditions necessary for health at individual, structural, social, and environmental levels through an understanding of the determinants of health: peace, shelter, education, food, income, a stable ecosystem, sustainable resources, social justice, and equity. For occupational therapists, the strategies used to promote health can also be seen to promote occupational development and achievement and ultimately, from a broader perspective, occupational justice as outlined by Townsend and Wilcock.[9]

From the outlook of those interested in the pursuit of occupational justice and those advocating a health promotion perspective, methods of knowledge creation are insufficient if they focus solely on individual level disease disability impacts on occupation.

As global forces, largely directed by multinational corporate interests, reshape international relations and power structures,[10] a growing disparity in resource allocation is becoming alarmingly apparent despite a growing understanding of the health impacts of social inequity.[11-13] Resource allocation inequities have a direct impact on the occupational opportunities available for individuals and communities around the world and are therefore of concern to occupational therapists.

Supported by an enormous pharmaceutical industry, Western approaches to health care and medicine predominate and increasingly influence the manner in which new knowledge is created and used.[14] This dominant perspective can blind us to the richness found in a diversity of cultural perspectives on healing, health, and client-centered practice. Diverse worldviews can challenge entrenched Western methods of knowledge creation and client-centered practice. For example, the tradition within current Western occupational therapy practice of focusing on occupational performance issues from the perspective of the individual may collide with cultural perspectives which value communal outlooks and responses to issues. Within such traditions, individuals are seen as integral parts of communities. Decisions made with individuals impact the community. The family or community may be the primary client. (For a detailed discussion on this issue, readers are referred to the discussion by Michael Iwama in Chapter 10 of this text). Accordingly, the concept of client has been expanded to include not only individuals, but also groups, communities, organizations, and governments as expressed in the Canadian occupational therapy guidelines.[15] The research process then, must also accommodate this expanded understanding of client. As occupational therapists who promote a relationship based on partnerships, however, we appreciate the problematic use of the term *client*, which brings with it Western notions of a business relationship.

The points discussed above – health promotion and the determinants of health, global economic pressures, shifting perspectives on the meaning of client in diverse communities – outline the need for a new and alternative way of creating knowledge. By incorporating these issues within an analysis of power relationships, participatory action research (PAR) engages citizens in their own change agendas. For occupational therapy practitioners and researchers, PAR provides an avenue for work oriented toward the creation of equitable occupational opportunities, i.e. occupational justice, while acknowledging associated power differences and diverse views within the research process.

WHAT IS PARTICIPATORY ACTION RESEARCH?

The Canadian Association of Occupational Therapists' guidelines, *Enabling Occupation*,[15] describe three main research paradigms: positivism, interpretive social science, and critical social science. Generally speaking, PAR practitioners embrace a critical social science perspective in their acknowledgement that existing social structures are unjust, benefiting privileged groups over marginalized groups, and are therefore in need of change. *Participatory action research* is a term that has several definitions and is often used interchangeably with the term *participatory research*, although some authors view these as two separate traditions.[2,16,17] PAR is a process of systematically examining issues from the perspectives and lived experiences of community members who are most affected by the issues under examination. Research from this perspective involves the process of collaborative information sharing, systematic inquiry, reflection, and action, with the expected outcome of meaningful social change.[18]

Change may come in the form of individual or group empowerment, greater community capacity to solve shared problems, or transformed organizational structures.[18] In PAR, broad theory development or empirical generalizations are of secondary importance.[19] Rather, PAR perspectives accept a postmodern understanding of 'knowing' as being a composite of multiple perspectives[20] where the collective reality that is known is understood to be socially constructed.[21] Distinguishing components of PAR in relation to conventional research are summarized in Table 33.1.

People who are marginalized due to barriers related to race, (dis)ability, age, socio-economic status, access to knowledge, gender, or geographic locations are often those who are included and involved in PAR. In this sense, PAR is very consistent with occupational therapy's concern for the elimination of environmental and contextual barriers to occupational performance[1,15] and in keeping with strategies aimed at overcoming occupational apartheid[23] as outlined by Kronenberg and Pollard (see Ch. 6) and in Townsend's[24] description of 'a spirituality of inclusiveness'. Occupational therapists have been involved in a variety of PAR projects with parents and children,[25] injured workers,[26] persons with mental health disorders,[27] people with physical disabilities,[28] and older adults.[2,29,30]

Although each PAR process is unique, there are some general and overlapping stages. These include:

- issue identification and initial planning
- planning and initial investigation
- cycles of action, reflection, and modification
- summarizing to create knowledge and change.[17,29]

Table 33.1 PAR compared with conventional research (adapted from Alary J (ed). 1992 Community care and participatory research.[22] With permission of Nuage Editions.)

Component	Conventional research	Participatory research
Naming the issue or problem	• The professional (OT)[a] identifies from personal interest or clinical observation or concern • Building on previous work (either individually or in literature)	• Identified by community group • Context specific • If from practitioner's perspective, usually in response to critical review of practice or connection with community
Purpose of the research	• To answer a question, to build knowledge • Develop generalizable information for larger population • Develop or demonstrate theories	• Knowledge that can be used by the community to improve a situation • Creation of new knowledge on change strategies • Not intended to generalize
Role of researcher (outsider/academic/professional)	• Assumes that the observer is objective with no impact on the process • Consultant, expert, or resource	• On a continuum, from outsider to insider, but is part of the process • Collaborator; co-researcher; one member of team • 'Tool' to be used by the community
Role of others	• Anyone with requisite skill and knowledge can be researcher (or assistant) on a project, no commitment to community, issue, or others on team required • Community members are subjects or participants but have no decision making power	• Each member plays important role throughout the research process, has opportunity to shape the project • The more the participants share their perspectives (researcher, as well as others) the more meaningful the project will be
Training	• Researcher holds specialized knowledge of techniques and methods, and of current theories in the field • Community does not have capacity to be trained	• Willingness to go beyond intuition and common sense to development of flexible, systematic, and critical analysis of practice • Often training in statistics, research methods part of the process • Experience with issues
Review of literature; hypotheses and variables	• Hypotheses defined at beginning • Literature review required to place research in context of current body of knowledge • Hypotheses must be tested • Variables controlled	• Questions (not hypotheses) developed from experiences or practice • Literature review informs practice and research • Questions and objectives defined to orient project • Recognition of many variables which cannot be controlled
Planning the research	• Detailed plan before project is started • Control procedures • Scientific measuring instruments	• General plan initially • Recognition that the process will affect the plan and project will evolve depending on the iterative nature of information gathered • Collective decision so not controlled by OT researcher

(Continued)

Table 33.1 (Continued)

Component	Conventional research	Participatory research
Analysis and information gathering	• Different methods, but usually validated using complex process (e.g. statistical)	• Quantitative or qualitative can be used, usually fairly simple • Qualitative may be more common • Flexible methods to meet needs of project
Results	• Academic language • Results to literature first, eventually to practice (if at all)	• In various forms (e.g. clear language documents, drama, art, advocacy work, organization change) • Results affect community and practice first, then theory and literature (if at all)
Usefulness of results	• Generalizable • Adds to knowledge and theory in field of research • Often difficult to transfer to practice	• Direct application in community, leads to social change • Participants may or may not have increased skill to tackle further research issues (skills may not generalize) • Practical use
Understanding of power	• Generally not addressed	• Key issue in all components (purpose, process, and actions) • Individual and social analysis
Time	• Theoretically predictable (in reality may not be) • Focused on research tasks	• Considerable time required for community building, familiarization, socializing • Often requires time commitment beyond apparent 'research' tasks
Compatibility with OT	• Researcher centered, not client-centered • OT needs to be an expert to engage in research	• More client-centered/client-directed • OT as ally and/or facilitator • Recognition of ability, not deficits • Research as viable occupation • Research/work at level of environmental change (not individual)
Funding	• Recognized and supported	• Often embedded in other community based work; not easily recognized by major funding sources

a OT–Occupational therapist

During the first stage, an individual or group of individuals identify a general issue. Anyone with sufficient knowledge of the PAR process and effective facilitation skills can lead the group of co-researchers. Occupational therapists who lead PAR processes often start with a group with whom the therapist has an existing relationship.[32,33] With facilitation support, the problem is further refined, research questions are articulated, and initial action plans developed.

Secondly, group members as co-researchers engage in preliminary information gathering, pose questions and hypotheses, and suggest solutions for the issues identified. This stage usually occurs over several weeks or months.

The PAR process then follows a continuous and emergent cycle of action, reflection, modification, and further action. The research group may choose to use a variety of occupational forms or change oriented projects, such as qualitative interviews, meetings, case studies, community focus groups, quantitative surveys, or educational workshops and events[19] to collect information. For example, in the older adult project outlined by Trentham[29] a falls prevention workshop and dramatization was used to gather prevention strategies from participants, which stimulated change initiatives, e.g. advocacy efforts to have fall hazards removed. Action is integrated with periods of reflection. Outcomes may include reports, dramatic or artistic events, community gatherings, or actions directed at policy makers.

Ideally, participants involved in a PAR process can expect to go through considerable learning, leading to personal transformation. Some PAR researchers argue that a project without this transformative change and without a recognition of the social implications for research is not truly PAR.[34–36]

A PARTICIPATORY ACTION RESEARCH STORY

To illustrate the application of PAR concepts, Case study 33.1 presents one PAR project – the Possibilities Co-op (pseudonym) This project story is told from the occupational therapists' perspective. However, it is understood that there may be as many variations to this PAR story as there are participants, each with significant limitations; presenting one does not present a full story.

CASE STUDY 33.1

The Possibilities Co-op research project began when a group of outpatients at an urban psychiatric hospital partnered with occupational therapists to create meaningful work for themselves.[37] The group crafted and sold a variety of items such as pillows, shopping bags, and candles. Following a description of the PAR process by the occupational therapist, members of the group decided to use it as a framework to address questions about the group's achievements and shortcomings, the barriers it had faced, and the actions that could be taken to continue to strengthen their work.

In this initial phase, the group had many discussions about what defines research. Several members who had been 'patients' in the mental health system for many years were enthusiastic about actually developing a research project from the beginning. Over several months, the group developed a proposal for a participatory, qualitative research project.

The therapist-researchers balanced roles as instructors (e.g. regarding research skills), advocates (regarding negotiating the institutional setting and ethical approval), group facilitators, and research collaborators. Many members commented positively on the experience of making contributions to the collective understanding of how the project would be carried out.[38,39] Members developed an interview guide, engaged in the interview process, and reviewed documents that the group had produced, for example meeting notes and posters. Regular meetings were held to reflect on the research process, including the effects on the members individually and collectively. Not all members of the group wanted to remain involved in the information gathering and analysis due to the significant amount of time required to carry out this aspect of the project adequately. A small group of interested members continued with a conventional qualitative analysis process that resulted in a report on the project, including key lessons and themes that became evident in the change process. This report was then shared and disseminated.

Change oriented actions were evident throughout the process. The group communicated with its institutional partners and presented at professional conferences, which increased awareness of the importance of both the nature of the group and the research work they were conducting. Funding was obtained to assist in completing the project, including the production of a written report.[40] The report described the research process, and was targeted to members of the group, the supporting organizations, and others who wanted to understand the outcomes of the project. Each of these actions represents significant occupational opportunities that were not available to members through other avenues. In addition, the research project contributed to the ongoing development of the day-to-day work of the group.

PROMOTING OCCUPATIONAL JUSTICE THROUGH PARTICIPATORY ACTION RESEARCH

PAR values the means (engagement in the research process) as well as the outcome (improvement of occupational opportunities) in the same way that occupational therapists view occupation as both a means and an end in the occupational therapy process. As illustrated in the research story in Case study 33.1, the research process itself can be seen as an opportunity for occupational engagement. Throughout the PAR process, facilitators encourage their co-researchers to reflect on their lived experience and to share solutions. This reflective approach to engagement in occupation has also been highlighted in the landmark Well Elderly study,[41] which provided evidence for the power of occupation to create change at the individual level. When people ask questions and *also* propose solutions, implement change, and disseminate new knowledge, they are participating in an occupational form (i.e. research) that helps to develop the skills and knowledge necessary to take greater control over their own lives; in so doing, they promote their own health as well as the health of other community members.

The outcome of the PAR process can also contribute to improved access to occupational opportunities and thus to improvements in occupational justice. The conventional research process fails to transfer new knowledge effectively and consistently to those who most need it.[3,42] By engaging front line workers, citizens, consumers of health services, or marginalized groups in creating change outcomes that facilitate greater occupational engagement, or, as it is described in the World Health Organization's International Classification of Functioning, Disability and Health terminology, social participation,[43] knowledge transfer is built into the PAR process. Direct involvement of those who are affected enhances the validity of the questions being asked. Questions are checked and rechecked in the reflective cycle of the PAR process, thus adding to the relevance of a study's findings.

CREATING CAPACITY FOR PARTICIPATORY ACTION RESEARCH

The PAR facilitator skill set has been outlined in our previous article[44] and is not discussed here in detail. However, it is important to highlight a requirement unique to the PAR facilitator – the ability to facilitate an empowering process with co-researchers. This skill should be second nature to most occupational therapists. However, unlike many therapists, PAR researchers make explicit the political aspect of their work.

As social change agents, PAR researchers must reflect on the political nature of their work. PAR researchers share the critical social science stance that existing power structures do not insure equitable opportunities for all citizens. An approach to research that is concerned with, in part, decisions on resource allocation amongst disparate and often opposing groups (i.e. politics) is needed.

A political skill set includes advanced skills in mediation and negotiation. In working with community citizens, we needed to be aware of the differing agendas of groups or individuals who had competing needs, interests, positions, or barriers. These may block the progress of a project and must be identified, articulated, and responded to. The researchers, including the facilitator, must attend continually to the power dynamics at play, to raise 'consciousness' in order to develop effective problem-solving strategies needed to balance opposing views. Our knowledge of group dynamics was essential in mediating and negotiating power imbalances. Being aware of who speaks and who doesn't, and noting any instances of participants being silenced by others, was often reason to encourage the members of the group to express their differences in order to stimulate better understanding. Frequently, less assertive individuals raised issues with the facilitator in private. These individuals were then supported in their efforts to raise these same issues within the group meetings, so they could be addressed with all members of the group. Such skills will remain ineffective without an attitude and value set that is consistent with PAR values. Humility, flexibility, and compassion are required. It may be uncomfortable, particularly for health professionals, to be in a place of 'not knowing', as a PAR path can often be unclear, requiring the input and wisdom from diverse PAR participants.

CHOOSING PARTICIPATORY ACTION RESEARCH: SOME CONSIDERATIONS

Increasingly, participatory action research is being recommended for more vulnerable communities who have been excluded from telling their own stories and contributing to knowledge creation. For example, as a result of the history of victimization and exclusion of aboriginal peoples, the Canadian Institute of Health Research has highly recommended that aboriginal people be full partners in research projects that concern them.[45] Responding to this challenge, one of our students has recently completed the initial phase of a PAR project with northern Ontario aboriginal youth.[46] Similarly, a discussion paper developed by the Centre for Independent Living in Toronto advised its members to seriously reconsider participating in research projects that are not participatory in nature.[47] As occupational therapists working with groups and communities who may be marginalized, vulnerable, or lacking in power, we should give serious and careful consideration to PAR.

As the authors' experiences with PAR projects expand and deepen, we find ourselves becoming increasingly cautious in embarking on projects. All therapists should consider, for example, that their ability to work in partnership could be challenged by the structural constraints imposed by social and professional locations. We need to anticipate these implications as we plan to engage in the PAR process.

The project setting must be supportive of PAR. Organizational settings that negate the value of participatory approaches to research could actually disempower those involved in the change process. Organizational systems that are highly bureaucratic with several layers of decision making may also limit the success of a PAR project. It is suggested that the organization's readiness or openness for change be assessed in light of the facilitator's PAR experience before a PAR project is considered. We are not aware of any formal screening tools to assess a group's readiness for a PAR process. It may be helpful to draw from the framework by Marullo et al.[48] This framework outlines questions that should be considered in the assessment of a community-based research initiative. Questions to be discussed include whether change is focused at macro, meso or micro levels, directed at enhancing capacity, increasing efficiency, empowering communities, or altering policies. Researchers must also consider how their outcomes relate to either process or impact objectives.

Potential PAR participants must be aware of the purposes, processes, and potential outcomes and consequences of a PAR project. There may be a need to develop basic skills (e.g. group decision making) to participate effectively in a PAR project. Participants must be willing to deal with the ambiguity of the process and be open to the large volume of frank and ongoing discussions, reflection, and dialogue required in every phase of the PAR process. Occupational therapists may struggle with what it means to be partners rather than experts[2] in the change process; their strong sensitivity to and experience of working with people of varying abilities strengthens their potential role as participatory researchers. The challenge for occupational therapy researchers is to facilitate the process and to recognize and make use of their own expertise in specific content areas without minimizing the expertise of others and dominating the process. For example, in the PAR project with older adults we described in Cockburn and Trentham,[44] the second author recalled his initial hesitation to share his knowledge regarding the causes and prevention of traumatic falls in the elderly, fearing that this would silence his co-researchers and discourage them from sharing their own experiences and ideas on fall prevention. Articulating this dilemma stimulated some discussion within the group on the kinds of expertise that participants brought to the project. It became clear that the other participants expected Trentham, as an occupational therapist, to share his knowledge on fall prevention. The older adult co-researchers saw themselves as experts in planning a fall prevention workshop process that would engage their fellow seniors. This exemplifies that it is imperative that occupational therapy facilitators demonstrate their credibility as knowledgeable professionals with a skill set that can be of use to a group of PAR co-researchers. Apart from specialized knowledge, Letts[49] identifies useful skills that she feels occupational therapists bring to community organizing, frequently a key component of a PAR process. These skills include small group facilitation, writing and information gathering, knowledge of evaluation, and other instrumental supports such as effective minute taking at meetings.

In situations where time restraints are dictated by an external source, e.g. thesis deadlines, caution should be taken in outlining a PAR process. The length and process of a project cannot always be predetermined and ideally should be under the control of the co-researchers. PAR projects can take years to complete and so participants should be made aware of the potential time commitments before embarking on a project. The time spent on reflecting on action, learning, and power issues varies significantly depending on the duration of the project and the motivations of the co-researchers. As PAR facilitators, we often felt that there was insufficient time spent on reflection, while others did not share that concern. This tension points to the need for continual reassessment and acknowledgement of the objectives and outcomes of the PAR process. Although the final outcome of PAR should express itself in meaningful change at the local level,[2,3,37,50] it is necessary to have ongoing learning and questioning of assumptions as to how that change should best take place.

Finally, PAR facilitators must also be aware of situations where the change process plays into the hands of more powerful and potentially self-serving groups within a community or organization. If the facilitator is not fully aware of the various power structures, the change agenda may serve only those who want to maintain their power over other marginalized groups.[51] This concern raises important ethical questions which are discussed below.

ETHICAL CONSIDERATIONS

Co-researchers and facilitators who may come to a project with a sincere desire for community driven change, but who lack sufficient skills and awareness of potential risks and consequences, may cause some vulnerable individuals to be further victimized. Co-researchers may become mere community tokens who give credibility to a PAR facilitator's change agenda in a way that is not truly participatory.

Highly politicized or polarized environments may also not be the first choice for a novice PAR researcher, given that the potential harmful impact to PAR researchers in such circumstances could be great. Changes made in any particular setting may have more repercussions on the PAR insider co-researchers. The PAR facilitator, who is very often an 'outsider' and an initiator of a PAR process, may have more options for retreat and therefore may not have to experience the unexpected consequences of the change process. For example, groups in war torn areas or those who live within repressive structures should carefully consider potential impacts.

Some of the projects that we have been involved with have been with occupational therapy clients. This raises the question: when are we doing therapy and when are we doing research? With most research projects, the distinction between therapy and research is clear. And for some, this concern may be limited to an academic discussion – except that there remains the question of professional accountability and responsibility to the clients for whom we are providing a service.[2,32]

One of the aims of PAR is to empower groups of citizens to make change, an objective shared with occupational therapy.[49] However, in Canada, as in many other countries, occupational therapy is a licensed and regulated profession where standards for appropriate assessment and intervention strategies are in place which structure the occupational therapy process. For example, the College of Occupational Therapists of Ontario publishes and requires adherence to standards of occupational therapy practice in the province of Ontario, Canada. Arguably, such standards may not always be consistent with the social change perspective of health promotion or PAR. According to these standards, the therapist is accountable for the provision of occupational therapy, and to a certain extent its outcomes. This expectation may raise an ethical dilemma. For example, in the PAR process, the PAR facilitator may use occupational therapy skills, but it is understood that there is shared accountability with co-researchers. In a PAR process, the perceived role of occupational therapists may be ambiguous: are they acting as researcher partners, or therapists, or both? In the situation where the co-researchers are also clients of the occupational therapist, who then is accountable should clients experience ill effects that they attribute to their involvement in the PAR process? The professional boundaries are considerably blurred in such situations. Occupational therapists as PAR facilitators must make explicit their roles and responsibilities, and these may need to be continuously renegotiated throughout the process.[2,3,37]

CONCLUSION

We remain committed to the use of PAR in creating new knowledge and making social change of importance to marginalized groups. PAR methods are useful for practitioners interested in making their practice more collaborative and client-centered while at the same time honoring the challenge to provide evidence-based service.

Participatory action research provides a useful framework for creating new knowledge that directly responds to the challenges outlined in this book, i.e. the empowerment of citizens who are marginalized due to social, structural, or environmental barriers. PAR, as an approach to occupational therapy research within the current reality of occupational injustice, requires a skill set and knowledge base that acknowledges the political processes involved in making change. PAR values the client-centered partnership approach espoused by occupational therapists and shares the profession's positive understanding of health as a resource for living; life, if it is to be lived successfully and joyfully, must abound with opportunities for engagement in purposeful and meaningful occupations. An occupationally just society is one where such opportunities exist for all individuals and groups regardless of abilities, conditions, ages, and socio-economic status.

References

1. Wilcock A. An occupational perspective of health. Thorofare, NJ: Slack; 1998.
2. Letts L. Occupational therapy and participatory research: a partnership worth pursuing. Am J Occup Ther 2003; 57:77–87.
3. Deshler D, Ewert M. Participatory action research: traditions and major assumptions. 1995. Online. Available: http://www.parnet.org/parchive/docs/deshler_95/
4. Jackson M. From work to therapy: the changing politics of occupation in the 20th century. Br J Occup Ther 1993; 56:360–364.
5. Griffin S. Occupational therapists and the concept of power: a review of the literature. Austr Occup Ther J 2001; 48:24–34.
6. Royeen CB. Occupation reconsidered. Occup Ther Int 2002; 9:111–120.
7. Kronenberg F. In search of the political nature of occupational therapy. Unpublished MSc OT paper. Linkoping University, Sweden. 2003.
8. World Health Organization (WHO). The Ottawa charter for health promotion. Ottawa, Canada: Canadian Public Health Association; 1986.
9. Townsend E, Wilcock A. Occupational justice. In: Christiansen C, Wilcock A, eds. Introduction to occupation: the art and science of living. Thorofare, NJ: Prentice Hall; 2004.
10. Ostry A, Cardiff K, eds. Trading away health? Globalization and health policy: report from the 14th Annual Health Policy Conference for Health Services and Policy Research, 9 Nov 2001. Online.

Available: http://www.chspr.ubc.ca/hpru/pdf/14thHPconf.pdf 15 Aug 2003.
11. United Nations Development Programme (UNDP). Human development report 2002: deepening democracy in a fragmented world. New York: Oxford University Press; 2002. Online. Available: http://www.undp.org/hdr2002/24 Feb 03.
12. Chappell N. Maintaining and enhancing independence and well-being in old age. In: Canada health action: building on the legacy. Papers commissioned by the National Forum on Health, vol. 2. Determinants of health – adults and seniors edition. Sainte Foy, QC: MultiMondes; 1998:89–135.
13. Frank J, Mustard F. The determinants of health from a historical perspective. Daedalus 1994; 123:1–19.
14. Hardon A. New WHO leader should aim for equity and confront undue commercial influences. Lancet, 2003; 361(9351):6.
15. Canadian Association of Occupational Therapists. Enabling occupation: an occupational therapy perspective. Ottawa: CAOT Publications ACE; 1997:17.
16. Hall B. Reflections on the origins of the International Participatory Research Network and the Participatory Research Group in Toronto, Canada; 1997. Online. Available: http://www.anrecs.msu.edu/research/hallpr.htm
17. Yeich S, Levine R. Participatory research's contribution to a conceptualization of empowerment. J Appl Soc Psychol 1992; 22:1904–1908.

18. Green LW, Georges MA, Daniel M, et al. Study of participatory research in health promotion: review and recommendation of the development of participatory research in health promotion in Canada. University of British Columbia; Vancouver: Institute for Health Promotion Research; 1995.

19. Reason P. Three approaches to participative inquiry. In: Denzin NK, Lincoln YS, eds. Handbook of qualitative research. Thousand Oaks: Sage; 1994.

20. Weinblatt N, Avrech-Barr M. Postmodernism and its application to the field of occupational therapy. Can J Occup Ther 2001; 68:164–170.

21. Gergen K. Introduction to social construction. London: Sage; 1999.

22. Alary J, ed. with Beausoleil J, Guédon M-C, Larivière C, Mayer R. Community care and participatory research. Montreal: Nuage Editions; 1992:243–245.

23. Kronenberg F. Street children: being and becoming, Research study. Heerlen, The Netherlands: Hogeschool Limburg; 1999.

24. Townsend E. Good intentions overruled: a critique of empowerment in the routine organization of mental health services. Toronto, Canada: University of Toronto Press; 1998:130.

25. Law M. Changing disabling environments through participatory action research. In: Smith S, Willms D, Johnson N, eds. Nurtured by knowledge: learning to do participatory action research. New York: Apex; 1997:34–58.

26. Injured Worker Participatory Research Project. Making the system better: injured workers speak out on compensation and return to work issues in Ontario. 2001. Contact: Dr. Bonnie Kirsh, Department of Occupational Therapy, University of Toronto, 500 University Avenue, Toronto, Ontario M5T 1W5.

27. Soult R, Anderson M, Gibson L. Let's have coffee: participatory evaluation of a community social support intervention. Paper presented at the thirteenth World Congress of Occupational Therapists. Stockholm, Sweden, 2002.

28. Stewart R, Bhagwanjee A. Promoting group empowerment and self-reliance through participatory research: a case study of people with physical disability. Disabil Rehabil 1999; 21:338–345.

29. Trentham B. Environmental factors in community capacity building with older adults. Paper presented at the twelfth International Congress of the World Federation of Occupational Therapists. Montreal, Canada. 1998.

30. Carswell A. Aging and health promotion; a participatory action research project with seniors (CHRU Publications No. M96–1). Ottawa,

Canada: Community Health Research Unit, University of Ottawa; 1995.

31. Hall B. Participatory research: an approach for change. Convergence 1975; 8:24–31.

32. Sherkin A. Occupational therapists' involvement in participatory research. Occupational Therapy Student Research Symposium Proceedings. Toronto: Department of Occupational Therapy, Faculty of Medicine, University of Toronto; 1999.

33. Takeda F. Experience of occupational therapists in participatory research. Occupational Therapy Student Research Symposium Proceedings. Toronto: Department of Occupational Therapy, Faculty of Medicine, University of Toronto; 1999.

34. Park P, Brydon-Miller M, Hall B et al. Voices of change: participatory research in the United States and Canada. Toronto: OISE Press; 1993.

35. de Koning K, Martin M. Participatory research in health: setting the context. In: de Koning K, Martin M, eds. Participatory research in health: issues and experiences. London: Zed Books; 1996:1–14.

36. Soltis-Jarrett V. The facilitator in participatory action research: les raisons d'être (methods of clinical inquiry). Adv Nurs Sci 1997; 20:45.

37. Cockburn L, Clark C, Nagle S, clients. Creating paid work: attempting collaboration in an institutional setting. International Association for Psychosocial Rehabilitation, Ontario conference. Barrie, Ontario; 1995.

38. Dinatolo M. Establishing a worker co-operative with mental health consumers: a participatory research project. Unpublished manuscript. Department of Occupational Therapy, University of Toronto; 1997.

39. Turack D. Establishing a worker co-operative with mental health consumers: a participatory research project. Unpublished manuscript, Department of Occupational Therapy, University of Toronto; 1997.

40. Productivity Plus Co-op. A look at Productivity Plus Co-op: voices from participants. [Booklet]. Toronto: 2001. Available from Lynn Cockburn.

41. Jackson J, Carlson M, Mandel D, et al. Occupation in lifestyle redesign: the well elderly study occupational therapy program. Am J Occup Ther 1998; 52:326–336.

42. Rappolt S, Tassone M. How rehabilitation therapists gather, evaluate and implement new knowledge. J Contin Educ Health Prof 2002; 22:170–180.

43. World Health Organization. The international classification of functioning, disability and health. Geneva, Switzerland: WHO; 2001.

44. Cockburn L, Trentham B. Participatory action research: integrating community occupational

therapy practice and research. Can J Occup Ther 2002; 69:20–30.

45. Institute of Aboriginal Health, Canadian Institute of Health Research. Five year strategic plan 2002–2007: Executive summary. Online. Available: http://www. cihr-rsc.gc.ca/institutes/iaph/publications/ strat_plan_2002_e.shtml. 25 Feb 2003.

46. Kiepek N. Exploring culture, occupation and health: a participatory action research project involving First Nations youth in northwestern Ontario. Paper presented at the 7th Annual Student Research Symposium, Department of Occupational Therapy, University of Toronto, 18 June 2003.

47. Woodill G, Willi V. Independent living and participation in research: a critical analysis: a discussion paper. Toronto: Centre for Independent Living in Toronto (CILT); 1992.

48. Marullo S, Cooke D, Willis J, et al. Community-based research assessments: some principles and practices. Michigan Journal of Community Service Learning 2003; 9(3):57–68.

49. Letts L. Enabling citizen participation of older adults through social and political environments. In: Letts L, Rigby P, Stewart D, eds. Using environments to enable occupational performance: Thorofare, NJ: Slack; 2003.

50. Chisholm F, Elden M. Features of emerging action research. Human Relations 1993; 46:275–298.

51. Krogh K. A conceptual framework of community partnerships: perspectives of people with disabilities on power, beliefs and values. Can J Rehabil 1998; 12:123–124.

Index

CPSIA information can be obtained at www.ICGtesting.com
Printed in the USA
BVOW061235270812

298782BV00005B/5/P